FOOD
Synergy

UNLEASH HUNDREDS OF POWERFUL
HEALING FOOD COMBINATIONS
TO FIGHT DISEASE AND LIVE WELL

FOOD *Synergy*

BY ELAINE MAGEE, MPH, RD

RODALE

Direct edition first published in 2007. Trade edition published in 2008.

© 2007 by Elaine Magee

All rights reserved. No part of this publication may be reproduced or transmitted in any form or by any means, electronic or mechanical, including photocopying, recording, or any other information storage and retrieval system, without the written permission of the publisher.

Rodale books may be purchased for business or promotional use or for special sales. For information, please write to: Special Markets Department, Rodale Inc., 733 Third Avenue, New York, NY 10017

Printed in the United States of America

Rodale Inc. makes every effort to use acid-free ♾, recycled paper ♻.

Front cover photographs © Isabelle Rozenbaum/Getty Images (left);
© Bill Arce/ Getty Images (right)

Book design by Tara Long

Library of Congress Cataloging-in-Publication Data

Magee, Elaine.
   Food synergy : unleash hundreds of powerful healing food combinations to fight disease and live well / By Elaine Magee.
      p.   cm.
   ISBN-13 978–1–59486–605–0 hardcover
   ISBN-10 1–59486–605–8 hardcover
   ISBN-13 978–1–59486–622–7 paperback
   ISBN-10 1–59486–622–8 paperback
   1. Functional foods—Popular works. 2. Diet therapy—Popular works. 3. Nutrition
Popular works. 4. Health—Popular works. I. Title.
  QP144.F85M34 2007
  613.2—dc22   2007014493

Distributed to the trade by Macmillan

2 4 6 8 10 9 7 5 3 1 hardcover

2 4 6 8 10 9 7 5 3 1 paperback

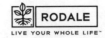

RODALE
LIVE YOUR WHOLE LIFE™

We inspire and enable people to improve their lives and the world around them

For more of our products visit **rodalestore.com** or call 800-848-4735

*To all the nutrition researchers around the world
who continue to unlock the synergy secrets within our food chain.
Thanks so much for all your hard work
(and your willingness to answer my many e-mails).*

CONTENTS

Introduction

Synergy is like adding 1 plus 1 and getting 4 instead of 2: The total is greater than the sum of the individual parts.

Sometimes we don't see the forest for the trees. And the field of nutrition is no exception. We can get so focused on the health benefits of a certain vitamin or nutrient that we miss a crucial link: Different components within a single food can work together for maximum health benefit, and certain components of different foods can produce amazing results when eaten together. For many years, the science of nutrition has focused on specific pieces of the puzzle instead of the power inherent in the whole picture.

This book will help you learn how to tap into that power.

For example, if you are a woman plagued by PMS, milk can be a powerful ally in combating symptoms. However, if we are to truly appreciate the dynamic healing power food has to offer, instead of saying "Drink your milk!" we need to shift our thinking to "Drink your milk fortified with vitamin D!" (Calcium plus vitamin D work synergistically to ease PMS symptoms.) Likewise, if you are a man, you need to shift from "Eat your broccoli—it's good for you" to "Eat your broccoli and tomatoes—that's even better for you!" (Components in broccoli work together with components in tomatoes to decrease prostate cancer growth).

The good news is that researchers are starting to pay more serious attention to the interaction among nutrients, even though the concept is hardly new. I remember sitting in Nutrition 101 about 20 years ago and learning that vitamin C enhances the body's absorption of iron. If you eat vitamin C–rich foods like citrus fruits and leafy greens and pair them with iron-filled foods like lean meats and fish, you absorb more of the mineral. Chances are you've been doing this unwittingly for years, but thanks to relatively recent scientific findings, researchers are increasingly applying their intellectual muscle to studying this phenomenon of "food synergy." The bottom line: Armed with the knowledge of what foods and food components go together for maximum favorable health effects, you can achieve the highest level of health possible.

WHY FOOD SYNERGY MATTERS

We all want the best value when we spend our money, right? And most of us over the age of 40 are very concerned about preventing cancer, stroke, and heart disease as we grow older. Well, food synergy is about getting the biggest health bang for your buck by pairing various foods and nutrients in meals and snacks. Think of it this way: Have you ever eaten a meal that was high in fiber and contained a sensible serving of protein and found that you actually ate less than usual but still felt satisfied? Have you ever noticed that when you include lots of calcium- and vitamin D–rich foods in your diet, your PMS symptoms seem to vanish? These are examples of food synergy in action.

But here's the caveat. Most of the health benefits derived from food synergy are long-term, and they're powerful, helping to prevent major chronic diseases like cancer, heart disease, and stroke. With baby boomers hitting their fifties (I'm a member of this distinguished group), this new way of looking at things through the lens of food synergy seems perfectly timed.

Of course, while the need to know more is strong and growing stronger, it's important to recognize that there's still a great deal to learn. Case in point: Over the past 10 years, scientists have identified hundreds of biologically active plant-food components called phytochemicals (also called phytonutrients). A decade ago, we didn't even know about phytochemicals, such as the powerful antioxidant *lycopene* (a red carotenoid found mainly in tomatoes), *anthocyanin* (a powerful antioxidant that gives berries their deep blue color), and *pterostilbene* (which appears to turn on a switch in cells that breaks down fat and cholesterol).

It's not that food synergy hasn't been studied over the years. Researchers, however, tend to isolate a nutrient or phytochemical and then study its effects without necessarily looking for relationships between foods or nutrients. But over the past 5 years or so, the veritable floodgates have opened, and now I see so much research about components in food and between foods working together for maximum health benefits that I can hardly keep up with it.

In the course of writing this book, I referred to an outstanding academic text titled *Food-Drug Synergy and Safety*, edited by Lilian U. Thompson and Wendy E. Ward, researchers with the University of Toronto. Top nutrition researchers from all over the world (including the Netherlands, Canada, Finland, France, New Zealand, Japan, and the United States) wrote the chapters. Reviewing their work and reading through the many examples of known and suspected food synergy, I definitely got the feeling that we've only begun to scratch the surface. You'll see this groundbreaking text cited often throughout this book, and I consulted with the editor and some of the chapter authors as well.

In writing *Food Synergy*, my goal was to create a scientific guidebook to boost awareness of the leading research, explaining it in understandable terms. But more important, I wanted to create a handbook with helpful solutions and advice for real people. It was my aim to not only give you the most up-to-date information available on food synergy but also show you how to put the power of food synergy into action in your own life. My hope is that you will also discover how all of this seemingly disparate scientific research actually comes together in a way that makes perfect sense.

10 Food Synergy Promises

By tapping into the amazing power of food synergy, you will:

✓ Absorb more nutrients from your food

✓ Experience fewer hunger pangs, thereby helping to control your appetite and lose weight for good

✓ Lower your risk of cancer, heart disease, stroke, and weight-related diseases like type 2 diabetes

Specifically, you can:

✓ Lose up to 20 pounds in 10 weeks by following the 1,500-calorie sample synergy menu plan and incorporating the food synergy weight-loss tips into your life

✓ Improve the health and elasticity of your arteries—keeping your arteries clear and plaque free

✓ Lower your blood pressure (without medication)

✓ Lower your unfavorable blood lipids as much as many drug therapies

✓ Reduce your risk of developing metabolic syndrome

✓ Enjoy relief from PMS symptoms

✓ Gain even more cancer prevention benefits from your diet because you have the power of food synergy working for you

HOW CAN I ACHIEVE FOOD SYNERGY?

We'll start off with a chapter about four big diseases (heart disease, stroke, cancer, and diabetes) to explain how food plays a role in preventing each of them and to make sure we are all on the same footing as we begin our discussion of food synergy. Then, chapter by chapter, we'll discover all the amazing suspected and known examples of food synergy, starting with vitamins and minerals, then phytochemicals, whole foods, food combinations, and food synergy within specific dietary patterns. In Chapter 7, we'll discuss how what we now know about food synergy can help us prevent the top diseases. And just in case your head is swimming with too many examples of food synergy, I've condensed the discussion in the previous five chapters into a section called "Achieving Food Synergy: 12 Rules to Live By." Unexpectedly, as I was researching this book, new examples of food synergy that help with weight loss and weight maintenance emerged, so I've added the summary section "Use Food Synergy to Work toward Weight Loss." Finally, I've offered sample daily menus that feature some of the food synergy connections presented in the book, so you can see what is possible for you at home. And let us not forget the recipes! Chapter 8 is packed with fun and easy-to-make recipes that help you begin to put the power of food synergy in action.

So, is it too early to write a book for the public on food synergy? Put it this way: I spent a year researching and writing this book and had plenty to write about—in many cases, too much! And even as I wrapped this up, there were examples of food synergy flooding in from scientific journals on an almost daily basis. We, my friends, are on to something here . . . something very special.

Sure, some examples might be considered only "suggested" or "possible" food synergy partnerships, requiring more research. But what you'll find as you take the food synergy journey with me is that even if some of the information is preliminary, *Food Synergy* basically brings us back to eating more whole foods, eating more plant foods, and eating more in balance. In a way, we are beginning to understand the amazing power that nature thoughtfully put on this planet with us and for us. And I, for one, am very grateful. I'm also grateful that you've decided to take this food synergy journey with me. So take my hand, and let's begin!

Chapter 1

Harnessing Food Power to Fight the Big Four: Heart Disease, Stroke, Cancer, and Diabetes

"I bought a book about food synergy to be inspired to eat better, not to focus on heart disease or cancer!" Is that what you thought when you read this chapter's title? After all, why would a book about food synergy begin with a discussion of diseases?

Actually, given the strong connection between food and health, it should come as no surprise that within the field of food synergy, most of the research thus far shows enormous benefits in reducing the risk of heart disease, stroke, cancer, and diabetes. If you are already well versed in the inherent role food plays in the development and reversal of these conditions, feel free to fast-forward to Chapter 2 and get started on your food synergy adventure. Otherwise, it's helpful to begin with a basic overview of these diseases and how diet can affect the risk of developing them. Whether we are talking about food pairs or food patterns, whole foods or combinations of nutrients or phytochemicals, there are countless examples of food synergy—when components within or between foods work together in the body for maximum health benefit.

DIET AND HEART DISEASE

Heart disease kills more men and women than any other disease. Close to half a million American women die of heart disease each year, more than from all cancers combined. While many factors besides food increase our risk of heart disease—including smoking, chronic stress, and an inactive lifestyle—a healthy diet's effect on both our blood chemistry and vascular system can help decrease our risk. Following the right eating plan can:

- Lessen the narrowing of the arteries by lowering the amount of fat in the blood that leads to plaque deposits
- Make components in blood less likely to stick together so clots are less likely to form
- Improve flexibility in artery walls so the circulatory system runs smoothly

With every passing year, there is more good news to report. For example, simply incorporating four cholesterol-lowering foods into your diet has been shown to lower cholesterol levels up to 30 percent, reducing the need for cholesterol-lowering drugs (statins) according to studies conducted at the University of Toronto. Researchers say we can benefit from eating:

- Soy, including soy-based meat substitutes and soy milk
- Sticky fiber (also known as viscous or soluble fiber), found in foods such as oats and oat bran and barley-based soups, as well as psyllium products

- Plant sterol–enriched margarine, such as Take Control, which was used in the study
- Nuts (participants ate a handful of almonds each day)

EVALUATING THE RISK FACTORS

In a landmark international study led by Canadian heart researcher Salim Yusuf, MD, which included almost 30,000 people from 52 countries, researchers concluded that close to 90 percent of first heart attacks can be attributed to nine risk factors, including five (identified in boldface type below) that have a direct link to what we eat.

1. Abnormal cholesterol
2. Smoking
3. Chronic stress
4. **Diabetes**
5. **High blood pressure** (Many lifestyle factors can lead to high blood pressure, including what we eat—like high-salt foods—and don't eat—like fruits and vegetables and low-fat dairy foods.)
6. **Abdominal obesity** (A waist circumference of more than 32 inches in women and more than 34 inches in men is linked to an increased risk of heart attacks. Measuring the waist is a better predictor of heart attack than is BMI—body mass index—because it measures abdominal fat, the fat most closely associated with heart attacks.)
7. A sedentary lifestyle
8. **Eating too few fruits and vegetables**
9. **Abstaining from alcohol** (Studies have shown that men who have up to two alcohol drinks a day and women who drink up to one a day have a lower risk of heart disease.)

So what's a more positive way of looking at this list of heart-attack risk factors? A good diet, regular exercise, and moderate alcohol intake reduced the risk of heart disease for the people in this study! According to Dr. Yusuf, poor diet as a whole accounts for about 35 percent of the risk of heart attack. "This includes too few fruits and vegetables and too many fried foods, meats, and salty foods," he explains. In this chapter, we'll cover what you need to know to harness the power of food synergy to fight high cholesterol, high blood pressure (also a leading risk factor for stroke), and diabetes.

The Six Steps to a Heart Attack

Step 1. **Cells that line the walls of the coronary artery are damaged.** These endothelial cells can be injured by debris (such as cholesterol), by a type of white blood cell that engulfs foreign matter, or from low or turbulent bloodflow in the arteries. (Narrowed arteries from atherosclerosis can cause turbulent bloodflow.)

Step 2. **Inflammation occurs in the artery.**

Step 3. **LDL cholesterol becomes oxidized and flows through the bloodstream.**

Step 4. **Plaque from cholesterol sticks to the lining of the arteries.**

Step 5. **Arteries constrict, and plaque ruptures and breaks off the artery wall. A blood clot forms.**

Step 6. **Arrhythmia, or a chaotic heartbeat, interrupts or stops the flow of blood and oxygen to the heart and body. This ultimately leads to:**

HEART ATTACK (also known as a myocardial infarction)

HEADING OFF HEART DISEASE

Of the primary risk factors for heart disease, high cholesterol is one of the most widespread conditions. Almost 54 million women and just over 48 million men have total cholesterol levels higher than 200 milligrams per deciliter (mg/dL). That's more than 100 million people! Even more alarming, most people who suffer a heart attack have only mildly elevated cholesterol levels. (Borderline high cholesterol is between 200 and 239 mg/dL; desirable levels are lower than 200 mg/dL.) These 100 million people can all benefit from even a 10 to 20 percent reduction in total cholesterol. Two simple steps to follow:

Take saturated fat down a few notches. The first thing many experts advise when you need to lower your cholesterol? Eat less saturated fat, which is found in animal products and dairy foods. This has long been known as an effective way to help lower your cholesterol because saturated fat raises harmful low-density lipoprotein (LDL) cholesterol levels.

Make the most of good fats. Next, boost your intake of healthful or "smart" fats, such as plant and fish omega-3s and monounsaturated fats (like olive and canola oil, ground flaxseed, and avocados), and your plant sterols and plant stanol esters—conveniently available in margarines such as Take Control or Benecol. When you use these in place of regular margarine, studies suggest, you can lower total cholesterol and LDL by about 10 percent. Plant sterols and stanol esters, which come to us courtesy of pinewood pulp and soybean extract, work by blocking cholesterol absorption in the digestive tract.

THE LOWDOWN ON BAD CHOLESTEROL

You may not know low-density lipoprotein by name; most people know it by its nickname, "bad cholesterol." LDL has a nasty habit of attaching to the artery walls as it travels through the bloodstream. As it builds up, it creates hard deposits that can restrict bloodflow and eventually lead to blockages associated with heart attacks and strokes. Therefore, if we are going to study the way diet influences heart disease risk, a good place to start is by evaluating how what we eat raises or lowers LDL and triglyceride levels. In addition to losing weight if you're heavy and increasing physical activity, you can lower LDL levels with some dietary changes.

Limit saturated and trans fats. Saturated fats, which we just discussed, are easy to identify because they're solid at room temperature (think butter). Trans fats, a once popular additive in many packaged foods, may be even worse for you than saturated fats. The good news is that new labeling laws let you know how much trans fat is in a product. And by limiting full-fat dairy products, higher-fat red meats, poultry skin, stick margarine (except cholesterol-lowering types), cookies, crackers, and fast-food french fries, you can significantly reduce your risk of heart disease. Try to keep saturated fat to less than 7 percent of your total calories per day (about 15 grams for a 2,000-calorie diet), and try to eliminate trans fats completely.

Size Matters When It Comes to Cholesterol

Canadian heart researcher Salim Yusuf, MD, suggests that cholesterol particle size also helps determine risk of heart attack. The smaller, heavier cholesterol molecules (a protein linked to LDL and other bad cholesterol particles) increase the risk of heart disease because they can more easily invade the artery wall, causing inflammation and atherosclerosis plaque, he explains. This factor alone may increase your risk of heart attack by as much as 54 percent. Blood tests such as the apoB (apolipoprotein B) can help measure the amount of these smaller, denser cholesterol particles.

Experiment with a vegetarian diet. A typical vegetarian diet includes many cholesterol-lowering foods, such as soy milk, soy burgers, oats, almonds, beans, and plenty of fruits and vegetables, all of which have been individually found to lower cholesterol levels. In one study, after 1 month, participants' LDL levels fell by 29 percent—a drop similar to that seen with some statin drugs. Other cholesterol-lowering benefits of a vegetarian diet include a higher consumption of plant stanols (2 grams a day is ideal) and soluble fiber (reaching the recommended 25 grams a day is relatively easy on a vegetarian diet). You don't have to become a full-fledged vegetarian to see results, however. Try to replace meat-based dishes with vegetarian entrées a few times a week.

Focus on flaxseed. According to Diane Morris, PhD, nutrition consultant to the Flax Council of Canada, clinical studies show that eating between 2 and 6 tablespoons of ground flaxseed daily for as little as 4 weeks lowers blood cholesterol 6 to 9 percent and LDL cholesterol by 9 to 18 percent. "However, I should point out that most clinical trials use amounts closer to 4 to 6 tablespoons of ground flax daily," notes Dr. Morris.

Enjoy almonds. A recent study found that when people with elevated blood lipids snacked on almonds, their coronary heart disease risk fell significantly, probably due in part to the fiber and monounsaturated fat components of almonds.

THE TROUBLE WITH TRIGLYCERIDES

Like measuring LDL cholesterol, taking note of triglyceride levels in the blood can shed light on heart health. People can have high triglyceride levels even when their cholesterol levels are normal. Blood triglycerides come mainly from the fat we eat in foods. But when we eat more calories than our body needs, no matter whether carbohydrate or fat, these excess calories are converted in the liver to triglycerides and stored in fat cells.

Higher blood levels of triglycerides increase the concentrations of two types of fat particles: chylomicrons and very low-density lipoproteins. These fat particles show up in the fat deposits in the arteries that eventually obstruct bloodflow. It's no surprise, then, that high triglyceride levels are a strong, independent predictor of personal risk for stroke. A study led by David Tanne, MD, with the Sheba Medical Center in Israel, followed more than 11,000 people with coronary heart disease and found that those with triglyceride levels of 200 mg/dL or higher had an almost 30 percent higher risk for stroke. High triglyceride levels are associated with higher rates of heart disease. The following shows what the numbers mean.

<150 mg/dL = normal
150–199 mg/dL = borderline high
200–499 mg/dL = high
500+ mg/dL = very high

If you want to lower your triglyceride levels, much of the same advice for lowering cholesterol applies. You should also consider the following:

Cut back on refined carbohydrates. Opt to enjoy sweets, soft drinks, and white bread only occasionally, and try to choose carbs that are lower on the glycemic index, or GI. (Choosing foods at least 12 points lower on the index reduced triglycerides by approximately 9 percent in 10 out of 11 studies.) Instead of processed carbohydrates, choose whole grain foods such as brown rice, whole grain cereals, and whole grain pasta.

Seek omega-3 fatty acids from fish. Start by eating fish a couple times a week. This may help lower triglycerides, especially if fish replaces other foods containing saturated and trans fats.

Add omega-3 fatty acids from plant foods, too. Switch to canola oil in your cooking. Other top plant sources of omega-3s are ground flaxseed, broccoli, cauliflower, cantaloupe, and red kidney beans. (Talk to your doctor about adding a tablespoon of ground flaxseed a day.) This may help reduce serum triglycerides along with total and LDL cholesterol.

Add soluble fiber. This strategy may rein in the potential increase in serum triglycerides and other blood fats in some people with diabetes who eat a high-carbohydrate diet. You'll find soluble fiber in beans, oats and oat bran, barley, psyllium products, some fruits (apples, mangoes, plums, kiwifruit, pears, berries, citrus, and peaches), and some vegetables (artichokes, celery root, sweet potatoes, parsnips, turnips, acorn squash, potatoes with skin, Brussels sprouts, cabbage, green peas, broccoli, carrots, green beans, cauliflower, asparagus, and beets).

THE KEY TO LOWER HOMOCYSTEINE LEVELS

Homocysteine is an amino acid in the blood that at high levels may be related to a higher risk of coronary heart disease and stroke. According to the American Heart Association (AHA), homocysteine may play a role in atherosclerosis (blood plaque deposits in the arteries) by damaging the inner lining of arteries and promoting blood clots. According to a report in *Stroke: Journal of the American Heart Association*, high levels of homocysteine may be significantly associated with an increased risk of stroke in people who already have coronary heart disease.

Two things are thought to influence homocysteine levels: genetics and diet. Some researchers suspect that folic acid and other B vitamins help break down homocysteine in the body. To help lower homocysteine levels:

- Get more folic acid by eating dark leafy greens, dried beans, asparagus, and spinach and drinking orange juice.

- Eat bananas, whole grains, nuts, and seeds for vitamin B_6.
- Take in B_{12} through low-fat dairy foods and fortified cereals.

A few other factors are also known regarding homocysteine levels.

- Men tend to have higher levels than women, and both sexes tend to show increasing levels as they age.
- Smoking is associated with higher levels.
- Higher coffee consumption is associated with higher homocysteine levels.
- Alcoholics have highly elevated homocysteine concentrations. Wine and hard liquor have been shown to raise concentrations—but there seems to be a loophole for beer, which seems to have no effect. Some researchers have suggested that the folate (folic acid) and B_6 in beer might help counteract the homocysteine-raising effects of the alcohol.

IS THERE REALLY "GOOD" CHOLESTEROL?

Recent advances in research have only brought more attention to the blood lipid awarded the nickname "good cholesterol," so known because high-density lipoprotein (HDL) cholesterol levels are associated with lower incidence of heart disease. Although many people still pay more attention to their LDL levels when they get a blood lipid test, there's growing evidence that HDL is just as important a factor in the development of heart disease.

"Boosting HDL is the next frontier in heart disease prevention," says P. K. Shah, MD, director of cardiology at Cedars-Sinai Medical Center in Los Angeles. Dr. Shah believes that if the new drugs that increase levels of HDL work, we could potentially reduce the number of heart attacks and strokes by 80 to 90 percent and save millions of lives.

Experts don't yet know for sure how HDL cholesterol helps reduce the risk of heart disease, but they are aware of a few possibilities. The National Cholesterol Education Program (NCEP) final report on high blood cholesterol states that in lab studies, high levels of HDL appear to protect against the formation of fatty plaques on artery walls (a process known as atherogenesis). Other studies suggest that HDL promotes the removal of cholesterol from lesions that have already begun to form on the walls. "Recent studies indicate that the antioxidant and anti-inflammatory properties of HDL also inhibit atherogenesis," adds the report.

Fast Facts about HDL Cholesterol

✓ HDL normally makes up 20 to 30 percent of the total cholesterol in the blood.

✓ Some evidence indicates that HDL cholesterol protects against the development of atherosclerosis (accumulation of plaque or fatty deposits in the artery walls), and as HDL levels increase, the risk for coronary heart disease decreases.

✓ A high HDL cholesterol value (greater than or equal to 60 mg/dL) remains a "negative" risk factor—meaning it subtracts one risk factor from the risk factor count.

✓ Epidemiological data signify that a 1 percent decrease in HDL is associated with a 2 to 3 percent increase in coronary heart disease risk.

✓ In prospective studies, HDL usually proves to be the lipid risk factor most highly correlated with coronary heart disease risk.

✓ In the general population, genetic factors account for about half of the variability of serum HDL levels.

✓ Women typically have higher HDL levels than men have; about one-third of men and one-fifth of women have levels below 40 mg/dL.

Nine Ways to Improve Good Cholesterol Levels

What many people don't know is that there are many ways we can increase our HDL cholesterol levels through diet and lifestyle.

1. **Orange juice:** Drinking 3 cups of orange juice a day increased HDL by 21 percent over 3 weeks, according to the results from a small British study of 25 healthy men and women with high total and LDL cholesterol. That's a nutritional commitment some people would be challenged to achieve, especially since it adds up to 330 calories and 75 grams of carbohydrate (plus about 240 milligrams of vitamin C and 1.5 grams of fiber). It's possible this study highlights an effect from high-antioxidant fruits and vegetables, so stay tuned for more news about this one in the years to come!

2. **Niacin:** There is some evidence that niacin (vitamin B_3) helps increase HDL. According to Michael Poon, MD, director of cardiology at the Cabrini Medical Center in New York, people with low HDL levels might benefit from taking 500 milligrams of niacin each day, building up to 1,000 milligrams a day. Supplemental niacin "can have some side effects and is not for everybody, particularly people who already have high HDL levels," cautions Dr. Poon, who recommends that people taking niacin be monitored by a doctor. The *Environmental Nutrition* newsletter reports that the preferred form of nicotinic acid is by prescription as Niaspan, an extended-release pill that's less likely to cause niacin's infamous flushing of the skin and is safer for the liver. These foods are also good sources of niacin.

Chicken, white meat (13.4 mg/3.5 oz)

Ground beef (5.3 mg/3.5 oz)

Mackerel (10.7 mg/3.5 oz)

Peanuts (5.3 mg/¼ c)

Trout (8.8 mg/3.5 oz)

Pork (about 4.8 oz/3.5 oz)

Salmon (8 mg/3.5 oz)

Chicken, dark meat (6.5 mg/3.5 oz)

Veal (about 8 mg/3.5 oz)

Peanut butter (4.4 mg/2 Tbsp)

Lamb (6.6 mg/3.5 oz)

Beefsteak (about 4.1 mg/3.5 oz)

Turkey, white meat (6.2 mg/3.5 oz)

3. **Glycemic load:** As glycemic load goes up, HDL cholesterol appears to go down, according to a small study that concluded that glycemic load is an important independent predictor of HDL in healthy people. Along these lines, the National Cholesterol Education Program (NCEP) recommends that most carbohydrate intake be in the form of whole grains, vegetables, fruits, and fat-free and low-fat dairy products. Carbs should be limited to 60 percent of total calories, even lower (about 50 percent of calories) for people with metabolic syndrome who have elevated triglycerides or low HDL cholesterol.

4. **Type of fat:** Replacing saturated fat with monounsaturated fat can help reduce levels of LDL and may increase HDL cholesterol.

5. **Soy:** Add "heart-healthy food" to the list of soy's potential health benefits. "The most recent published meta-analysis found that soy protein [plus isoflavones] raised HDL levels 3 percent, which could reduce coronary heart disease risk about 5 percent," says national soy expert Mark Messina, PhD. Other recent studies have shown a decrease in LDL (about 3 percent) and triglycerides (about 6 percent) with about three servings of soy a day (a total of 1 pound of tofu or three soy shakes). But give soy some time; another recent analysis of 23 soy studies found that HDL improvements were observed only in studies of longer than 3 months.

6. **Alcohol:** Consuming moderate amounts of alcohol, especially with meals, may reduce heart disease risk by increasing HDL levels and helping to move cholesterol deposits out of cells lining the artery walls.

7. **Aerobic exercise:** At least 30 minutes a day several days a week is the exercise prescription for raising HDL.

8. **Smoking cessation:** Kicking the habit may increase your HDL numbers a bit, too.

9. **Shedding excess pounds:** Being overweight or obese contributes to low HDL levels and is listed as one of eight causes of low HDL cholesterol by the NCEP. Although part of this effect can be explained by obesity's action of raising serum triglycerides, which lowers HDL cholesterol, there may be other mechanisms at work as well.

CRP—The New Blood Test

It happens quietly over time, over and over again. We can't feel it, but it may increase our risks of heart disease, stroke, diabetes, and even cancer. It's inflammation that flares in our blood vessels and arterial walls.

The blood test marker C-reactive protein (CRP) offers one way to measure this type of inflammation. People with high levels of CRP are at much greater risk for heart disease than those with low levels. New research suggests that people with elevated blood sugar and CRP levels may be at especially high risk, says Karen Collins, MS, RD, CDN, nutrition advisor for the American Institute for Cancer Research.

Knowing your LDL cholesterol levels is no longer enough. You need to know your CRP levels, too. Even if your LDL levels are in the safe range, you can have dangerously high CRP levels. In a recent study from the Center for Cardiovascular Disease in Women at Brigham and Women's Hospital in Boston, people who had desirable LDL levels (below 70) but CRP levels greater than 2 had a 45 percent increase in heart attacks and deaths from heart disease than those with normal LDL levels and CRP levels below 2.

In a second study, this one from the Cleveland Clinic Foundation's department of cardiovascular medicine, arterial plaque was measured in 502 people with heart disease before and after 18 months of statin (cholesterol-lowering medication) use. The people who experienced the biggest CRP drop had the smallest growth of arterial plaque buildup; in some cases, plaque even regressed. However (just when you thought we were on to something), researchers from the Atherosclerosis Risk in Communities study (ARIC) reported in the Archives of Internal Medicine that CRP adds no value to determining risk for heart disease. Even so, high CRP levels can at least alert your doctor to a potentially serious problem worth further investigation.

DIET AND STROKE

Many of the same blood vessel problems that can lead to heart disease can also cause a stroke. Similar to a heart attack, when bloodflow to the brain is interrupted due to a clot or hemmorhage, brain injury results. In fact, stroke is the number one cause of adult disability. But I'm going to give you the good news right now: Most strokes are preventable. How? By lowering high blood pressure, cutting cholesterol, and reducing the risk of blood clots.

But first, here's a quick review of the main types of stroke: An ischemic stroke, the most common type, occurs when a blood vessel in the brain gets clogged with plaque or a wandering clot lodges in the artery supplying blood to the brain. A hemorrhagic stroke is less common but more likely to end in death because, in this case, the weakened blocked vessels burst. A TIA, or transient ischemic attack, is a ministroke that often serves as an early warning of a more serious stroke.

EVERYTHING YOU NEED TO KNOW ABOUT HIGH BLOOD PRESSURE BUT ARE TOO STRESSED OUT TO ASK

High blood pressure makes your heart work harder than normal and renders both it and its arteries more prone to injury. High blood pressure also increases your risks of heart attack, stroke, kidney failure, eye damage, congestive heart failure, and fatty buildups in arteries. Almost one in three adults has high blood pressure!

If you're curious to see whether your readings place you in that group, know that the AHA defines high blood pressure as systolic pressure (the top number in a reading) of 140 mm Hg or higher or diastolic pressure (the bottom number) of 90 mm Hg or higher. People who have a systolic pressure of 120 to 139 mm Hg or diastolic pressure of 80 to 89 mm Hg are said to have prehypertension—and that includes about 28 percent of US adults, based on results collected by the Centers for Disease Control and Prevention (CDC) between 1999 and 2002.

(continued on page 18)

Eight Strategies to Reduce Stroke Risk

Besides the obvious healthy lifestyle habits, like exercising regularly and not smoking, what can you do? Take note of the following food-related strategies advised by the American Heart Association (AHA).

1. **Eat to lower your blood pressure and keep sodium in check.** Cut back on sodium by going easy on the processed stuff while upping your potassium with fruits and vegetables, beans, and low-fat dairy foods. People who took in more than 4,000 milligrams of sodium a day (no matter what their blood pressure) raised their risks of stroke by 90 percent, compared with people eating 2,400 milligrams or less, according to the results from Columbia University Medical Center.

2. **Manage your weight.** Abdominal fat is directly linked to increased risk of stroke, and the more you weigh, the greater your risk. Weight loss in general, though, will certainly help reduce your risk. An average weight loss of just 11 pounds resulted in a mean reduction of blood pressure of 4.4 mg Hg (milligrams of mercury) systolic and 3.6 mm Hg diastolic, according to an analysis of 25 research trials. Additional trials have found that modest weight loss can prevent hypertension by about 20 percent among overweight prehypertensive people.

3. **Reduce blood cholesterol.** Your risk of stroke rises with elevated total cholesterol and LDL cholesterol. And in men only, low levels of HDL cholesterol increase risk as well. (See page 12 for cholesterol-lowering strategies.)

4. **Control high blood pressure.** Keep your blood pressure out of the danger range (systolic pressure above 140 and diastolic above 90) using any means available—through diet, exercise, and medication, if necessary. This is a concern to the nearly one in three adults with high blood pressure. Here's the incentive: People with blood pressure of less than 120/80 mm Hg have about half the lifetime risk of stroke, compared with those who have hypertension, according to the AHA's "Heart Disease and Stroke Statistics—2006 Update."

5. **Keep blood sugar under control.** The risk for stroke is two to four times higher among people with diabetes, according to AHA statistics. This could be, in part, because if you have type 2 diabetes, you also face increased risk for two factors that can raise your risk of stroke: high blood pressure and elevated cholesterol levels. Rising blood pressure readings is no small matter either— about 73 percent of adults with diabetes have blood pressure values greater than or equal to 130/80 mm Hg or use prescription medication to help control high blood pressure. Keeping blood sugar levels steady will also help stabilize blood pressure and cholesterol problems.

6. **Eat six to seven servings of fruits and vegetables a day.** In a recent Danish study, the participants who did this were 28 percent less likely to suffer an ischemic stroke than those who ate only one or two servings a day. What's going on here? People who eat diets low in vitamin C or potassium are at greater risk of stroke, and fruits and vegetables are rich in both! And it's yet another example of how food works but supplements don't quite cut it. A Dutch study of women over age 55 revealed that while vitamin C–rich foods were protective against stroke, vitamin C supplements were not.

7. **Enjoy broiled or baked seafood.** Some research suggests that seafood slashes stroke risk, probably thanks to its omega-3s. But don't take that high–omega-3 fish and fry it; data from the Cardiovascular Health Study found that older people who ate fried fish had a higher risk of ischemic stroke than those who ate broiled or baked fish. The AHA recommends eating fish (particularly fatty types like salmon, sardines, mackerel, herring, and albacore tuna) at least twice a week.

8. **A little wine will do fine.** If you drink, enjoying a moderate amount of alcohol (one or two drinks per day) seems to have a beneficial effect on stroke risk, but excessive drinking (more than three drinks a day) actually raises the risk of stroke and the incidence of diabetes.

The systolic reading measures the pressure in the blood vessels during that split second when the heart pumps out the blood. The diastolic reading measures the pressure when the heart is at rest. Years ago, the diastolic measurement was considered the more important of the two. But we know now that the systolic reading is as—if not more—important in diagnosing and treating high blood pressure. While it is true that systolic blood pressure does tend to climb in most people as they grow older, it still shouldn't be considered normal, because it comes with an increased risk of stroke, heart disease, and kidney disease.

Because blood pressure readings are affected throughout the course of the day by changes in activity, stress, fluid levels, and diet, I think it's a good idea to have a reading taken as often as possible. It's a routine indicator of wellness

Can Folic Acid Lead to Fewer Stroke Deaths?

Some research suggests that foods fortified with folic acid might help reduce the deaths from stroke. Since 1998, when the United States and Canada started fortifying grain products with folic acid, one measurable result in large population studies has been increased blood levels of folic acid (folate) and decreased homocysteine levels. Researchers also noted a decline in stroke-related deaths in the United States between 1998 and 2002. In England and Wales, where grain fortification didn't take place, a similar decline in stroke death was not observed.

While other data suggest that B vitamins (including folic acid) offer no protection against the recurrence of stroke, some experts think these nutrients may help guard against a first stroke. Getting enough of three of the Bs—B_6, B_{12}, and especially folic acid—probably helps because one of their health benefits is breaking down homocysteine.

(like body temperature), so a doctor will take your blood pressure if you're in the office for just about anything—gynecological checkups, sick visits, and so on. If you can, keep track of the numbers for your reference. General recommendations, however, call for blood pressure screenings at least every 2 years. If your numbers are normal, you can stick with that schedule. But if either diastolic or systolic measurements are considered elevated, you should get a repeat measurement and, if necessary, begin treatment (possibly including counseling on diet, lifestyle changes such as exercise, and/or medication).

WHAT WE KNOW ABOUT DIET AND BLOOD PRESSURE

Here's a quick summary of the basic facts.

- Blood pressure tends to go up with higher intakes of sodium, alcohol, and protein.
- Blood pressure tends to go down with higher intakes of potassium, calcium, and magnesium.
- Salt intake may lead to an increase in blood pressure in people who are salt sensitive.
- Other risk factors for hypertension include obesity and lack of regular physical activity.

To review, then, given the above information about diet and blood pressure, the five habits you want to avoid and change are consuming too much salt, including too few potassium-rich foods, drinking a lot of alcohol, eating more calories than you expend, and being sedentary.

However, new research has brought our basic understanding of diet and blood pressure into sharper focus. Here's the latest news.

- Increasing potassium intake (remember, this mineral is in fruits and vegetables and low-fat dairy) may be even more important in fighting high blood pressure than reducing salt, especially in salt-sensitive people. Potassium may counter some of the bad effects of salt.

- Calcium in combination with potassium, magnesium, and moderate salt restriction seems to be much more effective at lowering blood pressure than calcium alone. Some experts recommend that to get all three minerals, you should drink one or two glasses of fat-free milk or eat one serving of low-fat yogurt a day.
- Eating more vegetable protein helps lower blood pressure, according to the results of a four-country study. For each 14 grams of vegetable protein (for a 2,000-calorie diet), participants experienced an average drop of 2.14 points in the systolic reading and 1.35 points in the diastolic.

WHO IS SALT SENSITIVE?

When it comes to salt and its effect on blood pressure, the connection exists only for people who are considered salt sensitive. This means that as they increase their salt intake, their blood pressure increases, too. There's no inexpensive or easy way to find out who is in that category and who isn't, but a number of factors increase the likelihood that you are salt sensitive. These include if you:

- Are female
- Are in your middle-age or golden years
- Have excessive abdominal obesity
- Have more than two drinks a day (for a woman) or more than three drinks a day (for a man)
- Are African American

- Have persistently high blood pressure (consistently high when measured by a professional)
- Have been diagnosed with isolated systolic hypertension (ISH), characterized by readings with systolic blood pressure of less than 140 mm Hg and diastolic blood pressure of less than 90 mm Hg
- Have impaired glucose tolerance
- Have diabetes
- Have kidney disease
- Have a family history of high blood pressure

Hey, my fellow baby boomers, guess what? We may be getting better, but we are also getting older: As age increases, so does salt sensitivity. Experts estimate that around 30 percent of people with high blood pressure are salt sensitive, but among African Americans, the number jumps to 75 percent. And as a general rule, the higher your blood pressure, the more likely it is that a high-salt diet will make it worse.

For those of you at risk for salt sensitivity, ask your doctor if you could try lowering your blood pressure with a lower-salt diet for 3 to 6 months before resorting to medication. Or, if you are the fast and furious type, drastically reduce the amount of salt you eat for a 2- to 3-week period. If this leads to a significant drop in blood pressure, you are probably salt sensitive.

DIET AND CANCER

Somehow the description "uncontrolled reproduction of abnormal cells" doesn't sound as frightening as the condition itself—cancer. Most people, including me, feel shock waves at the mention of the word. But there are many reasons to be hopeful and less fearful today.

Fast Facts about Cancer

✓ About 1.2 million Americans are diagnosed with cancer each year.

✓ One-third of the 500,000 cancer deaths in the United States each year can be attributed to poor diet and lack of exercise.

✓ Breast and prostate cancers are the most common types in the United States (excluding nonmelanoma skin cancer), followed by lung, colon, and bladder cancer.

✓ According to estimates from the American Institute for Cancer Research, if everyone ate at least five servings of vegetables and fruits per day, cancer rates could fall by as much as 20 percent.

Scientists have been gaining ground on this complex disease; specifically, we have a much better understanding of how cancer cells grow. In a nutshell, cancer comes down to this: DNA (the set of genetic instructions that tells body cells how to reproduce and grow) takes little punches over the years, eventually becoming so damaged that normal cell growth morphs, becoming uncontrolled and abnormal. We can avoid many of these everyday hits—such as exposure to tobacco and the sun's ultraviolet (UV) rays, overindulging in alcohol, or getting too few important nutrients in our diets—but cannot control others, such as certain viruses.

Because some cancers have a genetic link, if you have a family member who battled cancer, you may feel that there's a time bomb ticking inside you. Actually, it's estimated that only 5 to 10 percent of all cancers might be attributed to a genetic predisposition. However, lifestyle remains a significant factor. According to the American Institute for Cancer Research (AICR), 60 to 70 percent of cancers can be collectively attributed to lifestyle choices, including smoking, unhealthy diets, lack of physical activity, and excessive weight. In addition, scientists now estimate that approximately 35 percent of all cancers are attributable to what we eat. With some types of cancer, that number is even higher. For example, some experts assert that up to 90 percent of colorectal cancer in the United States could be avoided by choosing the right foods.

Granted, there are no guarantees to eating and living healthfully, but it sure does help put the odds in our favor.

FREE RADICALS 101

Though the term *free radicals* may suggest images of mutant aliens from deep space, it actually refers to naturally occurring oxygen molecules that contain unpaired electrons, which render them unstable. The body produces free radicals as part of its normal activity, but these substances can also enter us from outside, as a result of exposure to tobacco, sunlight, and pollution. Free radicals don't live long—just a few nanoseconds to 1 or 2 seconds—but they can cause considerable cell damage during that time, similar to the damage caused by radiation.

As free radicals roam the body, they scavenge electrons from other molecules. This only creates more instability, possibly setting the stage for cancer development. Here's a step-by-step breakdown of how free-radical damage occurs.

1. Free radicals damage cell walls by borrowing electrons from the LDL cholesterol on cell membranes (a process called *lipid peroxidation*).

2. Next, a free-radical "chain reaction" effect can take place: Once the lipids on the cell wall are oxidized, a door is essentially opened

that allows more free radicals to enter the cell, which leads to damage of the cell's internal components.

3. DNA, the genetic code that provides the cell with instructions on how to grow and reproduce, may become damaged.

4. The cell, receiving garbled instructions from damaged DNA, becomes more likely to grow incorrectly, thus setting the stage for cancer.

5. Free radicals can also trigger changes that increase the buildup of plaque in arteries and thicken arterial walls, which set the stage for heart disease and stroke.

Antioxidants are nutrients that help defend the body against free radicals and the damage they cause. When confronted by a free radical, an antioxidant will pair with the oxygen molecule's extra electron, thereby rendering it harmless. A healthy diet rich in a variety of plant foods provides a steady stream of powerful antioxidants, including:

- Beta-carotene (found in dark, leafy greens and bright red, yellow, and orange fruits and vegetables)
- Vitamin C (citrus fruits)
- Vitamin E (nuts, seeds, whole grains, wheat germ, and plant oils)
- Selenium (plant foods such as nuts and seeds—particularly Brazil nuts and sunflower seeds—whole grain pasta, oatmeal, and soy)
- Carotenoids (brightly colored fruits and vegetables like tomatoes, watermelon, and sweet potatoes)

THE ANTICANCER DIET

The way eating habits affect cancer risk comes down to a simple equation of imbalance. A diet that includes too much animal fat (mainly from red meat and high-fat dairy), alcohol, fried foods, refined carbohydrates, and sugars may increase risk. Likewise, a diet that lacks nutrient-dense plant foods may also raise risk.

In a recent diet analysis of the 90,000 premenopausal women enrolled in the Nurses' Health Study II, researchers found that the women who ate the most animal fat (23 percent of calories)—mainly from red meat and high-fat dairy foods—were 33 percent more likely to develop breast cancer, compared with women who ate the least (12 percent of calories) of those foods.

Randall Oyer, MD, chairman of medical oncology at John Muir Medical Center in Walnut Creek, California, isn't afraid to say that diet and nutrition play major roles in health and cancer prevention, but he resists applying the connection to a short time frame. "What a person has been eating a year before she was diagnosed with breast cancer probably isn't as relevant as what she'd been eating a decade or two before," explains Dr. Oyer.

Most cancer researchers admit that the scientific evidence that diet can reduce cancer risk is much stronger with colon cancer than it is with breast cancer. Even so, there are a few things we do know right now about diet and breast cancer, and there are a few strong possibilities for future treatment on the horizon.

WHAT WE KNOW ABOUT DIET AND BREAST CANCER

It might surprise you that the dietary factor most consistently associated with an increase in breast cancer risk is not animal fat—it's alcohol. "We know, for example, that alcohol increases the risk of breast cancer beginning at just a few drinks a week," explains Colleen Doyle, MS, RD, director of nutrition and physical activity for the American Cancer Society (ACS). A large-scale analysis of more than 50 studies suggests that imbibing two alcoholic drinks a day (no matter what type) increases the risk of breast cancer by approximately 25 percent.

So what about total dietary fat and breast cancer? The impact of food fat on breast cancer risk is unclear at the moment, with various studies reporting an assortment of results. Perhaps various types of fat may have different effects; if so, that makes future research even more complicated.

Meanwhile, don't order that bacon-and-egg breakfast. "We also know that postmenopausal women who gain weight are at increased risk for breast cancer," adds Doyle.

Perhaps the best course is simply to stick with a low-fat diet. In the recent Women's Intervention Nutrition Study, participants who followed a low-fat diet (around 20 percent of calories from fat) reduced their risks of recurrence from breast cancer during the next 5 years by 24 percent. It's possible, however, that the benefit came not from fat reduction itself but from another factor. For example, the women had been eating higher amounts of fruits and vegetables, which brought plenty of cancer-protective nutrients and fiber to the table. A lower-fat diet might also assist in weight loss, which also lowers cancer risk.

WHAT WE STILL DON'T KNOW: SOY'S EFFECT

Soy may be a double-edged sword in the fight against breast cancer. It's especially rich in natural plant estrogens (called isoflavones)—but some types of breast cancer are aggravated by high estrogen levels. The extra estrogen in soy may not be safe for women who've been treated for estrogen-positive breast cancer. On the other hand, soy may be helpful to some women trying to prevent breast cancer because when the body detects estrogen from the diet, it slows its own production of the hormone.

Johanna Lampe, PhD, RD, a researcher at the Fred Hutchinson Cancer Research Center, Seattle, believes it's most prudent for breast cancer survivors to use only moderate amounts of soy foods, eating them several times a week as part of a healthy plant-based diet. The ACS seconds that advice and also advises breast cancer survivors to avoid more concentrated sources of soy, such as soy-containing pills or powders or supplements containing isolated or concentrated isoflavones.

DIET AND PROSTATE CANCER

Breast cancer is by far one of the most studied of all cancers, but it shares a hormonal basis with cancers of the prostate, testes, uterus, cervix, and endometrium, notes Glen Weldon, communications director for the AICR. Scientists continue to debate whether circulating sex hormones encourage the growth of these cancers, or whether the link between diet and these "hormonal cancers" is indirect because these types of cancer are also strongly influenced by body fat.

While less studied, prostate cancer has begun to attract considerable attention in recent years. According to Weldon, in the last 15 years, advances in screening have revealed just how common prostate cancer actually is. "That realization triggered an explosion in human cohort studies into prostate cancer that, because prostate cancer is usually a slow-growing cancer, is only now beginning to see the light of day," explains Weldon.

It appears that a high intake of meat and dairy products is associated with higher prostate cancer death rates, according to William B. Grant, PhD, a researcher with the Physicians Committee for Responsible Medicine, who analyzed prostate cancer rates and diets in 32 countries. Daily intake of some vegetables (especially onions, leeks, and garlic) appears to help prevent prostate cancer as may cereals and grains, beans, and fruits.

Lycopene, considered the most potent antioxidant in the carotenoid family, is by far the most well-known food substance to show a protective role against prostate cancer, notes Weldon. "This finding was recently bolstered by the discovery that men who eat tomatoes and tomato products frequently have high levels of lycopene in the tissues of the prostate and testes," he says.

HOW STRONG IS DIET'S LINK TO CANCER?

POSSIBLE RISK FACTOR	CONVINCING LINK	PROBABLE LINK	POSSIBLE LINK
Obesity	Endometrial cancer	Cancers of the breast and kidney	Cancers of the colon, rectum, and gallbladder
Diet low in fruits and vegetables	Cancers of the mouth, pharynx, esophagus, lung, stomach, colon, and rectum	Cancers of the larynx, pancreas, breast, and bladder	Cancers of the liver, ovary, endometrium, cervix, prostate, thyroid, and kidney
Diet high in fat			Cancers of the lung, colon, rectum, prostate, and endometrium
Alcohol consumption	Cancers of the mouth, pharynx, larynx, liver, and esophagus	Cancers of the colon, rectum, and breast	Lung cancer
Diet high in red meat		Cancers of the colon and rectum	Cancers of the pancreas, breast, prostate, and kidney
Cured meats			Cancers of the colon and rectum
Grilled meats			Cancers of the colon, rectum, and stomach
Sugar			Cancers of the colon and rectum
Coffee			Bladder cancer

Scientific judgment of AICR (American Institute for Cancer Research) expert panel, "Food, Nutrition and the Prevention of Cancer: A Global Perspective"

THE OBESITY-CANCER CONNECTION

I always consider obesity the O-word I hate to mention. That's because I don't like the anxiety and feelings of self-loathing that many people have with obesity. But you'll notice it appears in the table above as a "possible risk factor" linked to six types of cancer. When it comes to eating to help prevent cancer, obesity is a necessary part of the discussion.

According to a recent study in the *New England Journal of Medicine*, overweight and obesity account for 14 percent of all deaths from cancer in men and 20 percent in women. Some researchers speculate that extra pounds

Discover Your Waist Circumference and Waist-to-Hip Ratio

Step 1: Use a nonstretchy tape measure. Make sure it's level around your waist and parallel to the floor.

Step 2: Measure your waist at its narrowest point, usually just above the belly button. Tighten the tape without pressing your skin. Write down this number.

Step 3: Measure your hips around the widest part of your hip bones. Tighten the tape without pressing your skin. Write down this number.

Step 4: Compare your measurements to the following guidelines.

FOR YOUR WAIST CIRCUMFERENCE:

A larger waist circumference is associated with an increased risk for type 2 diabetes, high cholesterol, hypertension, and cardiovascular disease in people with a high body mass index (BMI), between 25.0 and 34.9. For them, an unhealthy waist measurement is above 35 inches for women and above 40 inches for men.

FOR YOUR WAIST-TO-HIP RATIO:

Divide your waist measurement by your hip measurement.

A waist-to-hip ratio of 0.7 for women and 0.9 for men is considered safe.

A waist-to-hip ratio of 1.0 or more is considered high risk for heart disease, diabetes, and cancers of the breast and prostate.

raise levels of certain hormones (like estrogen and insulin), which may stimulate tumor growth.

The good news is that many elements of a cancer-prevention lifestyle, especially diet and regular exercise, are also major weapons in the fight against obesity. I admit that making these changes can be daunting, but if you focus on the health aspects, you'll be in a better place psychologically to maintain better eating habits and remain physically active. One of my nutritional mottos is "Eat and exercise for the health of it . . . and let the pounds fall where they may." Instead of focusing on numbers on the scale, turn your attention to the joy of living healthy because it's just plain good for you in both the short and long term.

Don't sweat a few extra pounds, either. Being a little overweight (according to those darn "weight for height" tables), if it's where your body seems comfortable while you are living this healthy life, might be fine for you. A more valuable guideline is to monitor your waist circumference because this measures the "extra" in the most dangerous place.

THE FOODS TO FOCUS ON

It's well established that fruits and vegetables are a big part of anticancer eating. Here's a sampling of some of the specific nutrients or foods that might offer valuable protection.

Flaxseed. This amber-colored, sesame-like seed has been around for hundreds of years, but taking a fresh look through the lens of food synergy, scientists suspect it can help fight cancer three different ways. First, ground flaxseeds contain soluble fiber, which is thought to help lower cancer risk by bulking up the stool and speeding bowel movements, thus ridding the body of possible carcinogens sooner. This fiber may also reduce the amount of bile acids, which may promote cancer in the intestinal tract.

Eat Your Way to Lower Cancer Risk

The following list represents the bottom-line advice for reducing cancer risk. However, experts I've talked to also urge us to stay tuned. More research is reported every month.

Curb alcohol consumption. If you drink alcoholic beverages, limit them to one a day; even better, cut down to fewer than three drinks a week. And if you drink alcohol, make sure you are meeting your folic acid requirements through food choices.

Load up on vegetables. Aim for 9 to 10 servings (about ½ cup each) of a variety of fruits and vegetables a day. Try to include a cup of dark green vegetables and a cup of an orange fruit or vegetable (for carotenoids, folic acid, fiber, and phytochemicals).

Savor seafood. Eat fish two to three times a week as a sub for red meat (or foods high in saturated fat) and as a source of omega-3 fatty acids.

Favor beans over meat. Three times a week, replace red meat with beans (including soybean products), a source of folic acid (lentils, pinto beans), fiber, and assorted phytochemicals.

Enjoy whole grains. Include several servings of fiber-filled whole grain foods each day. Along the same lines, limit refined grains and sugary foods because they contain empty calories.

Focus on dietary fat. For cancer prevention, some fats may be worse than others. While high-fat diets have been associated with an increased risk of colon and prostate cancer, it's the type of fat (rather than the total amount) that looks to be most important for preventing many types of cancer, including breast cancer. We may be adding ovarian cancer to that list, too. Although not definitive, a new study in *Cancer Causes and Control* found that women whose diets included large amounts of olive oil reduced their ovarian cancer risk by 30 percent. Choosing lean meats and low-fat dairy products and substituting olive and canola oil for butter, lard, and high-trans-fat margarines when possible is a great place to start.

Lose weight. Keep extra weight off as best you can by working out almost every day (consult your physician before starting an exercise program) and containing extra calories by limiting fat. If your favorite foods tend to be fattening, look for satisfying lower-fat substitutes that are higher in fiber.

Flaxseed also contains alphalinolenic acid (ALA), a plant form of omega-3 fatty acid. According to Weldon, ALA seems to possess potent anti-inflammatory effects that may help prevent the kind of long-term tissue and cellular damage that can spark the cancer process.

Finally, flaxseed is also the richest source of lignans on the planet. Basically, lignans—phytoestrogens that function like antioxidants—have a similar structure to estrogen, so they can bind to the same receptors in the body. Scientists believe that when lignans and similar plant substances bind to these receptors on cancerous cells, they prevent circulating estrogen from latching on, which helps discourage cancer growth: If the estrogen were to bind to the receptors, they would encourage the cancer cells to grow.

In 2000, encouraging results from the first human flaxseed and breast cancer study were presented at the San Antonio Breast Cancer Symposium. The study showed for the first time that adding a reasonable amount of flaxseed (the study used muffins containing 25 grams of flaxseed) for approximately 38 days reduced tumor growth in patients with breast cancer—similar to the benefits seen when the drug tamoxifen is given to patients before breast surgery.

Since then, many more studies have reported similarly favorable results. A randomized, double-blind, placebo-controlled clinical trial at the University of Toronto, for example, tested the effects of flaxseed in postmenopausal women with newly diagnosed breast cancer. The researchers concluded that "dietary flaxseed has the potential to reduce tumor growth in patients with breast cancer." In another study, mice were injected with human breast cancer cells and fed several different diets, one of which was supplemented with flaxseed. The researchers found that the cancer spread more slowly to the lungs and lymph node areas in the flaxseed-fed mice.

Although more research needs to be done, adding a tablespoon of ground flaxseed to your smoothies, muffin recipes, or meat loaf every day or a few times a week may be helpful. At the very least, it will raise the fiber and omega-3 fatty-acid content of your diet. Just don't confuse flaxseed with flaxseed oil, which doesn't contain the beneficial fiber or plant estrogens.

Conjugated linoleic acid (CLA). While the relationship between higher-fat diets and breast cancer may still be in question, the association between fat and other cancers remains fairly strong. The ACS states that high-fat diets are associated with an increased risk of colon, rectal, prostate, and endometrial cancer and that the consumption of meat, especially red meat, has been linked to colon and prostate cancer as well. Saturated fat specifically has been found to promote cancer development in laboratory studies. And gram for gram, fat in food contains more than twice the calories as carbohydrate and protein, making it a potential weight-gain promoter when eaten in excessive amounts day after day.

But there is a tricky fat found in very small amounts in meat and dairy fats—CLA, which may actually inhibit different types of cancer. Margot Ip, PhD, of the Roswell Park Cancer Institute in Buffalo, New York, has shown that CLA can exert a one-two punch to breast cancer. Here's punch 1: CLA inhibits the growth of breast cancer cells, as shown in laboratory (in vitro) studies. Punch 2: CLA inhibits the development of new blood vessels in the mammary or breast gland, which reduces the rate of mammary tumor growth.

How do we harness the potential power of CLA without the potential risks that come with eating too much animal fat? By eating small portions of meat and dairy as part of a mostly plant-based diet, says the AICR. I'll do you one better: Because dairy products contain the highest natural level of CLA among all dietary sources, how about we include a couple of servings of lower-fat dairy every day? Several other health programs already recommend this, including the DASH (Dietary Approaches to Stop Hypertension) diet for reducing heart disease and for osteoporosis prevention.

Folic acid (folate). Judith Christman, PhD, of the University of Nebraska Medical Center, is studying how diets lacking folic acid encourage the cancer process in general. "When diets lack folic acid," she explains, "the structure of the cell's genetic material becomes disrupted. If cells misread normal or read damaged genetic information and reproduce, cancer can develop."

If alcoholic drinks are a daily or weekly habit for you, you've got another good reason to eat folic acid–rich foods. A recent study from the Mayo Clinic, reported in the journal *Epidemiology*, revealed that women who consumed the least folic acid and the most alcohol had a 59 percent increased risk of breast cancer, compared with teetotaling women whose folic acid intake was above the median (294 micrograms per day, or 350 micrograms including vitamin supplements). Study author Thomas Sellers, PhD, a Mayo Clinic cancer epidemiologist, explains, "Alcohol is metabolized to acetaldehyde, a known carcinogen. People who have adequate folic acid intake, however, may have a better capacity to repair DNA damage caused by acetaldehyde." As long as you eat plenty of fruits and vegetables, beans and peas, and fortified breads and cereals, you should meet the recommended daily allowance for folic acid (400 micrograms).

Vitamin D. This powerful vitamin isn't just about boosting bones! There's so much more to vitamin D than enhancing calcium absorption; its anticancer benefit is just one other possibility. Most of 63 recently reviewed studies found a protective effect between vitamin D status and cancer risk. A study presented at the 2006 American Association for Cancer Research meeting suggested that an increase in vitamin D lowered the risk of developing breast cancer by up to 50 percent.

How might vitamin D help? It's the body's most potent regulator of cell growth, preventing cells from becoming malignant, explains Michael Holick, MD, PhD, head of the Vitamin D, Skin, and Bone Research Laboratory at Boston University School of Medicine. How much might be needed to help curb cancer risk? Research suggests around 1,000 IU. And where do you get it? Milk and milk products (and soy products) are often fortified with vitamin D (check the labels to be sure), but you can also find it in eggs and some seafood, like cod, shrimp, and chinook salmon. And don't forget good old-fashioned sun exposure. While experts say that in just 10 minutes you can soak up as much as 5,000 IU of vitamin D if you expose 40 percent of your body to the sun without sunscreen, given the link between skin cancer and sun exposure, you may be better off sticking to that glass of milk.

DIET AND DIABETES

Among all chronic diseases, diabetes best illustrates the power of food in ensuring good health.

One in every 20 people in the United States has diabetes, and the numbers keep growing each year. In fact, the typical high-fat, sedentary American lifestyle puts most of us at risk of developing type 2 diabetes.

Diabetes is closely connected to two other diseases discussed in this chapter—obesity and heart disease. If you are concerned about heart disease *and*

Fast Facts about Diabetes

✓ Diabetes afflicts more than 20 million people in the United States and is the main cause of kidney failure, limb amputations, and new-onset blindness in adults and a major cause of heart disease and stroke.

✓ Type 2 is the most common form of diabetes, representing more than 90 percent of cases and affecting about 7 percent of the US population age 20 and older.

diabetes, it may comfort you to know that many diet changes will help reduce the risk of both diseases.

The Diabetes Prevention Program, a major clinical trial comparing diet and exercise with Glucophage (an oral diabetes drug), was conducted on 3,234 people at 27 centers nationwide. Forty-five percent of the participants were from minority groups that suffer disproportionately from type 2 diabetes: African Americans, Hispanic Americans, Asian Americans and Pacific Islanders, and Native Americans. The study group also included other people known to be at higher risk for type 2 diabetes: those over 60, women with a history of gestational diabetes, and people with a first-degree relative with type 2 diabetes.

Participants who made lifestyle changes, including 30 minutes a day of exercise (usually walking or other moderate-intensity exercise) and a low-fat diet, cut their risk of type 2 diabetes by 58 percent. For people age 60 and older, these lifestyle changes reduced the development of diabetes by a whopping 71 percent. Most people in this group also lost 5 to 7 percent of their body weight, which computes to 9 to 12 pounds for a 180-pound person.

DIABETES 101

Diabetes is a disease in which the body does not properly produce or use insulin, a hormone secreted by the pancreas. At a cellular level, insulin helps the body use the glucose circulating in the bloodstream. In the liver and skeletal muscle cells, for example, insulin encourages the production of glycogen (the storage form of glucose). Insulin also encourages fat production, which is the body's long-term storage solution for excess glucose.

There are three basic forms of diabetes: type 1, type 2, and gestational. Type 1 is a form of diabetes that children get and is usually not associated with obesity. About 5 to 10 percent of Americans with diabetes have this form, which results when the pancreas literally stops making insulin. The lion's share of cases belongs to type 2 diabetes, which is mainly a metabolic disorder resulting from the body's inability to make or properly use insulin. With type 2 diabetes, the cells become increasingly resistant to insulin, brought on in many cases by a combination of genetic predisposition, obesity, and sendentary lifestyle. Gestational diabetes occurs during pregnancy and usually resolves with the birth of the baby.

While certain ethnic groups are at increased risk for diabetes, the following factors can raise anyone's risk: family history, being obese or significantly overweight, sedentary lifestyle, being over 45, having a history of gestational diabetes, or giving birth to a 9-pound or bigger baby.

FOODS THAT FIGHT DIABETES

In general, diabetes research has found that many of the basic elements of a healthy diet—whole grains, fruits and vegetables, beans and legumes, and low-fat dairy—may also have a significant impact on diabetes. The emphasis should be on choosing smart carbs (which contribute fiber and nutrients along with carbohydrate) and smart fats (monounsaturated fats and omega-3 fatty acids) whenever possible. In fact, people with diabetes who also have high triglycerides and high LDL cholesterol may benefit from including more monounsaturated fats (olive oil, canola oil, and avocados) and slightly fewer carbohydrates. (If you have diabetes, this is something you will want to work out with your dietitian or certified diabetes educator.)

With the recent popularity of the glycemic index (GI), the general public is more aware than ever of the type of carbohydrates in our food. The GI ranks various foods according to their ability to raise blood sugar: Low-GI foods have low impact; high-GI foods raise blood sugar quickly. And for people with diabetes, the American Diabetes Association (ADA) states that

Top Five Ways to Cut Diabetes Risk in Half

Several recent studies have shown that when people take the following five steps, they achieve greater weight loss and improve their glucose and insulin concentrations, compared with control subjects. One recent study led by Jaakko Tuomilehto, MD, of the National Public Health Institute in Helsinki, Finland, showed that key lifestyle changes reduced the risk of progression to diabetes by a striking 58 percent over 4 years in overweight people with impaired glucose tolerance.

1. **Get as close to your ideal weight as possible.** The low incidence of diabetes in people who lost at least 5 percent of their initial weight underscores the importance of even small weight loss when trying to prevent diabetes, according to results from the Helsinki study. Obesity is the most notable modifiable risk factor for developing type 2 diabetes; in fact, more than 80 percent of people with type 2 diabetes are overweight.

2. **Increase physical activity.** Both weight loss and improved fitness have been associated with the reduced incidence of type 2 diabetes. And even if it doesn't result in weight loss, regular exercise seems to pay off. For the study participants who did not lose weight, tallying more than 4 hours of exercise a week was still associated with significantly less diabetes risk.

"the use of glycemic index and glycemic load may provide a modest additional benefit over that observed when total carbohydrate is considered alone." Here are some highlights from the recent ADA recommendations regarding:

Fiber. People who are at risk for diabetes should aim for 14 grams of fiber for every 1,000 calories. This is about 28 grams for a typical 2,000-calorie intake or 35 grams for 2,500 calories. Fiber helps people with diabetes or at risk for diabetes in two ways: First, it seems to improve insulin sensitivity; second, it

3. **Eat less saturated and total fat.** Not only do saturated fats tend to raise blood levels of LDL cholesterol (and high LDL is associated with heart disease), but meals high in animal fat (much of which is saturated) stimulate higher blood sugar in some people. Some researchers think that in these people, fat-laden meals make insulin less effective. Avoiding high-fat meals also makes caloric sense because each gram of dietary fat contributes 9 calories, compared with the 4 calories contributed by each gram of protein or carbohydrate.

4. **Keep excess calories to a healthy minimum.** One of the keys to losing extra weight and maintaining a healthy weight is to keep excess calories to a minimum. It's when we eat more calories than we burn day after day that ensures the extra pounds will accumulate.

5. **Increase dietary fiber.** Eating too little fiber day after day has been associated with an increased risk of type 2 diabetes (as well as cancer, obesity, and heart disease). Fiber, particularly soluble fiber (the type that dissolves in water and forms a gel), helps regulate blood sugar, possibly by slowing down the absorption of other nutrients, including carbohydrates, eaten at the same meal.

appears to improve the body's ability to secrete enough insulin to overcome insulin resistance.

Saturated fat. Keeping saturated fat to less than 7 percent of total calories, avoiding trans fats, and limiting cholesterol to less than 200 milligrams a day are all recommended for people who already have diabetes. This may also help reduce diabetes risk by improving insulin resistance and possibly promoting weight loss. Lowering saturated fat is one of those diet recommendations that kills several birds with one stone. Saturated fat raises LDL

Eat Your Way to Better Diabetes Control

While it's vital that anyone with diabetes or prediabetes work with a doctor to develop a proper, personalized diet and weight loss plan, the following general tips can help.

1. Make fiber a part of almost every meal.

2. Count carbohydrates so you know how much your body can tolerate at different times of the day, taking into account your medication and exercise schedule.

3. Emphasize heart-protective fats.

4. Cut back on saturated fat and cholesterol.

5. Remember that calories do count.

6. Eat more fruits and vegetables.

7. Avoid eating large meals to minimize drastic spikes in blood sugar.

cholesterol and total cholesterol, increasing the risk of heart disease and stroke. Saturated fat may also increase the risk of certain cancers.

Weight loss. Why lose weight to help prevent or treat type 2 diabetes? Obesity influences insulin resistance. Short-term studies have demonstrated that losing 5 percent of body weight (about 10 pounds for someone weighing 200 pounds or 15 for a 250-pound person) helps decrease insulin resistance and improve high blood sugar, high blood lipids, and high blood pressure in people with type 2 diabetes.

Sugar. To eat sugar or not to eat it, that's the big question for people with diabetes. The answer: Go ahead and eat sugar, but follow the ADA's recommendations. Sugar-containing foods can be substituted for other carbohydrates in the individualized meal plan. Note that this recommendation is qualified by the urging to avoid excess calorie intake.

Here are some other worthy additions to your diet if you have type 2 diabetes.

Antioxidants. A new study supports the idea that the development of type 2 diabetes may be held off with the intake of antioxidants in the diet. Vitamin E (we'll talk more about food sources in Chapter 2), as well as one of the carotenoids (B-cryptoxanthin), was associated with a reduced risk of type 2 diabetes.

Omega-3 fatty acids. These may be especially helpful for people with type 2 diabetes who are at increased risk of heart disease. The ADA recommends eating at least two servings of nonfried fish per week. (More on omega-3s throughout the book but specifically in Chapter 5.)

Soy. Available in many forms, soy has been shown to make cells more responsive to insulin, which may help control blood sugar. (More on soy in Chapter 4.)

Buckwheat. New research shows that extract of buckwheat lowered meal-related blood sugar levels by 12 to 19 percent when given to rats.

Chapter 2

When Two or More Nutrients Are Better Than One: Vitamins and Minerals

For decades, most headlines from the field of nutrition research simply focused on specific parts of our diet. Nutrients like vitamin C and calcium were discovered, and signs of nutrient deficiencies like scurvy or rickets were uncovered. We accumulated knowledge in pieces rather than taking a look at how our diet relates to food habits or eating patterns. Such an approach hardly provides an opportunity to gaze at the whole picture. In some ways, it's like looking into a rearview mirror to try to gauge your hem length.

But in the past decade or so, more research has led to a better understanding of synergy that exists between nutritional components, and along the way this research has revealed quite a bit about the power of whole foods and dietary patterns. And now that a true picture of nutrition is starting to take shape, it seems there is a lot more to the story. "There is increasing interest in this broader approach, since with all the efforts we made during the last years to approach nutrition-related problems, we did not really solve the problems," says Ingrid Hoffmann, PhD, of the Institute of Nutrition Science, University of Giessen in Germany. To create effective solutions, we need a more integrative and encompassing approach, she says.

This logic makes perfect sense. After all, the human diet is a highly complex mixture of foods, each comprising a unique blend of components and natural chemicals. As researchers have begun to see patterns emerge that show how various food components actually work together to yield even greater health benefits, the study of nutrition has been taken to a higher level. It's almost as if a new language is being spoken. From my perspective, looking at nutrition with an eye toward synergy takes us closer to the truth. And isn't that what the study of nutrition is all about? "The past and ongoing research illustrates that the whole may not be obtained by solely investigating its parts and adding up this knowledge but, rather, that the whole is more than the sum of the parts," explains Dr. Hoffmann.

We now know that synergy does exist at the micronutrient level, in various combinations of vitamins and minerals. These nutritional partnerships also explain, in part, why some research that has focused on only one nutrient may not have had the expected health results.

A CHANGE IN PERSPECTIVE

One clear-cut example of a study that shifted the way scientists think about nutrition was the landmark CARET study (Carotene and Retinol Efficacy Trial), published in 1996. Beta-carotene, the phytochemical supplement once thought to reduce the risk of cancer, was found to actually increase the risk of lung cancer in smokers. The results from large, controlled trials of beta-carotene supplementation provide striking evidence of adverse effects in smokers (more lung cancer than expected, as well as overall mortality). But the harm may be in taking large amounts of beta-carotene all by itself, via supplements; numerous past studies indicated that people who eat the most vegetables and fruit and foods rich in carotenoids have the lowest risk of lung cancer.

A similar story cropped up a few years later with vitamin E supplements. "High doses of vitamin E were found to raise the risk of dying," read the headlines in 2004. According to a pooled statistical analysis of 19 studies, people taking 400 IU or more a day had about a 5 percent higher death rate than those who didn't take that much vitamin E. The researchers noted that the higher the dose, the greater the risk.

Then the largest clinical trial to study the effects of vitamin E on the prevention of cardiovascular disease and cancer—the Women's Health Study— had surprising results. Among 20,000 women taking 600 IU of natural vitamin E every other day for 10 years, there was no apparent significant reduction in risk for cancer or major cardiovascular events (heart attack, nonfatal stroke, and death from cardiovascular disease). Another recent study found that 400 IU or more of vitamin E a day might actually increase the risk of heart failure, causing some experts to caution people to limit or stop taking vitamin E altogether.

How could this popular antioxidant increase such risks, much less fail to offer hoped-for protection? The scientific community is still trying to find answers to that question, but some point to the fact that many of the studies used alpha-tocopherol supplements, which are one particular form of vitamin E. Apparently, alpha-tocopherol supplements decrease levels of another form of vitamin E, gamma-tocopherol, which some researchers suspect may play a big role in many processes in the body. In other words, the magic of vitamin E may arise from the mixture of its various forms (found in food); thus, focusing on one type misses the combined effect. For example, in one recent study, researchers compared two groups to see how vitamin E affected the clumping together of blood particles that can lead to blood clots, a process known as platelet aggregation. In one group, participants took supplements of a mixed tocopherol preparation that more closely resembles the blend of nutrients found in food sources of vitamin E (100 milligrams of gamma-tocopherol, 20 of alpha-tocopherol, and 40 of beta-tocopherol). The other group took alpha-tocopherol only. The group receiving mixed tocopherols experienced less platelet aggregation.

Reviewing these studies, I can't help but think that sometimes in the field of nutrition what seems unconnected at first glance is actually connected.

VITAMIN SYNERGY

Current developments in nutrition seem to beg the question that if we are popping supplements high in one particular vitamin or mineral, are we disrupting the beautiful and beneficial synergy that exists in nature? I think it wise to consider supplement choices carefully because the truth is that we just don't know about all the relationships that occur among nutrients.

One recent study, for example, compared how the body responds to lutein (a type of carotenoid) when it's taken as a supplement versus as a food source. It found that although lutein supplements decrease beta-carotene concentrations in the body, lutein from food (like yellow carrots) actually increased measurable lutein levels in the body without affecting beta-carotene levels. In my opinion, our best source of nutrients and phytochemicals has always been and will always be, quite simply, food.

This chapter will explain the synergy that we currently know about or suspect between various vitamins and minerals. And the potential food partnerships that these synergies suggest will inspire many a tasty recipe in Chapter 8!

FIGHT HEART DISEASE WITH THE THREE BS

Three B vitamins—folic acid, B_6, and B_{12}—appear to work together to decrease the risk of heart disease, but they seem to have more of an additive effect when it comes to homocysteine. (At high levels, homocysteine is thought to damage artery linings, leading to heart attack and stroke, as well as contribute to blood clots.) In other words, they each work independently to help lower homocysteine

B Vitamins: How Much Do I Need Each Day?

The 1998 Dietary Reference Intakes recommend the following:

FOLIC ACID

✓ 400 mcg (dietary folate/folic acid equivalents)/day for men ages 19+

✓ 400 mcg (dietary folate equivalents)/day for women ages 19+

VITAMIN B_6*

✓ 1.3 mg/day for men ages 14–50

✓ 1.7 mg/day for men ages 51+

✓ 1.2 mg/day for women ages 14–18

✓ 1.3 mg/day for women ages 19–50

✓ 1.5 mg/day for women ages 51+

VITAMIN B_{12}

✓ 2.4 mcg/day for men ages 14+

✓ 2.4 mcg/day for women ages 14+

These intakes may not be sufficient for people who eat a high-protein diet with 100 grams of protein or more per day.

levels. But put them together, and the benefit becomes even greater.

Some researchers theorize that these three B vitamins may help reduce the risk of cardiovascular disease independent of and in addition to lowering homocysteine concentrations. For example, this nutritional trio may encourage regression of plaque in the carotid artery (the large artery on either side of the neck that supplies blood to the brain). Here's a quick summary of each:

Folic acid. Essential for the formation of DNA and RNA (our genetic blueprints at the cellular level), folic acid is particularly important for body tissues that have fast cell production and turnover, such as bone marrow and the intestinal tract. It's also required for the synthesis and breakdown of amino acids. A deficiency of folic acid can affect the nervous system and brain function.

Vitamin B_6. The body needs B_6 to produce both red and white blood cells, as well as to convert stores of carbohydrate (glycogen) into glucose. Nerve cells need B_6 in order to function properly; this vitamin may also be involved in the metabolism of polyunsaturated fats.

Vitamin B_{12}. I call B_{12} the enzyme-assistant vitamin because it is required for several enzymatic reactions. It helps protect against heart disease by helping to control homocysteine levels and thus reduce the risk of heart attack and stroke. Like B_6, B_{12} has an important role in building and maintaining the sheaths that protect nerve fibers. B_{12} is needed, together with folic acid, for cell formation and growth and to help manufacture red blood cells.

So it should be simple enough to whip up a meal including these three Bs and reap the health benefits, right? Not quite so easy, folks—it gets a bit tricky. Even though the different types of vitamin B provide many common benefits, they actually come from very different sources. B_{12} is found in animal products, for example, while folic acid is found in plant foods.

So what's the ideal solution? Turn to Appendix B for a list of top food sources. But if you want to consider some easy ways to get all three in a meal or snack, try the suggestions in "12 Smart Ways to Get Your Three Bs" on pages 50–51.

VITAMIN E: THE SYNERGY WITHIN

Vitamin E is an intriguing nutrient because while it is an antioxidant, it is also a fat—a fat-soluble vitamin, to be exact. As if that weren't enough, there are eight forms of vitamin E (alpha-, beta-, gamma-, and delta-tocopherols and -tocotrienols).

Years ago, the most active form of vitamin E was thought to be alpha-tocopherol, and that's the form you find in many supplements. However, as mentioned earlier in this chapter, there are studies that have demonstrated unpredictable health benefits from alpha-tocopherol alone. As a result, some researchers hypothesize that alpha- and gamma-tocopherol or a mixture of tocopherols may be more effective together. This is what we know so far.

There is evidence that if you supplement with one form of vitamin E, it may affect the levels (positively or negatively) of another form in the body. It is well known, for example, that high doses of alpha-tocopherol supplements decrease gamma-tocopherol concentrations in the blood, according to Sridevi Devaraj, PhD, an associate professor with the Laboratory for Atherosclerosis and Metabolic Research at the University of California, Davis, Medical Center. That may be undesirable, as gamma-tocopherol may help reduce free radicals and be more potent than alpha-tocopherol in inhibiting inflammation associated with heart disease. And gamma-tocopherol appears to have a different set of protective properties, such as helping the body eliminate extra sodium, which may be helpful for people with high blood pressure.

So if you do decide to use vitamin E supplements, should you go au naturel? Natural E is more likely to contribute E compounds other than alpha-tocopherol, such as gamma-tocopherol, and when equivalent amounts are compared, synthetic vitamin E is half as effective as natural. Some experts suggest not exceeding 200 IU of all-natural, mixed-tocopherol vitamin E. No study has found doses this low to be harmful.

12 Smart Ways to Get Your Three Bs!

After looking at "B Vitamins: How Much Do I Need Each Day?", your head is probably swimming with a veritable banquet of assorted food sources but no idea of how to put them together into a meal or dish. No worries. Here are 12 surefire ways to blend your three Bs into a high-synergy meal.

1. Enjoy Mexican meals that contain pinto or black beans with chicken, beef, or pork.

2. Drink orange juice when you eat fish or meat. You'll get the possible synergy between folic acid, B_6, and omega-3s, too!

3. Enjoy crab whenever possible; it has all three B vitamins, plus omega-3s.

4. When you make an omelet or scrambled eggs (B_{12}), add some spinach and broccoli (folic acid) and have a side of low-fat breakfast potatoes (B_6).

5. Consider spinach salad more often (folic acid and B_6), and add chopped egg, fish, meat, or cheese (B_{12} and, if using fish, omega-3s).

6. Make a smoothie with banana (B_6); yogurt (B_{12}); and orange juice, papaya cubes, or tofu (folic acid).

7. Enjoy dishes that feature avocado (folic acid and B_6) with any of the top B_{12}

Vitamin E should always be taken with a meal so that it will be properly absorbed, according to Maret Traber, PhD, a professor of nutrition with the Linus Pauling Institute at Oregon State University, Corvallis, Oregon. Ideally, take it with dinner to avoid any possible interference with drugs that you may be taking in the morning.

Vitamin E and lycopene reduce heart disease and prostate cancer risk. Vitamin E seems to have a nice synergistic relationship with lycopene, a phytonutrient found in red foods, including tomatoes, watermelon, pink

foods, such as fish, meat, or dairy products. A shrimp and avocado salad would, for example, give you all three Bs plus omega-3s.

8. Warm yourself up with a hearty lentil soup or lentil salad that includes any fish or meat . . . or enjoy the soup or salad with yogurt or a glass of milk (B_{12}).

9. Make a broccoli-and-cheese potato, and you'll get folic acid from the broccoli, B_6 from the potato, and B_{12} from the cheese. Top it with plain yogurt for even more B_{12}.

10. Whip up a Caesar salad with grilled chicken (B_{12}) and romaine lettuce (folic acid), and dress it up with sunflower seeds and/or avocado (folic acid and B_6).

11. At your next barbecue, when grilling your lean steak or pork tenderloin (B_6 and B_{12}), throw some high–folic acid veggies on the grill, like asparagus, okra, broccoli, or Brussels sprouts.

12. When tossing a pasta salad together, add some pieces of lean meat—such as skinless roast chicken or turkey, beef (B_6 and B_{12}), or salmon (omega-3s)—to the pasta (enriched with folic acid). Add some kidney beans and/or avocado, and you'll crank the folic acid up a couple notches.

grapefruit, and dried apricots. Together they provide several important examples of food synergy.

First, they help reduce low-density lipoprotein (LDL) cholesterol oxidation, and this is most definitely a good thing. The more LDL cholesterol that's oxidized, the higher the risk you'll collect plaque inside the walls of your arteries, which can be a precursor to a heart attack.

Second, in recent lab studies, a combination of lycopene and vitamin E suppressed the growth of prostate cancer cells by 73 percent and increased survival time by 40 percent. In the control group, neither lycopene nor vitamin E alone significantly reduced cancer cells. What mechanism might enable lycopene and vitamin E to have synergy in reducing prostate cancer growth? Nobody knows the answer yet, but "most likely the mixture acts by optimizing the mechanisms of both compounds alone," explains Wytske van Weerden, PhD, the lead researcher of the study at Erasmus University in Rotterdam, the Netherlands.

Vitamins C and E work with beta-carotene to lower LDL cholesterol. In a recent study, vitamins E and C appeared to hook up with another famous antioxidant, beta-carotene, to help reduce LDL cholesterol oxidation. Vitamins E and C have also been observed as having synergy with a particular phytochemical found in almond skins, possibly protecting LDL cholesterol from oxidation, according to a recent lab study from Tufts University, Medford, Massachusetts.

BETA-CAROTENE–RICH FRUITS AND VEGGIES ALSO RICH IN E AND C

An impressive number of fruits and vegetables contribute a good or great amount of beta-carotene. Since there is a suspected synergy between beta-carotene and vitamins E and C, these values are also listed in the table below. Quite a few fruits and vegetables boast fair amounts of all three antioxidants—killing three birds with one stone. These foods are indicated by an asterisk (*).

	BETA-CAROTENE (MCG)	VITAMIN E (IU)	VITAMIN C (MG)
FRUIT			
*Mango slices, 1 c	3,851	2.8	46
Cantaloupe cubes, 1 c	3,072	0.4	68
Apricots, 3 each	1,635	0.9	10.5
Watermelon, diced, 2 c	674	0.7	29
Peach slices, 1 c	452	1.8	11
Grapefruit, pink, 1 c	359	0.9	88
Orange juice, fresh, 1 c	92	0.3	124

	BETA-CAROTENE (MCG)	VITAMIN E (IU)	VITAMIN C (MG)
VEGETABLE			
Carrot slices, ¾ c, cooked	14,404	0.5	8.2
Sweet potato, 1 small	7,864	0.3	17
Kale, 1 c, cooked	5,772	1.7	53
*Greens (beet, collard, mustard), 1 c, cooked	3,568	2.5	35
Spinach leaves, 2 c	2,393	1.7	17
Romaine lettuce, 2 c	1,747	0.7	27
Broccoli pieces, 1 c, cooked	1,359	1.1	123
Pumpkin, raw cubes, ¾ c	822	1.4	8
*Tomato sauce, ½ c	704	2.6	16
Tomato paste, 2 Tbsp	468	2.1	14
Tomato, 1 medium	446	0.7	23
Acorn squash, ¾ c cubes, baked	393	0.3	17
Tomato juice, 1 c	293	0	20
Red bell pepper, chopped, ¼ c	212	0.4	71

Red wine helps boost the effects of vitamin E. Wines contain a large number of polyphenols, compounds that, according to researchers from the Heart Research Institute in Australia, may enhance the antioxidant activity of vitamin E in our bodies. In a lab study, mice were fed a diet supplemented with alcohol-free red wine, which increased antioxidant concentrations in the blood while significantly decreasing plaque buildup in the heart. Another laboratory study in France examined how red wine polyphenolic compounds affect LDL cholesterol oxidation. The researchers found that the polyphenols worked with vitamin E to effectively lower oxidation, but most interesting was the fact that polyphenols stopped working once the vitamin E supply ran out—leaving researchers to speculate that this interaction makes good use of extra vitamin E first and helps preserve what the body has already stored on its own. To use a wine metaphor, it's like the wine ensures the body makes good use of all available vitamin E, just as it's wise to cook dinner with the leftovers from last night's bottle of wine instead of opening a new one.

Sesame seeds may improve the immune-functioning power of vitamin E. Sesame seeds contain a special phytoestrogen called sesamin that may play a role in helping vitamin E curb the production of inflammation-causing eicosanoids. When the body has too many omega-6 fatty acids and not enough omega-3s, it tends to produce eicosanoids, which in turn affect immune function. So look for opportunities to add sesame seeds to your meals, especially when you are eating something high in vitamin E, such as sunflower seeds, almonds, peanut butter, canola oil, Swiss chard, or broccoli.

Vitamin C boosts the effectiveness of phytoestrogens. Vitamin C may boost the effectiveness of certain phytoestrogens' ability to inhibit the oxidation of LDL cholesterol, according to researchers at the University of Southern California. In lab experiments using LDL isolated from adult blood samples, they found that increasing amounts of three phytoestrogens (genistein, daidzein, and equol) inhibited LDL oxidation; this protective effect was even more powerful when ascorbic acid (vitamin C) was present, too. Genistein and daidzein are the isoflavones found in soy and soy products. Pairing soy with citrus sounds like a partnership that can't miss.

SMART FATS AND VITAMINS

You might be wondering, *Are there actually fats that are smart?* Smart fats, as I fondly refer to them, are dietary fats that offer health benefits without harming the body like the other "bad" fats (namely, saturated and trans fats).

In this book we'll focus on two smart fats in particular: omega-3 fatty acids and monounsaturated fats.

Monounsaturated fats lower LDL cholesterol levels and reduce the risk of heart disease. They may also increase high-density lipoprotein (HDL, or "good") cholesterol levels, reduce blood pressure, and improve insulin sensitivity. Good sources include olive oil, canola oil, peanut oil, avocados, and some nuts, such as almonds.

Omega-3 fatty acids, on the other hand, especially those found in fish, may reduce the risk of blood clots, lower triglyceride levels, and promote normal blood pressure. There's also some evidence that omega-3s may lower heart disease risk, and scientists continue to study their role in reducing cancer risk. Great sources include fish (especially coldwater fish like salmon, tuna, mackerel, trout, herring, and bluefish), ground flaxseed, and canola oil. Plant food sources include broccoli and other green leafy vegetables, kidney beans, cantaloupe, walnuts, soy, and pecans.

Omega-3s, vitamin E, and niacin help lower cholesterol. Here's a perfect snapshot of food synergy. A recent Italian study suggests that a combined

The Omega Basics

There are two main families of polyunsaturated fat: omega-3s and omega-6s. While each is essential to health, most experts don't consider omega-6s part of the "smart fats" category. When we eat omega-6s in excessive amounts (and most Americans do), they can spur the production of hormonelike substances called eicosanoids that can lead to inflammation and damaged blood vessels. Excessive omega-6 has been associated with blood clots and constricted arteries and can interfere with the body's natural conversion of plant omega-3s to the more powerful omega-3s, like those found in fish.

supplement composed of a smart fat (omega-3), an antioxidant vitamin (E), and a B vitamin known to be a heart helper (niacin) helps limit the amount of cholesterol produced in the body. In the study, one group of people received a placebo (an inactive pill), another group took a supplement combining omega-3 and vitamin E, and a third group received that combo plus niacin. The latter trio best improved cholesterol profiles and helped protect against inflammation and oxidative stress to the point that lower doses of the supplements could be given.

How could these three seemingly different supplements demonstrate such powerful effects in the body? First of all, they aren't the strange bedfellows you might think. Niacin is very effective at decreasing triglycerides and LDL cholesterol and raising HDL cholesterol. Fish oil with omega-3s makes cholesterol particles larger and less likely to stick to artery walls and has been shown to decrease triglycerides, too. Vitamin E is well known as an antioxidant, meaning it may prevent the oxidation of cholesterol, rendering it less likely to encourage plaque and fatty deposits in the artery walls. All these effects build on each other in combination therapy, according to Penny Kris-Etherton, PhD, RD, nutrition professor and researcher at Pennsylvania State University in University Park. The bottom line in this case: "It's more effective to have lower doses of multiple agents acting in different ways than a lot of one agent acting by one mechanism," explains Dr. Kris-Etherton.

Fish omega-3s may up the need for vitamin E. To prevent heart disease, a number of experts recommend aiming for about 0.5 gram per day of EPA and DHA (eicosapentaenoic acid and docosahexaenoic acid) omega-3s in fish. When heart disease is already present, 1 gram per day is recommended. While eating fish (preferably fatty fish) a couple times a week is a great way to achieve half a gram a day, reaching a whole gram a day may require eating foods enriched with fish omega-3s or taking fish oil supplements. And there's the rub.

According to some omega-3 experts, vitamin E isn't as critical when you get your omega-3s from natural food sources like canola oil or ground flaxseed. "No need to add vitamin E to increasing fish intakes," says Richard Deckelbaum, MD, a lipid researcher and director of the Institute of Human Nutrition at Columbia University in New York.

However, if you decide to boost dietary intake of EPA and DHA through supplements, experts advise taking an optimal intake of vitamin E (400 IU) as well. In fact, the fish oil supplements now add vitamin E. The incredible dynamic between omega-3s and vitamin E is a great illustration of food synergy at work. Just like any oil, omega-3s easily combine with oxygen molecules (the process of oxidizing), rendering the fats useless to the body. Antioxidants like vitamin E step in on behalf of the omega-3s, slowing down oxidation and allowing the omega-3s to do their good deeds longer.

This example also illustrates how dietary supplements operate differently than natural foods in the body. Plant sources of omega-3 also contain their own antioxidants—built in by nature and found in the foods' pigments or seeds.

Take ground flaxseed and walnuts, for example. Both are rich sources of plant omega-3s (ALA) and are also naturally rich in antioxidants. But, according to Dr. Kris-Etherton, when you strip out the omega-3s (EPA and DHA) from fish tissue and isolate the pure oil, the omega-3s can more easily oxidize, just like any oil exposed to oxygen. The theory here, and the reason supplement manufacturers add vitamin E to their fish-oil products, is that this vitamin helps prevent oxidation of fatty acids. So what's the take-home message? According to Dr. Kris-Etherton, well-designed, long-term studies on people have not shown clearly that vitamin E supplements help prevent heart disease. However, she believes there is a consensus that diets with a favorable fatty acid composition that are also rich in food-derived antioxidants are effective in this role. So, perhaps when taking fish-oil supplements, it's even more important to make sure the diet also contains antioxidant-rich foods like citrus and lycopene-rich tomato products.

Pears and green tea may enhance vitamin E. Actually, the real heroes may be two components in pears and green tea—caffeic acid and catechins, respectively—that may extend the effectiveness of vitamin E (as well as vitamin C). Caffeic acid is also found in grapes, blueberries, and apples. Green tea catechins may help recycle vitamin E! So you might want to enjoy your afternoon cup of green tea with a handful of vitamin E–rich almonds, peanuts, or Brazil nuts.

MINERALS ARE A SYNERGY MUST!

Minerals matter, too! We'll start with the mineral we hear about most often—calcium—then work our way to some of the less popular and perhaps undervalued minerals.

CALCIUM SYNERGY BOOSTS BONE MASS

Calcium is the mineral du jour when it comes to bone development; vitamin D seems to get short shrift, despite its importance to a strong skeleton. Vitamin D improves the amount of calcium that gets absorbed in the intestines and is required for normal bone growth. But that's only the beginning. Recent results from the Women's Health Initiative (WHI) trial, involving more than 36,000 women ages 50 to 79, taught us a few important lessons about calcium and vitamin D. Here's a quick summary:

More calcium helps only if you don't get enough. When researchers compared hip-bone density of women getting 1,000 milligrams of calcium a day with women getting 2,000, they found that taking in more calcium improved bone density only slightly, and the risk of fractures was the same between the groups.

You may need more vitamin D than you think. The study involved 400 IU doses of vitamin D, but new research suggests that 700 to 1,000 IU of vitamin D a day may be the ideal amount to prevent fractures.

Where's the D?

The adequate daily dietary intake for vitamin D for adults is:

    200 IU for ages 19–50

    400 IU for ages 51–70

    600 IU for ages 71+

The body is designed to synthesize and regulate the amount of vitamin D when skin is exposed to sunlight, so this is a naturally easy way to get some D. The other way is through food, but very few foods naturally contain vitamin D—only fish liver oils, fatty fish, and egg yolks from chickens that have been fed vitamin D. The rest of the foods that contain D generally have been fortified—milk, yogurt, margarine, and cereal.

FOOD	VITAMIN D (IU)
Cod liver oil, 1 Tbsp	1,360
Oysters, Pacific, 3.5 oz, cooked	640
Mackerel, 3.5 oz canned	360
Milk, fortified, 1 c	100
Fish (most types), 3.5 oz	88 (average)
Egg, 1, cooked	26
Beef, chicken, turkey, pork, 3.5 oz	12
Butter, 1 Tbsp	8
Cheese, 2 oz	8
Yogurt, 1 c	4

You need consistently high nutrients for benefits. At the end of the trial, only 59 percent of the women were still taking their pills as instructed by the researchers. What about the women who actually took their calcium and vitamin D supplements correctly and consistently? Well, they had 29 percent fewer hip fractures than those who'd not followed precise instructions.

There could be a calcium–vitamin D cancer connection. Keep in mind that short-term studies are simply not long enough to see definitive effects on cancer incidence. Cancer is a disease that typically develops over 10 to 20 years. From this trial, though, certain interesting results were noted. The women who started the study with low blood levels of vitamin D developed colorectal cancer twice as often as those with the highest levels. This evidence supports the idea that long-term vitamin D status may affect our risk for this cancer, according to Karen Collins, MS, RD, CDN, nutrition advisor for the American Institute for Cancer Research.

In another large study, this time with Swedish men, calcium was found to be potentially protective for colon cancer. The men in the top half of calcium consumption were 27 to 32 percent less likely to develop colorectal cancer than the men in the bottom half.

CALCIUM, VITAMIN D, AND A LOW-FAT DIET TO EASE PMS DISTRESS

Got PMS? Many of you will answer yes because, according to some estimates, about two-thirds of women report regular premenstrual discomfort, with about one-third seeking help from a health care provider. And about 3 to 8 percent of women experience severe impairment called premenstrual dysphoric disorder.

These pesky and sometimes debilitating PMS symptoms occur between ovulation and the start of your period. Here's the bad news for all you twenty-somethings: PMS becomes increasingly more common in women as they move through their thirties, and symptoms can worsen over time as well. What kinds of symptoms are ascribed to PMS? Consider this cornucopia of complaints: breast swelling and tenderness, bloating or water retention, headaches, irritability and moodiness, depression, food cravings, and more!

PMS symptoms may be aggravated by a high-fat diet. It's been suggested that a high-fat diet may have something to do with PMS breast pain. Researchers at the University of Milan surveyed 34 women complaining of severe breast pain and 29 women without breast pain (with a mean age of 34 years). The researchers found that women with soreness tended to have a higher fat intake (38 percent calories from fat versus 34 percent) throughout their cycles, compared with women without pain. The way I see it, this is yet another reason to avoid eating a high-fat diet.

Got milk? Or Tums? Probably the most effective potential PMS helper is calcium. Some researchers suggest a daily calcium intake of around 1,200 milligrams a day. Several studies have suggested that PMS patients have altered calcium balance and are at increased risk for osteoporosis. Adding fuel to this fire, other recent studies have linked lessening PMS symptoms with adequate calcium and milk intakes. In a Columbia University study, women with moderate to severe PMS who took two Tums E-X tablets twice a day (for 1,200 milligrams of calcium) reported a 48 percent reduction in PMS symptoms (pain, water retention, negative affect, and food cravings). And a Turkish study of PMS symptoms in adolescent girls found that drinking more milk was associated with less bloating, cramps, and cravings and less increased appetite.

VITAMIN D–FORTIFIED FOODS

Since vitamin D is hard to get, especially in winter, but is much needed for several synergistic reasons, here are some of the food products I found that are fortified with vitamin D. The first two sections of this chart include fiber and sugar data. The last section, which focuses on margarines and spreads, includes data about the fat content of each.

PRODUCT	VITAMIN D (% DV)	CALCIUM (% DV)	CALORIES	FIBER (G)	SUGAR (G)
Breakfast Cereals					
GENERAL MILLS					
Basic 4, 1 c	10	25	200	3	5
Wheat Chex, 1 c	10	10	180	5	5
Total Raisin Bran, 1 c	10	100	170	5	19
Total Whole Grain, ¾ c	10	100	100	3	5
Total with Strawberries, 1 c	10	100	180	4	13
KELLOGG'S					
Smart Start Antioxidants, 1 c	10	0	190	3	14
Yogurt (6 oz)					
WEIGHT WATCHERS					
Strawberry, Vanilla	30	30	100	3	12
DANNON LIGHT & FIT					
Cherry Vanilla	20	20	60	0	8
Vanilla, Raspberry	20	20	60	0	7
YOPLAIT ORIGINAL					
Blackberry Harvest, French Vanilla, and other flavors	20	20	170	0	27
YOPLAIT LIGHT					
Apricot Mango and other flavors	20	20	100	0	14
Lemon Cream Pie	20	20	110	0	15

PRODUCT **Yogurt Smoothies and Drinks**	VITAMIN D (% DV)	CALCIUM (% DV)	CALORIES	FIBER (G)	SUGAR (G)
YOPLAIT					
Yoplait Nouriche, 11 oz	25	30	170	5	18
Yoplait Smoothie Light (with Splenda), 8 oz Strawberry Light and other flavors	20	20	90	3	9
DANNON					
Dannon Frusion Smoothie, 10 oz Wild Berry Blend and other flavors	35	25	270	<1	48
Dannon Light & Fit Smoothie, 7 oz assorted flavors	15	15	70	0	12

PRODUCT **Margarine (1 Tbsp)**	VITAMIN D (% DV)	CALCIUM (% DV)	CALORIES	FAT (G)	SATURATED FAT (G)
Canola Harvest	15	10	100	11	1.5
Fleischmann's Original	15	0	70	8	1.5
Country Crock Plus Calcium & Vitamins	15	10	50	5	1
Promise Buttery Spread	15	0	80	8	1.5
Smart Balance 67% Buttery Spread	15	0	80	9	2.5

HIDDEN CALCIUM IN FOOD PRODUCTS

You expect to find calcium in the dairy aisle, but the cereal aisle? Certain cereal products contain impressive amounts of added calcium. Here's what I found in my cereal aisle.

PRODUCT	CALCIUM (% DV)	CALORIES	FIBER (G)	SUGAR (G)
Cereal Bars				
QUAKER BREAKFAST COOKIES				
Oatmeal Raisin, 1	30	180	5	15
Apple Cinnamon, 1 *(also contain 15% Daily Value for vitamins E, A, and the B vitamins)*	30	170	5	15
Hot Cereal				
QUAKER INSTANT OATMEAL (LOWER SUGAR)				
Apples & Cinnamon, 1 packet	10	110	3	6
Maple & Brown Sugar, 1 packet *(also contain 20% vitamin A, folic acid, and the B vitamins)*	10	120	3	4
Cold Cereal *(see "Vitamin D–Fortified Foods" on page 62 for cereals that contain vitamin D plus calcium)*				
GENERAL MILLS				
Fiber One Honey Clusters 1¼ c *(3 grams of the fiber are soluble)*	10	170	14	5
QUAKER				
Cinnamon Life, ¾ c	10	120	2	8
Oatmeal Squares, 1 c	10	210	5	10

So excited about soy and calcium. In lab studies, calcium in combination with soy isoflavones was found to preserve bone mineral density to a greater extent than either did alone. So it seems that in this case, two nutrients were actually better than one. However, if you want to reap similar rewards, note that not all soy products are calcium fortified. The only way to know for sure is to check the nutrition information label. Look toward the bottom of the label, where it lists the percentage Daily Value of various vitamins and minerals. I rolled up my sleeves and read labels in my supermarket; in the box below, I list the soy products with more than 10 percent of the daily value for calcium.

WHICH SOY PRODUCTS ARE TOPS IN CALCIUM?

FOOD	CALCIUM (% DV)	SOY PROTEIN (G)	VITAMIN D (% DV)
Swiss Flavor, 1 slice	15	3	10
Yellow American Flavor, 1 slice	20	3	10
Pepper Jack Flavor, 1 slice	20	3	10
Cheddar Flavor, 1 slice	20	3	10
Mozzarella Flavor, ¼ c	30	6	25
Gimme Lean! Ground Beef Style, 2 oz	10	8	0
Meatless Chick'n Nuggets, 4	20	11	0
Extra firm tofu, 2.8 oz	15	7	0
Firm tofu, 2.8 oz	15	7	0
Ayazuma Lite extra firm tofu, 2.8 oz	15	7	30
Black Bean Chipotle Wrap, 1	25	13	0
Garden Veggie Patties Veggie Burgers, Cheddar Burger, 1	15	13	0
Meatless Lasagna, 1 pkg	15	20	0
Meatless Burgers, 1	15	14	0

MAGNESIUM MAY HOLD METABOLIC SYNDROME AT BAY

We all know calcium is vital to our health, but magnesium deserves some respect, too. This mineral is involved in biochemical reactions that keep our bones strong, our heart rhythm healthy, and our nervous system functioning smoothly. Eating a magnesium-rich diet may also help reduce your risk of developing metabolic syndrome (a collection of risk factors leading to heart disease, stroke, and diabetes). Researchers from a huge multicenter study called CARDIA (Coronary Artery Risk Development in Young Adults) that followed thousands of adults over 15 years found that those who took in the most magnesium in food were 30 percent less likely to develop metabolic syndrome than those with the lowest magnesium intakes.

That's all pretty important, don't you think? But only about 32 percent of the US population met the recommended daily intake for magnesium, according to data from the Agricultural Research Service Community Nutrition Research Group.

You can actually meet almost your entire magnesium requirement with a healthy handful of roasted pumpkin seeds! Just ¼ cup contains about 300 milligrams (95 percent of the Dietary Reference Intake). For other foods considered to be "rich" in magnesium, see the list on page 353.

ZINC FOR IMMUNE FUNCTION

Many enzymes that help the body run smoothly, including those involved with energy metabolism, require zinc. This mineral is also important for the proper functioning of the immune system—which you definitely want in top working order! Zinc also aids in the regulation of blood pressure and the mineralization of bone.

Daily intakes recommended for zinc are around 15 milligrams for men and 12 milligrams for women age 11 and older. Only a few foods contain at least half this amount; most zinc sources (meats, nuts, and grains) range from 1 to 4 milligrams per serving.

POTASSIUM FOR HYPERTENSION

An intake of around 3,500 milligrams a day—the amount believed to help reduce incidence of hypertension—would also closely match the government recommendations to eat more fruits and vegetables.

Chapter 3

When Two or More Nutrients Are Better Than One: Phytochemical Edition

Admittedly, the amazing world of phytochemicals can be confusing. The lengthy word itself, phytochemical, is derived from the Greek word for "plant" (phyto). Simply put, phytochemicals are active components naturally found in plants that provide health benefits and disease protection in the human body.

From my perspective, it's hard to believe how far we've come in understanding phytochemicals—in fact, 20 years ago, when I first began to study nutrition, we didn't know most of these nutrients even existed! The number of known phytochemicals in foods is now estimated at roughly 8,000, according to Cornell University food scientist Rui Hai Liu, PhD. Eight thousand different nutrients working together in the food we eat—the implications for human health are simply staggering.

Within the plant world, phytochemicals perform many important duties. Some help protect the plant from various types of stress, while others serve as antibiotics. And some are best known for giving plants their signature color.

Beta-carotene, for example, lends a yellow-orange hue to carrots and sweet potatoes, while the red in tomatoes comes from the phytochemical lycopene.

These same nutrients confer a wide variety of health benefits to humans as well. Perhaps most exciting, new avenues of research are leading scientists to better understand the complex interaction among phytochemicals, as it seems some combinations provide even more benefits when consumed together than alone. This synergism is one of the key reasons many experts advise eating plant foods in "whole" form whenever possible. In this way, we partake of all the nutrients a food has to offer and reap the rewards of those phytochemicals in their nature-made combinations.

A DECADE OF NEW KNOWLEDGE

Because scientists have so much yet to learn about phytochemicals, some experts are guarded about offering advice on which food combinations might be most effective in fighting disease. They might be grouped into the "glass half empty" experts. But wherever food is concerned, I tend to see the glass as half full. I think we certainly know enough about phytochemicals to make some smart suggestions. To me, plants (fruits, vegetables, whole grains, beans, nuts, and seeds) are really "packages" containing beneficial nutrients, fiber, and phytochemicals in ideal amounts and ratios to each other, in most cases delivering powerful protection against many diseases.

To learn more, I asked several phytochemical experts in the United States to share their perspectives on what we've learned in the past 10 years of research and what lessons they think the next 10 years might bring. "There are tens of thousands of compounds in plants that may not have nutrient value but may have a significant impact on reducing risk for chronic disease and/or optimizing health," answers Clare Hasler, PhD, executive director of the Robert Mondavi Institute for Wine and Food Science at the University of California, Davis.

In fact, phytochemical expert Rick Weissinger, MS, RD, believes that past research helped uncover the knowledge that many benefits previously attributed to vitamins and minerals are derived instead from phytochemicals. "We've realized that most of the antioxidant power in foods comes from phytochemicals, not vitamins and minerals," says Weissinger, noting that these recent revelations are largely due to the efforts of scientists like Dr. Liu and Ronald Prior, PhD, and Prior's colleagues at the USDA's Agricultural Research Service. "This nicely explains at least one reason why we need to get our nutrition from plant foods before we reach for any supplements."

What I find most enlightening about phytochemical research is the accumulating evidence that synergy exists among different phytochemicals as well as between phytochemicals and other natural compounds. Jeffrey Blumberg, PhD, FACN, CNS, director of the Antioxidants Research Laboratory at Tufts University in Boston, agrees. "Research studies indicate that phytochemicals may have their actions not only directly but indirectly by acting in synergy with other phytochemicals as well as with essential nutrients," affirms Blumberg.

"Some exciting examples of phytochemical synergy include the ways that green tea, soy foods, and fruits and vegetables reduce cancer risk," notes Weissinger. Want examples of phytochemical synergy? "Look at how much lower the risk for cancer is in a population that combines these foods, especially when you contrast them with Western populations subsisting on soda pop, cheese puffs, and cheeseburgers," he says.

LOOKING TO THE FUTURE

We can look forward to finding new phytochemicals within plant foods that enhance health, predicts Dr. Hasler. For example, the benefits of flavonoids in dark chocolate for heart health is a relatively recent research phenomenon. Dr. Hasler is confident that over the next decade, other phytochemical synergies will be discovered for other diseases, too.

Dr. Blumberg explains that it is difficult to know how many biological functions and health benefits phytochemicals may ultimately be shown to influence. "But studies are ongoing about their potential to benefit Alzheimer's and Parkinson's disease, cancer, diabetes, heart disease, immunodeficiency states, osteoporosis, and many more conditions," he adds.

Weissinger thinks that the next 10 years will probably produce many studies that explore drug forms of various phytochemicals, most of which he predicts will be disappointing, much like the research into antioxidant vitamins. "As old-fashioned and unscientific as it sounds," he says, "we should have some faith in Mother Nature, and just eat more foods that contain phytochemicals, rather than looking for yet another pharmaceutical shortcut."

PHYTOCHEMICAL FAMILIES

Many of the phytochemicals described in this section have strong antioxidant effects. In fact, a few are actually thought to be more powerful antioxidants than vitamins C and E. For example, a recent US population study suggested that drinking at least three glasses of fruit or vegetable juice a week could cut the risk of Alzheimer's disease by 75 percent, compared with having less than one serving per week. The researchers suspect that much of the protection comes from a group of phytochemicals known as polyphenols, because the results persisted after they accounted for intake of other known Alzheimer-fighting nutrients, including vitamins E, C, and beta-carotene. Other laboratory studies have also confirmed that some polyphenols from juices appear to offer brain cells stronger protection than antioxidant vitamins do.

How could polyphenols protect against Alzheimer's disease? The development of the disease isn't fully understood, but some researchers believe it's related to a buildup of plaque from deposits of a protein called beta-amyloid. The antioxidant properties of polyphenols may help protect brain cells from the damage and death from oxidative stress associated with these deposits.

This is just one example of food synergy in action—the more we study, the more it becomes clear that food is nutritious not because of any one isolated ingredient but because of the complex interaction of all these components that offers disease-fighting potential. In Appendix C, you'll find a master table that groups the phytochemicals and summarizes their food sources and functions wherever possible. To be honest, I need this table myself just to keep things straight!

Antioxidants: Fighting Disease at the Cellular Level

What do antioxidants do in your body? Antioxidants oppose oxidation, a natural process that occurs when a substance or chemical combines with oxygen molecules and becomes a free radical. So an "anti" oxidant protects against cellular damage caused by free radicals. Without antioxidants, what would free radicals do to us? Favorite targets of these molecular assassins include the unsaturated fatty acids on cell membranes. Free radicals begin by causing cell wall damage through the oxidation of LDL cholesterol on the cell membranes. Later, they may wreak havoc by damaging the cell membrane itself (a process called lipid peroxidation). Once inside the cell, free radicals may damage DNA and other parts of the cell that help it function properly. Similar to the DNA damage associated with radiation, free-radical damage has been associated with cancer.

POLYPHENOL FAMILY

Polyphenols are the mother of all phytochemical families, containing a whopping 2,000-plus compounds. Polyphenols give many fruits and vegetables their blue, red-blue, or violet colors. This amazing family is basically divided into two subgroups, phenolic acids and flavonoids.

Phenolic acids include, among others, ellagic acid, found in raspberries and strawberries (and other fruits); p-Coumaric acid, in citrus fruits; and resveratrol, in red grape skins, wine, and nuts. Ellagic acid is believed to reduce damage caused by carcinogens in tobacco smoke and air pollutants, while resveratrol has shown powerful antioxidant action, potentially offering protection from heart disease.

Flavonoid phytochemicals are thought to reduce the risk of cardiovascular disease, possibly by reducing blood pressure and strengthening the antioxidant defense systems that protect the heart. Flavonoids also help maintain healthy capillaries, the extremely narrow blood vessels that connect small arteries throughout the body with small veins, by reducing the activity of certain enzymes that naturally break down the supporting structures of blood vessels.

Catechins may fight heart disease and cancer. Catechins, one member of the flavonoid family, offer an impressive list of benefits and may play a role in fighting cancer and heart disease, as well as stimulating the immune system and spurring weight loss. Tea is the best source of catechins, and green tea contains about three times the amount found in black tea. Researchers in Sweden recently examined the health habits of 60,000 women and found that drinking at least 2 cups of tea a day cut the risk of ovarian cancer by nearly 50 percent. There's a lot more about the benefits of tea on pages 132–35.

Quercetin and catechin improve platelet function. Platelets are small particles in the blood that play an important role in the clotting process. In lab studies, quercetin and catechin have been shown to act synergistically to guard against platelets' tendency to clump together, a dangerous condition that can lead to the clots and blockages associated with stroke and heart attack. Quercetin is found in red grapes, cherries, kale, lettuce, garlic, onion, apples, pears, yellow-fleshed nectarines and peaches, and broccoli, while catechin is found not only in tea but also in grapes, cocoa, lentils, black-eyed peas, and white-fleshed peaches and nectarines.

Flavonol-rich red grapefruit reduces cholesterol. Remember the grapefruit diet? Well, nix the diet but keep the grapefruit. Two new studies place red grapefruit at the front of the line of health-promoting fruits we should be eating. Researchers from the Hebrew University of Jerusalem's Medical School in Israel studied the antioxidant effects of red and white grapefruits, which, along with other citrus fruits, contain high amounts of antioxidants like vitamin C and a number of polyphenols, particularly flavonoids. The lab studies showed

(continued on page 76)

Flavonol-Rich Foods

What three foods contain the most flavonols (the group of phytochemicals that includes quercetin, along with mycertin and kaempferol)? Why, it's onions, apples, and tea! For more on each of these powerful foods, turn to pages 86, 118, and 132.

The flavonoids anthocyanin and proanthocyanidins provide color and antioxidant activity to many fruits and vegetables. Often, we can let our eyes guide us to the fruits and vegetables highest in flavonoids—the ones with the most color! You'll find them in these fruits and vegetables.

Top fruit sources: Blackberries, cranberries, raspberries, grapes, and elderberries

Top vegetable sources: Eggplant and red cabbage

Other top sources: Wine and black and green teas

Who doesn't absolutely love when those beautiful berries start hitting the super-markets in spring! Berries are brimming with nutrients and phytochemicals. Black-berries, raspberries, and strawberries, for example, contain several types of bioflavonoids and—along with blueberries—some phenolic acids. Both of those phyto-chemical families have powerful antioxidant duties in the body and help protect against disease in several different ways.

Cancer-fighting compounds. Berries have been named a "food that fights can-cer" by the American Institute for Cancer Research (AICR). Berries are loaded with vitamin C and fiber, and diets high in both of these substances have been consis-tently linked to lower cancer risk. But they also contain ellagic acid (especially promi-nent in strawberries and raspberries) that laboratory studies have shown may help prevent cancers of the skin, bladder, lung, esophagus, and breast. "This phyto-chemical seems to use several different anticancer methods at once: It acts as an antioxidant, it helps the body deactivate specific carcinogens, and it helps slow the reproduction of cancer cells," notes the AICR. And blueberries contain a family of phenolic compounds called anthocyanosides, which seem to be among the most potent antioxidants yet discovered.

Ample antioxidants. Raspberries possess 50 percent more antioxidant power than strawberries, 10 times more than tomatoes, and three times more than kiwifruit, according to a recent study by Dutch scientist Jules Beekwilder, PhD, with Plant Research International in Wageningen, the Netherlands. The study suggests that while vitamin C makes up about 20 percent of the total antioxidant activity in rasp-berries and red anthocyanins account for 25 percent, the lion's share—more than 50 percent—comes from phytochemicals called ellagitannins. "These special tannins usually occur in leaves and bark, but in the raspberry they also end up in the edible parts—the fruit," says Dr. Beekwilder. "Besides being antioxidants, these compounds work against intestinal infections like salmonella."

Assorted nutrients. Berries are at the top of my product list, not only because they have such a unique sweet taste and come in beautiful shades of red, blue, and purple, but also because they are "berry" nutritious. A serving supplies a nice dose of fiber, vitamin C, and assorted other vitamins and minerals in addition to its impressive lineup of phytochemicals. Check out the nutrition profile of the four most popular berries.

BERRY (1 CUP SERVING)	CALORIES	FIBER (G)	VITAMIN C (% DV)	FOLIC ACID (% DV)	VIT. B_6 (% DV)	VITAMIN B_{12} (% DV)	CALCIUM (% DV)	MAGNESIUM (% DV)
Strawberries (sliced)	50	3.8	125%	7%	8%	10%	2%	5%
Raspberries	60	8.4	41%	8%	5%	10%	3%	7% (also 8% of niacin)
Blackberries	75	7.6	40%	12%	6%	5%	5%	9%
Blueberries	81	3.9	25%	2%	4%	7%	1%	2% (also 6% of thiamine)

ENJOY BERRIES AT THEIR BEST

I love almost all types of fruit, but my absolute favorites are strawberries, raspberries, and blackberries! My favorite jam is triple berry. Favorite pie? You guessed it—berry! One of the food products that gets me through winter is frozen berries; we blend smoothies year-round in the Magee house! And to me, summer hasn't really begun until I've gone to the farmers' market in my town and made a batch of triple berry jam (using less sugar, of course). I hold the jar up and announce, "The first jam of summer!" not unlike when the conductor shouts, "The first gift of Christmas!" in The Polar Express.

Just in case you are timid about buying and storing berries, here are four basic tips.

- Avoid buying bruised or oozing berries. Turn the clear baskets over to check the berries on the bottom.

- Look for firm, plump, full-colored berries.

- When you bring berries home, cover and refrigerate them until they are ready to be served.

- Use berries quickly, because if they are perfectly ripe the day you buy them, they can deteriorate and become soft and moldy within a couple days. The exception to the rule is blueberries, which can be stored for about 5 days or so.

a 10 percent higher free-radical-scavenging activity for red grapefruit. This was followed by a human trial of postoperative bypass patients with high triglyceride levels who were put on a very low-fat diet (the standard for fighting heart disease), but one group was given red or white grapefruit every day for 30 days. The grapefruit eaters, in general, had lower total and low-density lipoprotein (LDL) cholesterol levels. However, only those eating the red grapefruit enjoyed a 17 percent decrease in serum triglycerides, compared with the control group. The researchers suspect that we can thank the antioxidants in red grapefruit for these desirable blood lipid benefits.

More recently, UCLA scientists performing a lab study noted that naringenin, a flavonoid found in grapefruit and oranges, helped repair damaged DNA in cancer cells. This knack for repairing DNA may also help *prevent* cancer because it is thought to prevent rapid spreading of mutations in these cells.

Caution: Grapefruit may interact with some drugs for cholesterol, blood pressure, heart rhythm, depression, anxiety, HIV, immunosuppression, allergies, impotence, and seizures, possibly due to its natural phytochemicals called furanocoumarins. If you are under treatment for any of these conditions, check with your doctor or pharmacist before adding grapefruit to your diet.

Resveratrol reduces oxidative stress. A polyphenol found in grapes, resveratrol belongs to another subclass of antioxidant phytochemicals called phytoalexin. Plants that produce resveratrol do so in response to stress, so this phytochemical serves as a natural antibiotic for the plant. In humans, its protective effects may contribute to the Mediterranean paradox—the protective effect of red wine drinking on cardiovascular health.

Isoflavones fight cancer. Abundant soy products, isoflavones are plant-based estrogens and antioxidants that have shown the ability to inhibit the growth of cancer cells in numerous lab studies. As if that's not enough, isoflavones also show promise in protecting us from heart disease by inhibiting the deposit of platelets on damaged blood vessel walls. For more on soy benefits, check out the Synergy in Action sidebar on pages 106–108.

HOW MUCH ISOFLAVONE IS IN THIS SOY PRODUCT?

Isoflavone content varies widely among different types of soybeans and from product to product, depending on the manufacturing; thus, all the values here are approximates. You might want to look to specific brand and product labels to find specific amounts.

FOOD	ISOFLAVONE (MG)	PROTEIN (G)	CALORIES
Whole soybeans, ½ c, cooked	88	14	149
Roasted soybeans, ¼ c	84	15	202
Tempeh, 4 oz	61	17	204
Soy flour, defatted, 3.5 oz	44	47	329
Soy milk, regular, 1 c	40	10	140
Tofu, firm, 4 oz, uncooked	38	9	120
Textured soy protein, ½ c, cooked	35	11	59
Soy milk, light, 1 c	20	4	100
Isolated soy protein, ¼ c	14	6	30
Soy concentrates, 1 oz, dry	12	17	94

CAROTENOID FAMILY

You may have heard news bites about a particular carotene, beta-carotene, in recent years. Well, it turns out that we probably should be inviting the whole family of carotenoids to dinner! Some researchers suggest that mixtures of carotenoids exhibit more antioxidant activity than each of the carotenoids does by itself.

For example, even though lycopene appears to have some effect on its own against prostate cancer, scientists have found that tomatoes also contain a variety of other ingredients that are likely responsible for lowering cancer risk. A shared concern among nutritionists and many scientists is that people will take lycopene supplements rather than eat lycopene-rich foods like tomatoes and

(continued on page 82)

This fruit that acts like a vegetable is locked and loaded with food synergy potential. It first grabbed headlines when researchers discovered that it's loaded with lycopene (thought to have the highest antioxidant activity of all the carotenoids), which has synergy with vitamin E and other food components. But upon closer inspection, it's a standout among fruits and vegetables because it actually contains all four major carotenoids (alpha- and beta-carotene, lutein, and lycopene) and all three high-powered antioxidants (beta-carotene, vitamin E, and vitamin C), also thought to have synergy together.

Tomatoes are also well known for containing antioxidants that inhibit the cellular damage that can lead to cancer. But recent lab research suggests that tomatoes may also help combat cancer at its later stages. In several studies, tomato components have stopped the growth of several types of cancer cells (in the breast, lung, and endometrium). Other lab studies have linked a tomato-rich diet with lower prostate cancer risk. According to the American Institute for Cancer Research (AICR), a few small clinical studies have investigated how tomato-rich diets influence the health of prostate-cancer patients during treatment, and the preliminary results are encouraging.

Tomatoes may decrease risk of heart disease and prostate cancer. Eating foods rich in lycopene has been linked to a lower risk of heart disease; a serving a day may add up to as much as a 30 percent lower heart disease risk. Eating two to four servings of tomato sauce a week was associated with a 35 percent risk reduction of prostate cancer, according to a large prospective study of male health professionals.

Tomatoes may prevent or treat skin cancer. According to the AICR, epidemiological (population) studies suggest that people who consume more lycopene have less skin cancer. If you commit to regularly eating tomato products, such as tomato paste and sauce, over several weeks, you'll find yourself 40 percent less sunburned than those who skimp on those foods. Of course, continue to slather on the sunscreen. But who wouldn't want to boost protection with such a tasty kitchen staple?

A team of German researchers conducted a fascinating study about sunburn protection from two antioxidant-rich foods—olive oil and tomatoes—with impressive results. Half of all the participants consumed 10 grams of olive oil (about 2 teaspoons) and 40 grams (about ¼ cup) of tomato paste daily for 10 weeks. The other half didn't get the additional tomato paste and olive oil. As the study moved along, the researchers used a sunlamp to measure how much exposure produced skin reddening in each subject. By the end of the study, those who ate tomato paste and olive oil were experiencing 35 percent less reddening than the other group. While this didn't amount to a great deal of extra skin protection, the ability of olive oil and tomato paste to make a measurable difference in such a short time was significant.

ENJOY TOMATOES AT THEIR BEST

When it comes to maximizing the synergy and nutrients from fresh tomatoes, two food-prep rules run counter to many recipes: 1. Don't peel them. 2. Never toss out the seeds. Most of the antioxidant power of the tomato actually lies in the peel and seeds, so the best way to cook fresh tomatoes is au naturel, whenever possible. Of course, there's no harm in using already cooked or processed tomatoes; in fact, once cooked, the phytochemicals are rendered more available and thus more likely to be absorbed.

No one has to ask me twice to eat more tomatoes. I'll get them any way I can. Here are some of my favorite ways to enjoy tomatoes.

- Toss cherry or grape tomatoes in green or pasta salads.
- Stick tomato slices in a sandwich or have them sitting pretty on an open-faced grilled cheese.
- Chop and add tomatoes to an egg dish or vegetable sauté.
- Enjoy dishes featuring tomato-based sauces, such as marinara or salsa.

Broccoli is one of those standout vegetables because it has so many powerful components, each offering wonderful health benefits. But recent research suggests that several of those components are working together, too. Matthew Wallig, DVM, PhD, professor of comparative pathology at the University of Illinois at Urbana-Champaign, discovered that crambene, one of the phytochemicals in cruciferous vegetables (like broccoli), is more active when combined with another better-known cruciferous phytochemical, indole-3-carbinol. There's also evidence that components in broccoli have synergy with components in other plant foods. For example, subjects in lab studies fed a combination of tomatoes and broccoli had markedly less prostate tumor growth, compared with groups who ate either food alone or a fourth group fed a diet containing the specific cancer-fighting substances isolated from tomatoes and broccoli.

Broccoli may help reduce cancer risk. Several components commonly found in the cruciferous family (cauliflower, cabbage, Brussels sprouts, bok choy, and kale, as well as broccoli) have been linked to lower cancer risk. In lab studies, cruciferous components have shown the ability to stop the growth of cancer cells in tumors in the breast, endometrium, lung, colon, liver, and cervix. And studies that track the diets of people over time have found that diets high in cruciferous vegetables are associated with drastically lower rates of prostate and bladder cancer. For example, men who ate three servings of these vegetables a week reduced their prostate cancer risk by 41 percent, as reported in the September 2006 issue of *Environmental Nutrition*.

Lab studies suggest that many important phytochemicals in broccoli fight tumor growth at different stages of the cancer process, making it a true powerhouse vegetable. Broccoli is rich in sulforaphane (a member of the isothiocyanate family of phytochemicals), which stimulates enzymes in the body that detoxify carcinogens before they have a chance to damage cells in the first place. Through different mechanisms, indole-3-carbinol and crambene activate enzymes that help the body eliminate carcinogens before they can harm our genes.

In Dr. Wallig's recent study, his team exposed the detoxification enzymes to both indole-3-carbinol and crambene at the same time. They found that the two compounds performed better together, offering greater protection against liver cancer, than either did alone. "If the effect of these two phytochemicals on activating the phase two enzymes was simply additive, we would have gotten two plus two equals four. But what we found was that two plus two equals more like six," says Dr. Wallig. The dose of the phytochemicals used in his animal study weren't comparable to amounts that would be reasonable in human diets, but the results suggest there is some potentially important synergy within broccoli.

Broccoli may help combat heart disease, stomach ulcers, and macular degeneration. Researchers theorize that sulforaphane, which is abundant in broccoli, may combat heart disease and perhaps stomach ulcers by inhibiting the presence of *Helicobacter pylori* (*H. pylori*) infection. Broccoli does indeed contain two phytochemicals thought to help eye health, lutein and zeaxanthin, and fend off macular degeneration (an age-related eye disease).

Broccoli may help reduce inflammation and joint pain. Laboratory studies show that sulforaphane may also block an enzyme that triggers inflammation and joint pain. This is great news for those who suffer from arthritis or give their bones and joints a beating by running on hard surfaces or playing contact sports. Prolonged pressure on the joints can suppress the function of helpful phase two enzymes, but sulforaphane may regenerate and reenergize these wonderful enzymes. Your knees and elbows will thank you for eating broccoli!

ENJOY BROCCOLI AT ITS BEST

When buying fresh broccoli, look for firm florets with a purple, dark green, or bluish hue on the top; they are likely to contain more beta-carotene and vitamin C than florets with lighter green tops. Broccoli that's tinged with yellow or is limp and bendable is too old; I wouldn't recommend buying it. Instead, pick up some broccoli from the frozen section.

Chopped broccoli makes a great addition to soups, stews, and casseroles. Cook it until it's bright green and tender, but take care not to overcook it—broccoli can produce a strong sulfur odor and become quite unappealing.

Of course, no raw veggie platter is complete without those dark green florets! And tossed into a green salad, they offer a huge nutrient boost.

watermelon. The possibility of another "beta-carotene scenario" (that is, in which a greater cancer risk is found with the supplements in spite of a lower expected risk) should make us wary of opting for supplements instead of foods. Overall, the evidence of lycopene's prostate-saving effect (and anticancer effect in general) is more evident in people who eat plenty of tomato products than in those who take supplements. Eating combinations of fruits and vegetables rich in carotenoids—a sweet potato and a carrot and a mango, for example—automatically offers you a nature-made mixture and possibly the best protection.

In the meantime, the research on this amazing phytochemical family just keeps stacking up. Here's what we know about the potential health benefits of some key carotenoids, along with even more exciting news about the benefits they offer together.

Lutein and zeaxanthin may slash the risk of non-Hodgkin's lymphoma. The results of a new study in the *American Journal of Clinical Nutrition* suggest that high daily intake of the carotenoids lutein and zeaxanthin cuts the risk of non-Hodgkin's lymphoma by almost 50 percent. (Whenever something decreases risk by half, that gets my attention.) The researchers found that people with the highest intake of lutein and zeaxanthin had a 46 percent lower risk, compared with people with the lowest intake. The researchers also found that people with a higher number of weekly servings of all vegetables had a 42 percent lower risk than those with the lowest intake of vegetables. What could be going on here? Weissinger suspects that the carotenoids (or other compounds linked to them by virtue of being in the same foods) could be protecting T cells from DNA damage, a known means to developing this form of cancer. Carotenoids seem to protect DNA, so this makes sense. "If the DNA in T cells is damaged, faulty programming can be passed on and a mutated line of cells created, resulting in a lymphoma," explains Weissinger. Want to know what fruits and vegetables are rich in the carotenes/carotenoids besides carrots and sweet potatoes? Check out "Food Sources of Standout Carotenoids" on page 84. There might be some surprises!

Lycopene fights a range of diseases. The fat-soluble red pigment found primarily in tomatoes is thought to have the highest antioxidant activity of all the carotenoids and antioxidant compounds and may reduce the risk of an assortment of diseases, from Alzheimer's to cancer. Lycopene concentrations can be measured in certain areas of the human body, including the blood plasma, liver, lungs, prostate gland, colon, and skin, so it probably isn't too surprising that many researchers think the health benefits of lycopene look very promising.

Carotenoids may help prevent stroke. As a group, the carotenoid family appears to play a significant role in boosting heart health by lowering the amount of plaque that collects in the arteries. Numerous studies have observed that people who eat a lot of carotenoid-rich foods tend to have lower incidence of fatty deposits in their carotid arteries. This finding could be especially important for stroke prevention because the carotid artery delivers oxygenated blood to the brain.

Top Lycopene-Rich Foods

Bright-red tomatoes may be a top source of lycopene, but they're not the only one. The red and pink pigments in watermelon, guava, and red and pink grapefruit signal the presence of lycopene, too. You should try to regularly include lycopene-rich foods in your diet because this natural antioxidant can neutralize unstable molecules that might otherwise damage cells. Several studies link a greater consumption of foods high in lycopene with a lower risk for prostate cancer and possibly other cancers. More research is needed before firm conclusions can be made. While lycopene is available in supplements, keep in mind that studies associated the possible benefits with eating whole foods.

Lutein and beta-carotene protect against colon cancer. Lutein, an antioxidant found in avocados, oranges, and most leafy green vegetables, appears to protect against colon cancer, especially tumors in the large intestine and in people who developed tumors when they were young, according to a recent University of Utah School of Medicine study. Even after the researchers adjusted for dietary fiber (which otherwise might contribute to the results of the study), more lutein was associated with less colon cancer. Some researchers propose that beta-carotene might work at early stages of colon tumor development, whereas lutein may work later in the disease process.

From my perspective, this sequence of protective effects suggests that the presence of several carotenoids in many foods is purposeful, not accidental; it seems to me that nature may have intended for us to eat this way for a reason.

FOOD SOURCES OF STANDOUT CAROTENOIDS

	ALPHA-CAROTENE	BETA-CAROTENE	LUTEIN	LYCOPENE
Fruits				
Apples	X			
Apricots		X		X
Avocados			X	
Cantaloupe	X	X		
Grapefruit				X
Guavas				X
Mangos		X		
Oranges			X	
Papayas		X		
Persimmons				X
Plantains		X		
Watermelon				X

	ALPHA-CAROTENE	BETA-CAROTENE	LUTEIN	LYCOPENE
Vegetables				
Broccoli		X	X	
Carrots	X	X	X	
Celery		X	X	
Dark green leafy vegetables (in general)		X	X	
Green peas	X			
Kale		X	X	
Lettuce			X	
Okra				X
Parsley			X	
Peppers				X
Pumpkin		X		
Spinach		X	X	
Sweet potatoes		X		
Tomatoes	X	X	X	X
Vegetable juice	X	X		X
Winter squash	X	X		

ORGANOSULFUR FAMILY

I call this the smelly family of phytochemicals because you find them in odiferous allium vegetables, including garlic, onions, leeks, scallions, and chives, as well as equally noticeable cruciferous vegetables like cabbage and broccoli. In general, these phytochemicals are thought to help reduce cancer risk by increasing enzyme activity that can detoxify carcinogens and prevent nitrosamines and other carcinogenic compounds from forming. It's worth noting that several phytochemicals in this family may help prevent heart disease, too.

(continued on page 89)

Loaded with phytochemicals, onions and garlic are members of the allium family of plants (other members include scallions, leeks, and chives), which produces organo-sulfur phytochemicals, including allicin and diallyl disulfide (DADS). (The members of this veggie family can thank these phytochemicals for their notoriously pungent aroma.) How do garlic supplements stack up against the real thing? According to the experts at *Environmental Nutrition*, eating fresh garlic regularly is still the best advice. An independent testing firm analyzed 16 brands of garlic supplements and found that few products clearly label how much active compound they contain; even when they do, it's often not accurate.

It's probably not one component in garlic and onions that holds the wealth of health benefits, either, but a combination of substances. For example, originally researchers focused on allicin, the compound that can be blamed for garlic's taste and smell. But now researchers are looking at the other sulfur compounds in garlic (including DADS and SAC, S-allylcysteine), as well as nonsulfur components like the phytochemicals saponins. I suspect that, as with many plant foods, the many differ-ent compounds in whole garlic and onions offer better protection because they inter-act with each other in complex ways that are not yet known or understood. According to the American Institute for Cancer Research, some research suggests that four to five cloves of garlic a week may be ideal for health. That's definitely doable without resorting to supplements.

Garlic may help lower blood lipids. The studies done over the years on garlic's lipid-lowering effects have been, in a word, inconsistent. But a recent review of garlic research by the Albert Einstein College of Medicine in New York City concluded that garlic does indeed have modest lipid-lowering effects when consumed for 6 months.

Studies on a particular form of supplement, AGE (aged garlic extract), have some encouraging results to report. Two small studies from Pennsylvania State University in University Park and UCLA found that AGE reduced total cholesterol by 7 percent and 3 percent, respectively, and reduced LDL cholesterol by 8 percent and 22 percent. Levels of high-density lipoprotein (HDL, or "good") cholesterol increased only in the

UCLA study, which also reported that AGE did three other beneficial things to lower the risk of heart disease: lowered homocysteine levels, stimulated circulation, and inhibited dangerous plaque formation in arteries. Another benefit to consider: AGE is formulated with S-allylcysteine, not allicin, so the characteristic garlic odor is absent.

Onions may help protect against heart disease and stroke. Onions are one of the richest sources of quercetin on the planet. This potent antioxidant is suspected of helping protect against heart disease, stroke, and certain cancers, according to *Environmental Nutrition*. Red and yellow onions possess higher levels of quercetin than white do. The sulfur compounds in raw onions (the ones that, no matter what you do, make you cry) appear to have a blood-thinning effect, according to animal studies from the University of Wisconsin–Madison. Other studies link these compounds with lowering blood pressure and cholesterol, although more research needs to be done.

Onions may help the gut. In addition to all the beneficial components already discussed, onions contain fructooligosaccharides (FOS). This nondigestible type of fiber encourages the growth of helpful and healthful bacteria in the digestive tract, thus producing probiotics! Consumption of onions and garlic, therefore, might reduce your risk of suffering from traveler's diarrhea or diarrhea due to oral antibiotic use and may ease the terrible discomfort of Crohn's disease, ulcerative colitis, and irritable bowel syndrome (IBS). In addition, probiotics can help fend off yeast infections and other bacterial overgrowth.

ENJOY GARLIC AND ONIONS AT THEIR BEST

Some experts say that to get the most health benefits, you need to eat one or two cloves of raw garlic daily. No matter whom you listen to, though, the bottom line is that garlic and onions are good for you, so eat more. When shopping for onions, keep this basic information in mind.

(continued)

- Mild-flavored onions include the white or yellow Bermuda onion, yellow Spanish onion, red onion, and pearl onion, along with specific sweet onions like Vidalia and Maui.

- Strong-smelling onions have probably been bruised, so pass them up.

- Choose onions that seem heavy for their size (that means they have plenty of water in them) and have papery, dry skin.

- If the onion has started to sprout, it's past its prime.

Some experts say that heating garlic right after it's been peeled and crushed causes it to lose most of its active ingredients, but a Penn State study found that allowing chopped or crushed raw garlic to stand for 10 to 15 minutes before heating helps preserve most of its anticancer activity. Personally, my garlic product of choice is bottled minced garlic. It's always in the refrigerator, so whenever I need some garlic, I just measure out a tablespoon or so. Here are some ideas for adding more garlic to your recipes.

- Slip a couple of extra cloves (freshly chopped or roasted) in entrées, from meat loaf to stir-fry to pasta.

- Instead of making plain vegetables, give them a quick stir-fry with a little bit of olive oil or canola oil and some minced garlic.

- Don't be a potato purist; add garlic (fresh or roasted) to your favorite potato dishes.

- Simmer sauces with a teaspoon or two of minced or roasted garlic.

- Dress up dips and dressings with a teaspoon of minced or roasted garlic.

My other favorite way to enjoy garlic is roasted! I love how the flavor mellows and deepens at the same time. To roast, I follow these steps.

Preheat the oven to 350°F. Cut off the tops of two or three garlic bulbs, exposing the cloves.

Set the bulbs in a large square of foil, and drizzle about ½ teaspoon of olive oil over each bulb. Let them sit for 15 minutes.

Wrap the cloves with the foil, so they are inside the foil pouch. Roast for 45 minutes. Squeeze the roasted garlic out of each bulb, clove by clove, and enjoy in your recipe or dish.

The four "big guns" in the organosulfur family are DAS (diallyl sulfide) and DADS (diallyl disulfide), which are both fat-friendly compounds, and SEC (S-ethyl cysteine) and NAC (N-acetylcysteine), which are water-friendly. DADS has been shown to possess the strongest antioxidant activity to prevent LDL cholesterol oxidation. SEC and NAC are linked to cardioprotective activity, along with antioxidant and (especially SEC) antiglycation properties. In the body, glycation is a process that begins when sugars attach to proteins and other structures, rendering them nonfunctional; because glycated substances are slow to leave the body, they may accumulate and wreak havoc until the immune system is triggered.

Garlic and onions may help prevent some cancers. Italian researchers, using data from several Italian and Swiss cancer studies, found that people whose diets are rich in onions, garlic, and other allium family vegetables have a much lower risk of several types of cancer, compared with those who avoid those veggies. Moderate consumption of onions appeared to reduce the risk of colorectal, laryngeal, esophageal, and ovarian cancers, with the protective effect being greatest in people who ate the most onions.

People who ate the most garlic had a lower risk of all cancers studied except breast and prostate cancers, and again, the anticancer benefits were highest in the people who ate the most garlic. The protective effect of onions and garlic didn't disappear after the researchers controlled for the total amount of vegetables eaten, which suggests that there is some definite effect apart from simply eating more vegetables.

The most promising findings, according to *Environmental Nutrition*, have been for stomach, colon, and prostate cancers. Several large population studies have suggested that garlic eaters have significantly lower rates of these three cancers compared to non–garlic eaters—about 50 percent less risk for stomach and prostate cancer and about 33 percent less risk for colorectal cancer. The AICR names garlic as one of 11 foods that fight cancer and reports that laboratory research suggests diallyl disulfide helps protect against cancers of the skin, colon, and lung. Components of garlic have also shown the ability to slow or stop the growth of tumors in the prostate, bladder, and stomach tissue, and animal studies have shown that components in allium vegetables slow the development of cancer in several stages at various body sites: stomach, breast, esophagus, colon, and lung.

How might these smelly veggies be helping? In general, the group of allium vegetables appears to help block cancer-promoting enzymes, promote DNA repair, and regulate the cell life cycle. We definitely need more questions answered, but some researchers suspect that garlic may suppress the formation of carcinogens beyond its antioxidant contribution, possibly by inhibiting tumor cell growth, influencing hormones, or controlling blood vessel formation. As for onions, they boast impressive amounts of lignans, phytochemicals that are thought to be cancer-fighting compounds. Onions also contribute the flavonoid quercetin, which acts as a powerful antioxidant, possibly protecting against certain cancers as well, according to *Environmental Nutrition*.

Chapter 4

Whole Foods: Tapping the Synergy Within

What do Heath Ledger, Johnny Depp, and Denzel Washington all have in common? Besides being top movie actors, they don't just look good, they *are* good. What does this have to do with whole foods, pray tell? Well, when we go to the box office, we are buying their "total package." They rarely disappoint, what with their top-shelf acting abilities and stunning good looks. Okay, this example is a bit of a reach, but it's sort of the same with whole foods. We are buying the total package, and it rarely disappoints us nutritionally.

"Whole foods" is a term used to describe ingredients—like fruits, vegetables, whole grains, nuts, and seeds—that have not been refined or processed, so original nutrients remain intact. Taking a dietary supplement simply does not provide the same benefit. I know it's easier to pop a pill than to choose whole grain bread or whole grain–blend pasta, or to remember to add ground flaxseed to your fruit smoothie, or to make a point each day to eat a bunch of fruits and vegetables. It's easier to grab chips or cookies than to choose yogurt and nuts for a snack. But there is magic in the packaging! Just remember that.

WHY WHOLE FOODS ARE THE ANSWER

The more we know about nutrition and health, the more it seems we need to eat the way we did a hundred years ago. Recent research is pointing us in the direction of eating mostly whole foods or food in as close to its natural form as possible. Wondering whether you'll enjoy eating this way? It's not hard. Consider the following whole food switches.

- Whole grains instead of refined grains whenever possible
- Fruits, vegetables, and beans instead of a supplement containing fiber or vitamins
- A skinless chicken breast cooked with healthful ingredients instead of chicken nuggets made from processed chicken with added fats, flavorings, and preservatives
- A baked potato with chopped green onions and light sour cream instead of sour cream–and–onion potato chips
- Fresh berries for a naturally sweet breakfast instead of berry-flavored pastries or breakfast bars
- A smoothie made with blueberries, yogurt, and frozen banana instead of a blueberry slush or flavored drink

Eating more whole foods is one of the easiest routes to improving health and preventing disease. Whole foods retain fiber, as well as a host of beneficial phytochemicals and nutrients often removed in processed foods. Vegetables, fruits, whole grains, nuts, and legumes are great examples of foods that offer a powerful combination of important vitamins, minerals, fiber, protein, and antioxidants. Here are the top six reasons why you should eat more whole foods starting, like, yesterday!

1. Nutrient shortages are nationwide. According to a USDA survey in the report "What We Eat in America," almost everyone in this country is coming up short on a few key nutrients. The survey showed that almost a third of us get too little vitamin C, almost half get too little vitamin A, more than half get too little magnesium, and 92 to 97 percent get too little fiber and potassium. I'm doing the math here, and that means only 8 percent of us are getting enough fiber and potassium! According to the American Institute for Cancer Research, these particular nutrients are important because they help lower the risk of cancer, heart disease, high blood pressure, and diabetes.

What's the easiest way to correct this nutrient shortage? Two words: *whole foods*. "Almost all of the shortfalls identified by this survey can be corrected by eating a balanced, mostly plant-based diet," notes AICR nutrition advisor Karen Collins, MS, RD, CDN.

2. Whole foods offer good fats. When you concentrate on eating whole foods, it becomes easier to cut bad-for-your-health fats (trans fats and saturated fats) from your diet because these fats are often added to processed foods and fast food. Likewise, emphasizing the good fats (omega-3s from fish and plants and monounsaturated fat from plants) should be a snap. (Well, maybe not a snap, but it'll be a little bit easier.)

3. Fiber, fiber, fiber. Whole plant foods contain beneficial amounts of fiber, whereas processed foods often do not. Fiber helps your health in all sorts of ways: It keeps the gastrointestinal tract moving, helps you feel full faster, and helps fight heart disease and diabetes. "Foods are a better way to get fiber than supplements. You get the whole package," says Martin O. Weickert, MD, of the German Institute of Human Nutrition in Potsdam-Rehbrücke, referring to the fact that most plant foods have both types of fiber (soluble and insoluble). Foods rich in fiber are related to the control of blood glucose, blood lipids, and weight in adults, according to researchers from the Georgia

Prevention Institute who recently conducted a study on whole grain foods and abdominal fat deposits in teenagers.

4. The benefits extend beyond fiber. "Whole grains are rich in a myriad of vitamins, minerals, and phytochemical compounds that alone or in combination are likely to have significant health benefits beyond those from dietary fiber," notes Simin Liu, MD, ScD, researcher and professor of epidemiology at UCLA.

Want to lower your risk of developing type 2 diabetes? Want to lower blood levels of insulin and glucose after a meal? Want to improve your serum lipid levels? Want to lower oxidative stress? Then get ready to switch to whole grains. Whole grain foods have recently been linked to smaller after-meal glucose and insulin levels. And according to Dr. Liu, consistent research strongly supports the premise that eating more whole grain foods can lower the risk of type 2 diabetes.

More whole grains may lead to less VAT (visceral adipose tissue) fat. This is the type of abdominal fat deposited between the organs and the abdominal

"Whole Foods" as a Business?

One supermarket chain in particular believes so much in the "whole foods" movement, they named their company after it! The now ubiquitous and booming Whole Foods Market grocery chain started in 1980 as one store in Austin, Texas. Their mission was simple: "to provide a more natural alternative to what the food supply was typically offering at the time." First and foremost stated in the company philosophy is a dedication "to food in its purest state." So how's business? Well, let's just say Whole Foods is now the world's leading retailer of natural and organic foods, with 184 stores in North America and the United Kingdom. Their 2005 revenue was $4.7 billion, and they have 78 new stores in the pipeline between now and 2009.

muscle and, in excessive amounts, is associated with an increased risk for a number of health problems. Researchers from the Georgia Prevention Institute measured the abdominal fat and food intake of 460 teenagers and concluded that whole grain foods may protect against VAT fat accumulation in teens who have higher levels of subcutaneous abdominal tissue (fat deposits just beneath the skin).

5. Whole foods include fewer extras. Whole foods are basically as nature made them, without added fat, sugar, or sodium. Eating more whole foods makes it easy to cut down on extra calories when they replace processed foods, which contain so many added fats and sugars. According to a USDA survey in "What We Eat in America," roughly half the adults in this country keep their dietary fat intake in the recommended range of 20 to 35 percent calories from fat; 44 percent of us exceed that. For a person eating 2,000 calories a day, the acceptable range requires eating no more than 78 grams of fat (about what's found in 7 tablespoons of butter).

If you look at our sodium consumption, the picture is more grim. An analysis of the 2001 to 2002 data found that more than 97 percent of men and women between ages 19 and 50 were taking in more than the suggested 1,500 milligrams a day, and that's not including salt added at the table.

6. Whole foods provide phytochemical insurance. Over the past 10 years, scientists have identified hundreds of components in our food system called phytochemicals (also called phytonutrients). We still don't know all of them, but these health-promoting components are there in abundance in plant foods. A decade ago, we knew much less about phytochemicals, such as the powerful antioxidant lycopene (a red carotenoid found mainly in tomatoes), anthocyanins (potent antioxidants that give berries their deep blue color), and pterostilbene (which appears to turn on a switch in cells that breaks down fat and cholesterol) in blueberries and two grape varieties—Gamay and Pinot

Noir. And the bioflavonoids are actually thought to have more antioxidant power than vitamins C and E. The only way to make sure you are getting the phytochemicals we know about and the ones we haven't yet discovered or named is to eat plant foods in their whole, unprocessed form (grinding is fine for grains or seeds).

WHOLE GRAINS = COMPLETE NUTRITION

According to a recent national survey, only 8 percent of American adults eat the recommended three servings of whole grains a day. How easy is it? Consider that if you use 100 percent whole wheat bread for your sandwich each day, plus enjoy a bowl of whole grain cereal as a snack, you net three servings without so much as having to boil water.

Once you start opening your mind to the "brown" options (whole grain breads and cereals are usually brown instead of refined-grain white),

Whole Grain History

When the industrialization wave hit the United States in the late 1800s, a new way of milling and mass refining took hold in the grain business and never let go. Removing the bran and germ seemed like a good idea at the time because it meant that grain products could sit on store shelves much longer without spoiling. Wrong!

The worldwide epidemic of B-vitamin deficiencies (pellagra and beriberi) that followed was only the beginning. Frankly, we are just realizing the nutritional fallout from minimizing whole grains in our diet. Now, more than 100 years later, we are coming full circle and learning how to make products and create recipes that keep the grain the way nature made it—whole!

opportunities abound. For example, there are tasty, higher-fiber whole wheat hot dog and hamburger buns now at most supermarkets, including national chains like Trader Joe's and Whole Foods Markets. Or when you're having hot or cold breakfast cereal, reach for one that has plenty of whole wheat. When a Chinese restaurant offers you a choice between brown and white rice or an Italian restaurant offers the option of whole wheat pasta (some do here in California), take the whole grain ball and run with it.

Whole grains (and legumes) are unique to other whole foods because they are naturally low in fat and cholesterol free; contain 10 to 15 percent protein; and offer loads of fiber, resistant starch and oligosaccharides, minerals, vitamins, antioxidants, phytochemicals, and, often, phytoestrogens. With all those nutrients in one package, it's no wonder whole grains provide so many health benefits, including protection from cardiovascular disease, stroke, diabetes, insulin resistance, obesity, and some cancers.

THE WHOLE TRUTH ABOUT WHOLE GRAINS

Want to statistically reduce your risk of death from all causes? You'll need to make only one dietary change. According to results published in the *American Journal of Clinical Nutrition*, choose whole grains whenever possible.

About the only refined-grain products I eat are the occasional pizza crust or sourdough and French bread (in restaurants) and sometimes pasta (which I always cook al dente because it has a lower glycemic index this way). I used to think I could never accept whole wheat noodles as "pasta." Never say never! In developing the recipes for this book, I used a whole wheat pasta blend and really started to like it (so did my family—which includes two picky teens).

Here's a quick list of all the ways that whole grains benefit your body. After reading it, you may ask yourself, "What *don't* they do?"

Improve your blood sugar. Whole grains are digested more slowly than refined grains, which have beneficial effects on blood sugar and insulin (keeping levels of both down). A recent study found that the more whole grains men and women ate, the lower their fasting insulin levels were. And this is a good thing.

Lengthen your life span. After analyzing data from more than 15,000 people ages 45 to 64, researchers from the University of Minnesota School of Public Health found that as whole grain intake went up, total mortality (the rate of death from all causes) went down. The people who ate the most whole grains had a 23 percent lower risk of all-cause mortality than those who ate fewer whole grains.

Reduce the risk of type 2 diabetes. The Nurses' Health Study found that women who ate more than 5 grams of fiber from whole grain cereals daily had about 30 percent less risk of developing type 2 diabetes than those who got less than 2.5 grams a day. Other research found that women who ate a diet low in cereal fiber and high on the sugar (glycemic) index doubled their risk.

Improve weight control. One study found that women who ate three or more servings of whole grain foods a day had significantly lower body mass indexes (BMIs) than those eating less than one serving a day. (This was found in men, too, but the link was more significant in women.) Another study found that women whose diets included the most whole grains were half as likely to gain a lot of weight over a 12-year period than those who ate the least whole grains. This slimming effect was seen even in teens.

Avoid metabolic syndrome. Research has found that metabolic syndrome— a condition that raises the risk of diabetes, heart disease, and stroke—was found less often in people who ate the most cereal fiber and whole grains, compared with those who ate the least.

Reduce the risk of heart disease. At least 25 studies have found that people who regularly eat whole grains have a lower risk of heart disease. One study suggests that we can probably cut our risk for cardiovascular disease mortality in half with a high intake of whole grains. When studying people age 60 and older, researchers found that the people who ate the most whole grains had a 52 percent lower death rate from heart disease than people with the lowest intake. "These findings are supported by studies of cardiovascular disease incidence in younger populations," explains Paul Jacques, DSc, a researcher at Tufts University in Boston. "For example, Simin Liu and colleagues observed a 25 percent lower cardiovascular disease incidence among high whole grain consumers, compared with those with low intakes in women age 38 to 63 years old." The researchers found the drop in heart disease was even greater (50 percent) when smokers weren't included in the analysis.

"The evidence is quite consistent and convincing that people who eat at least one serving of whole grains a day have a lower risk of heart disease and stroke," reports Mark Pereira, PhD, a nutritional epidemiologist at Harvard Medical School.

In studying the dietary habits of male health professionals, researchers found that for every 10 gram increase in cereal fiber eaten each day, the risk of heart attack was reduced by nearly 30 percent. A more recent study found that this beneficial effect is even stronger in women.

Cut cholesterol levels. Researchers at Northwestern University's Feinberg School of Medicine in Chicago found that adding oats to an already low-fat diet helped women cut their blood cholesterol by an additional 8 or 9 mg/dL after only 3 weeks. That came on top of the 12 mg/dL reductions seen with the low-fat diet alone! Antioxidants in oats cut cholesterol by suppressing the molecules that make blood cells stick to artery walls. When these cells stick to artery walls and cause inflammation, plaque deposits build up and narrow the passageways where blood flows, leading to "hardening of the arteries."

(continued on page 102)

While getting more fiber is a good reason to reach for that packet of oats in the morning, there's a lot more to oats, nutritionally speaking. Half a cup will give you a nutritional boost beyond the 4 grams of fiber. You also get some protein; smart fats (from monounsaturated and polyunsaturated fat); and a host of vitamins, minerals, and phytochemicals to boot! In fact, the health benefits of oats are so solid that in 1997, the FDA approved a heart health claim for oats. Here's a brief rundown on the science behind the claim that oats can:

Block harmful effects of "bad" cholestrol. Oats contribute two important antioxidant phytochemicals to your diet: avenanthramides (a member of the polyphenol phytochemical family) and phenolic acids (found in most fruits, vegetables, and whole grains). More needs to be known about oat phytochemicals, but researchers from Tufts University in Boston completed a clinical trial using an avenanthramide-rich oat extract and found that the oat phytochemicals worked synergistically with vitamin C to protect LDL cholesterol from oxidation. Oxidized LDL becomes a lot more harmful and more likely to encourage plaquing (or fat deposits) in the arteries.

Lower blood pressure. In many studies, eating oats has been shown to help reduce blood pressure, too. One particularly interesting study at Tufts observed what happened when 43 people consumed low-calorie diets with or without oats for 6 weeks. To control results, the researchers provided the participants with all their food and caloric beverages. The study began with a 2-week weight-maintenance phase, followed by a 6-week weight-loss phase. During the weight-loss phase, one group consumed oats with every meal, while the other did not. While both groups lost comparable amounts of weight and improved their diastolic blood pressure readings (the second number in a reading, which reflects arterial pressure when the heart is at rest), only the oat eaters also saw significant decreases in their systolic readings (the top number that measures arterial pressure when the heart beats).

ENJOY OATS AT THEIR BEST

Oats can be easier to eat than you might think. Of course there are baked goods, like muffins, breads, and certain desserts. Crisps, for example, traditionally call for oats. And granola usually includes plenty of oats, too. But one of the easiest ways to enjoy oats is as instant oatmeal. Usually instant oatmeal is prohibitively high in sugar, but there are now some choices in the supermarket that keep the convenience and lose some of the sugar. For information on instant oatmeal and other ways to enjoy oats, check out the next five tips.

Choose healthier instant oatmeal. Most people prefer some sweetness in their oatmeal. But the amount in all those fun-flavored packets is more than is needed, that's for sure. How do I know? I've sampled the new less-sugar options, and they taste great! Quaker Instant Oatmeal offers Apples & Cinnamon or Maple & Brown Sugar with less sugar, plus my personal favorite—Take Heart Blueberry. A packet (34 grams) of Quaker's Lower Sugar Maple & Brown Sugar contains 4 grams of sugar (13 percent calories from sugar), along with 3 grams of fiber (1 gram of which is soluble). Take Heart Blueberry (a larger 45-gram packet), with added oat bran and flaxseed, contains 6 grams of fiber (4 grams soluble), 9 grams of sugar (22.5 percent calories from sugar), and 130 milligrams of plant omega-3 fatty acids.

Make muffins. Look for recipes that call for oats and whole wheat flour; you'll get a nice balance of soluble fiber (from oats) and insoluble fiber (from the whole wheat). Oats add texture and a mild nutty taste to muffins. Use either quick or old-fashioned oats; most brands of instant oats usually include added sugars, which may affect your finished dish.

Substitute oats for other ingredients. Replace bread or cracker crumbs in meat loaf or meatball recipes with oats. When baking breads, cakes, pancakes, or muffins, you can replace up to one-third of the flour with oats. A quick whirl in the food processor will render it almost as fine as white flour.

Toast oats for added flavor. Toasted oats can be added to trail mix or sprinkled on top of yogurt, frozen yogurt, or fresh fruit. In cookie dough, toasted oats make a great lower-fat replacement for a portion of the nuts. To toast oats: Add about ½ cup of quick or old-fashioned oats to a nonstick skillet coated lightly with canola-oil cooking spray. Spray the tops lightly, too, if desired. Keep stirring the oats gently over medium-high heat as they lightly brown, about 3 minutes. Store in a covered container or sealable plastic bag.

Eat oatmeal raw. Oatmeal can even be eaten uncooked, which means you can add oats to yogurt, salads, sandwiches, soups, cold cereal, and trail mix. Two tablespoons of oats adds a gram of fiber.

Reduce blood pressure. Eating barley has been shown to decrease blood pressure and improve several other risk factors for heart disease. (Other studies of high-fiber, whole grain foods have reported significant reductions in blood pressure.) Researchers have also observed a 21 percent decrease in total and low-density lipoprotein (LDL, or "bad") cholesterol in people eating lots of soluble fiber, such as that found in barley and oats. Levels of high-density lipoprotein (HDL, or "good") cholesterol either increased or did not change.

Decrease your risk of stroke. A recent Harvard study linked a diet heavy on whole grain foods with a decreased risk of stroke in women. Many studies have looked at whole grains in combination with other healthful food choices and the reduction of stroke. A Mediterranean diet, which is high in whole grains, fruits, vegetables, and beneficial oils (see Chapter 6), has been shown to reduce stroke and heart attack by 60 percent, notes J. D. Spence, MD, with the Stroke Prevention and Atherosclerosis Research Centre in London, Ontario. And a recent review of 121 scientific publications all researching

Four Ways Oat Fiber Helps Your Body

1. Slows down digestion, so it takes longer for the stomach to empty into the small intestines, which helps you feel fuller longer

2. Reduces the amount of insulin the pancreas releases after meals, helping steady blood sugar levels

3. Forms a gel that binds bile acids in the intestinal tract, so they're excreted faster, reducing the amount of cholesterol absorbed in the intestine

4. Gets fermented by bacteria in the colon, which may have an anti-inflammatory effect and improve metabolism of dietary fats

dietary factors and the risk of stroke or high blood pressure concluded that a diet low in sodium; high in potassium; and rich in whole grains, cereal fiber, fruits and vegetables, and fatty fish will likely reduce the incidence of stroke.

Reduce cancer risks. More than 40 studies looking at 20 types of cancer have suggested that regularly eating whole grains reduces the risk of many gastrointestinal cancers, such as stomach and colon, along with cancers of the oral cavity, pharynx, esophagus, and larynx. Whole grains may accomplish this by blocking DNA damage, suppressing the growth of cancer cells, providing antioxidant protection, and preventing the formation of carcinogens. The particular components of whole grains that offer such protection include fiber, antioxidants including vitamins (like vitamin E) and minerals (like selenium), and various phytochemicals.

Ready to start adding more whole grains to your life? Just say yes.

BEANS, GROUND FLAXSEED, AND NUTS: EASY ADD-INS

How can you crank up your nutritional intake and score big on fiber, key phytochemicals, smart fats, and more, without drastically changing what you eat? By turning to nutrition-boosting "add-in" ingredients, that's how! These foods are so easy to toss into your favorite dishes, you'll hardly notice that they are there.

To qualify as an add-in, these chosen foods had to be tops in nutritional attributes and easy to work with in the kitchen. I'll admit it may take a pinch of practice and a dose of diligence to remember to add these nutritional boosts in. Keep visible reminders of these ingredients on your kitchen counter or at the front of your refrigerator to help you remember to use them.

THE WHOLE GRAIN LINEUP!

Here's a complete rundown of my favorite grains and the reasons I think they're great. I've also indicated whether the grain contains gluten, a protein that can be problematic for people with certain allergies.

	PERSONAL ENDORSEMENT	NUTRITIONAL SELLING POINTS	GLUTEN?
Amaranth	Amaranth flour has a sweet, spicy, nutty flavor. It's best used as an accent flour in waffles, pancakes, or muffins.	¼ c dried amaranth: 200 calories, 7 g protein, 3 g fiber	No
Barley	Hulled barley has the bran, so that's the one you want to buy. But even if you purchase pearl barley, which has the bran removed, you'll get around 50% of the original fiber because barley's fiber is found throughout the grain (unlike the wheat kernel). Barley has a nutlike flavor and can be used instead of rice or added to soups and stews.	½ c whole cooked barley: 135 calories, 6.8 g fiber, 8% Daily Value for vitamin E, 7% B_1, 10% B_3, 6% B_6, 8% magnesium, 33% selenium	Yes
Brown rice	It's actually not very brown once you cook it. I've made light fried rice with brown rice, and nobody noticed that the rice wasn't white. Switching to brown rice will boost your fiber from 1 g to 3.5 g per cup of steamed rice.	1 c cooked long-grain brown rice: 216 calories, 3.5 g fiber, 5% Daily Value for vitamin E, 17% B_1, 20% B_3, 18% B_6, 30% magnesium, 35% selenium	No
Buckwheat groats	Groats, the hulled kernels of buckwheat, come whole or cracked. You might find a side dish recipe or two calling for groats, or you can use them in soups and stews. (Don't confuse them with buckwheat flour, which is very dark and dense and usually added to pancake recipes in fairly small quantities.)	¾ c cooked buckwheat groats: 136 calories, 3.4 g fiber, 5% Daily Value for vitamin E, 9% B_3, 7% B_6, 12% folic acid, 27% magnesium	No
Bulgur	Bulgur is wheat in disguise. It's just been steamed and dried, so you generally have to soak it to make it tender. It's used in Middle Eastern dishes like taboulleh and pilaf.	See whole wheat flour (next page).	Yes
Millet	You'll find millet hulled in cracked or pearled form. It can be sweetened and used as a cereal or pudding and can take the place of bulgur in recipes.	¾ c cooked millet: 214 calories, 2.3 g fiber, 17% Daily Value for vitamin B_1, 11% B_2, 16% B_3, 12% B_6, 19% folic acid, 28% magnesium	No

	PERSONAL ENDORSEMENT	NUTRITIONAL SELLING POINTS	GLUTEN?
Oats	One of my favorite whole grains, oats can be the star attraction (hot oatmeal) or an ingredient (cookies, cakes, crisps). I like to use oat bran in combination with whole wheat and unbleached white flours for baking. That way, I get soluble and insoluble fiber from the two grains.	½ c dry rolled oats: 156 calories, 6% Daily Value for vitamin E, 26% B_1, 21% magnesium, 25% selenium	Yes
Rye flour	The two rye flour products you're most likely to find are bread and crackers. Try both for a change of pace from your usual choices. Rye bread is particularly tasty paired with tuna salad, sliced turkey, or provolone or other mild cheese.	¼ c dark rye flour: 104 calories, 7.2 g fiber, 11% Daily Value for vitamin E, 9% B_1, 9% B_3, 9% B_6, 11% folic acid, 28% magnesium, 21% selenium	Yes
Quinoa	Not as well known as the other whole grains, quinoa is a mild-flavored grain that can be baked into breads and casseroles or paired with vegetables and beans.	¼ c dry quinoa: 140 calories, 4 g fiber, 5 g protein, 26% Daily Value for vitamin E, 12% B_2, 8% B_3, 12% folic acid, 32% magnesium	No
Whole wheat flour	I tend to use part whole wheat flour and part unbleached white; otherwise, the texture is too dense and the color too brown to pass muster with the rest of the Magee clan. Don't forget you can include whole wheat in your day just by buying 100 percent whole wheat bread.	¼ c whole wheat flour: 102 calories, 3.5 g fiber, 2% Daily Value for vitamin E, 12% B_1, 13% B_3, 7% folic acid, 15% magnesium, 39% selenium	Yes

BEANS: THE MAGICAL FRUIT

I call beans protein pellets because they are big on plant protein (a half-cup serving packs around 9 grams of protein—15 percent of the recommended intake for a woman), and these perfect packages also include a healthy supply of complex carbohydrates (around 27 grams) and fiber (11 grams). Certain beans even add some plant omega-3s into the equation—with soybeans and red kidney beans leading the list.

Try adding a can of beans, rinsed and drained, to green salads as well as rice, pasta salads, soups, stews, and casseroles. They're a natural fit with

(continued on page 108)

Soybeans are a unique member of the legume family: They contain a large amount of natural plant estrogens (isoflavones), as well as all the essential amino acids and a number of antioxidant phytochemicals. Genistein, the main isoflavone in soy, has possible antitumor activity, but soy possesses other cancer-fighting components. Researchers suspect that these powerful anticancer components work at different stages of the cancer process. This means there is value in eating your soy in close to whole form so you are sure to get all of the aforementioned components versus just one in a soy supplement.

It's also probably better to get your soy in food form to fully benefit from the cholesterol-lowering properties of its protein. Processing can reduce the isoflavone content of some soy protein products by as much as 80 percent, warns soy expert Mark Messina, PhD, and isoflavone supplements alone may be ineffective. "Conceivably, isoflavones and soy protein work cooperatively to reduce cholesterol," he says.

If you require further convincing, here's one more reason to eat your soy in close to whole form: Soy contains "inactive" components along with the "active" ones we've just discussed. It's possible that some of these inactive components are required for the active ones to be useful. Plus, dietary soy has been shown to improve blood pressure by preventing blood vessels from constricting in the presence of two hormones (angiotensin II and phenylephrine).

More mood-enhancing than hot flash–banishing? Over the past few years, a great debate has ensued in the research community: Will eating more soy during menopause keep hot flashes away? A recent Italian study suggests soy isoflavones perhaps don't actually minimize hot flashes but instead have the ability to improve mood, thereby rendering women less inclined to care about their hot flashes. The theory makes sense, given that estrogen receptors exist in the mood area of our brain, and soy is rich in natural plant estrogens.

Soy good for the heart? The definitive news on how soy affects heart health has not yet been reported because researchers are still looking into whether—and how—it helps. A few years ago, a meta-analysis of 34 trials reported that soy protein lowered blood cholesterol, and the mean decrease in LDL cholesterol was 12.9 percent; shortly thereafter, the FDA proposed a health claim for soy protein and heart disease. But in 2006, the American Heart Association issued a statement questioning whether soy protein really does lower cholesterol, although it was suggested that soy foods can play an important role in the diet by displacing foods high in saturated fat.

In the meantime, recent lab data have shown that isoflavones in soy can reduce plaque buildup in the arteries. And in studies comparing diets based on soy versus animal proteins, a soy-filled diet has also been associated with larger LDL cholesterol particle size (remember, the smaller particles become more problematic because they more easily lodge in the artery walls). Each gram of soy protein from soybeans and traditional soy foods contains about 3.5 milligrams of isoflavones.

Soy synergy as a tool in radiation therapy? Here's a benefit that might surprise most of us: Under certain conditions, it seems that eating soy may make radiation more effective during prostate cancer treatment. According to new research by Gilda Hillman, PhD, an associate professor of radiation oncology with the Karmanos Cancer Institute in Detroit, soy foods appear to render cancer cells more susceptible to radiation (or more radiosensitive). But here's the fascinating news that suggests to me that soy has synergy from multiple components in this mighty bean, and the best way to get soy is probably as a whole food: In lab studies, when Dr. Hillman isolated the soy isoflavone, genistein, it boosted the cancer cells' sensitivity to radiation, but it also showed the potential to help tumor cells spread from the prostate to the lymph nodes. However, when she switched to more complete soy powder, she got the same exciting radiosensitive effect on the cancer cells but without the negative effect of the tumor spreading. "It's intriguing that whole soy did not stimulate prostate cancer cells to metastasize, while a single soy component did," says Dr. Hillman.

(continued)

First of all, that's over-the-top exciting. But second, more clinical data in human subjects are needed before advice about soy and supplements during treatment can be made, advises Dr. Hillman. So we'll just have to stay hopeful while we await more research.

ENJOY SOY AT ITS BEST

In my supermarket, you can buy edamame in the frozen vegetable section in two ways: as a 16-ounce bag of shelled edamame (boiled green soybeans without their pods) or as a bag of edamame in pods. Both are already cooked and ready to be thawed and eaten! I have both in my freezer because I like to snack on edamame in pods—you have to work harder to get to each soybean—and I like the shelled edamame for use in cooking casseroles, soups, stews, noodle and rice dishes, and so on.

At the very least, you can keep edamame in pods around for a low-maintenance finger food; just thaw and keep in the refrigerator for a quick snack, perfect for when you (or a family member) are hungry but it's an hour or more until dinner. One and one-eighth cup of edamame in pods adds up to only 120 calories, and the high amount of protein and fiber with a touch of smart fat makes it satisfying and longer lasting, too.

Mexican foods like salsa, quesadillas, enchiladas, and burritos. Beans offer a number of nutritional benefits and may help you:

Fight diabetes. An eating plan that emphasizes whole grain cereals and legumes (beans and peas) has been associated with improved blood sugar control in people with diabetes and who are insulin resistant. Soy protein appeared to moderate hyperglycemia (high blood glucose levels) and hyperinsulinemia (high insulin levels) in studies on people with or without diabetes, but more and larger studies need to be done to confirm this benefit. Other research suggests that when plant protein replaces animal protein, as beans do in vegetarian dishes, it may reduce the risk of developing kidney disease in people with type 2 diabetes.

Beat cancer. Several new studies suggest that beans help lower the risk of developing noncancerous tumors (adenoma) in the colon, which can progress into colon cancer. For example, the Nurses' Health Study found that women eating four or more servings of legumes a week were 33 percent less likely to develop these colorectal adenomas than those eating one serving or less. Perhaps this is partly why beans are named specifically in the AICR advice for lowering cancer risk as part of a healthy lifestyle.

Lose weight. A current theory of appetite control suggests a beneficial synergy between fiber and protein, and beans offer both. High-fiber foods tend to fill us up so that we stop eating sooner, and moderate amounts of protein keep us feeling full longer. "This combination of an abundance of high-fiber foods and a moderate amount of protein offers an eating pattern that can help us cut back on how much we eat so we can lose weight," says Collins. What's one of our most impressive food sources of fiber and plant protein? In one word—*beans!* Try a lunch or dinner entrée featuring beans, and see for yourself if you seem to eat less during the meal and stave off hunger for hours afterward.

ARE YOU NUTS?

Nuts are probably one of the most misunderstood foods. Because they are relatively high in fat, they were often relegated to the "limit" or "avoid" columns in our dietary lists of yesteryear. After all, a food must be terribly high in fat when they make "oil" or "butter" from it—like walnut oil, soy oil, and peanut butter.

Yes, nuts are high in fat, but theirs is for the most part a combination of monounsaturated fat and polyunsaturated fat, which are known to have a favorable effect on cholesterol levels. And this fat comes to us in a nice little package that includes some fiber, protein, and phytochemicals, too. Some nuts contribute other valuable nutrients.

NUTRIENT DENSITY OF COMMON NUTS

NUTRIENT	SOURCE
Plant omega-3s	¼ c walnuts: 2.7 g plant omega-3s
Selenium	2 Tbsp Brazil nuts: 4 times the daily requirement
Vitamin E	2 Tbsp Brazil nuts or ¼ c peanuts: ⅓ of the recommended daily intake (RDI); ¼ c almonds: 24%
Magnesium	¼ c almonds: 38% of RDI; ¼ c peanuts: more than 20%; ¼ c walnuts and macadamia nuts: almost 15%
Folic acid	¼ c peanuts: almost 30% of RDI
Protein	¼ c peanuts: 9 g protein; ¼ c Brazil nuts: 5 g; ¼ c other nuts: 2–4 g

"Frequent nut consumption is associated with lower rates of coronary artery disease," explains Joan Sabaté, MD, MPH, DrPH, a professor of nutrition at the Loma Linda University School of Public Health in California. And according to Dr. Sabaté, nut-rich diets improved the cholesterol levels of participants in dietary intervention trials. Epidemiological studies have linked nuts not only to a significantly reduced risk of dying from heart disease but also to overall longevity. As a baby boomer who is closing in on 50, that sounds pretty good to me.

Antioxidant-rich almonds. It's practically common knowledge that fruits and vegetables are rich in antioxidants, but did you know that many nuts are, too? A recent study concluded that in terms of antioxidant content, almonds are right up there with produce. Researchers from the Antioxidant Research Laboratory at Tufts University tested the skins and kernels of eight common varieties of California almonds and found that their principal flavonoids (catechin, epicatechin, and kaempferol) provide more protection against oxidant-induced cell death than any other flavonoid. Ounce for ounce, the total flavonol content of almonds is similar to what's in red onion, the kaempferol and quercetin amounts compare with broccoli, and the catechin content is between the amounts in brewed black and green tea.

Natural phytosterols in nuts and seeds. Phytosterols are plant-based fats with a chemical structure similar to cholesterol. You may have heard of phytosterols in margarines like Benecol or Take Control. Consumed in sufficient

Nut Butter Wisdom

When buying nut butter, look for brands that don't have any added sugar or fat. The ingredient label should say "nuts" and nothing else, except maybe "salt." Remember that a little goes a long way—around 120 milligrams of sodium per 2 tablespoons usually does the trick!

If buying commercially made nut butter, read the label and avoid any that contain hydrogenated or partially hydrogenated oil—these are surefire sources of the dreaded trans fats. Refrigeration is usually recommended for nut butters to stem the growth of a fungal contaminant called aflatoxin. But if your family blows through peanut butter like mine does (we go through a 16-ounce jar in a few weeks), this probably won't be a problem.

If you like freshly ground nut butter, buy it in a 2-week supply because it has a very short shelf life. To reap the rewards of nut butters, consider the following uses.

- ✓ Spread nut butter (instead of butter or cream cheese) on whole grain toast or bagels for breakfast or a snack.
- ✓ Replace the butter or margarine with nut butter in muffin or pancake batter; a little nut butter in homemade granola bars adds extra flavor and helps bind ingredients.
- ✓ Add nut butter to smoothies, especially chocolate- or banana-flavored ones.
- ✓ Use nut butter to flavor and thicken stir-fry sauces.
- ✓ Give fat-free or light salad dressing more body with nut butter. Beat until smooth using an electric mixer, a small food processor, a blender, or a whisk.
- ✓ Smear nut butter on wheat crackers for a snack.
- ✓ Use nut butter and a less-sugar jam for an even healthier PB&J.

amounts, phytosterols seem to offer three important protective qualities: They may reduce blood cholesterol, enhance the immune system, and decrease the risk of certain cancers.

But before you stock up on margarine, consider this: As a group, nuts and seeds are a rich source of phytosterols, too. A recent analysis of 27 nut and seed products found that sesame seeds, wheat germ, pistachio nuts, and sunflower seeds have the highest concentration of phytosterols. Per 100-gram serving, sesame seeds and wheat germ contain more than 400 milligrams of phytosterols; pistachios have 279 milligrams, and sunflower seed kernels have 270 milligrams. Brazil nuts and English walnuts followed with around 100 milligrams.

Want to know what effect nuts have on cholesterol? Well, so did a team of South African researchers from North-West University in Potchefstroom. After analyzing 23 dietary intervention studies on the independent effect of nuts on lipid levels, they concluded that eating between 50 and 100 grams of nuts five or more times a week, as part of an overall diet with total fat content around 35 percent of calories (and high in mono- and/or polyunsaturated fats), may reduce total cholesterol between 2 and 16 percent and LDL cholesterol between 2 and 19 percent.

How much is 50 to 100 grams of nuts? The bottom of the range, 50 grams, is around ⅓ cup, an amount in line with the FDA-approved qualified health claim from 2003 that eating 1.5 ounces (around 43 grams) of nuts a day may reduce the risk of coronary heart disease. That adds up to around 270 calories, though, and 23 grams of fat (depending on the nut).

If you're worried about gaining weight on a nut-rich diet, consider that several recent studies suggest that eating nuts doesn't automatically correlate to weight gain or increased BMI (body mass index). In fact, preliminary data from Sabaté indicate that people on nut-rich diets seem to excrete more fat in stools, meaning less fat is absorbed into the bloodstream.

Which nut is best? In my opinion, the answer is to go nutty with all types of nuts. Each has good points. One is highest in vitamin E (sunflower seeds), another is rich in omega-3s (walnuts), while another bursts with B vitamins (pistachios). In fact, every nut and nutlike legume studied so far seems to present health benefits. Consider the following:

- Several analyses of data from large-scale studies have consistently shown that regular consumption of small amounts of nuts leads to a 30 to 50 percent reduction in the risk of cardiovascular disease. For example, eating an ounce of nuts more than five times a week could reduce the risk by 25 to 39 percent, according to Penn State researchers who recently reviewed 16 major studies on nuts and heart disease.

- At least 5 ounces a week of nuts and peanut butter might even lower the risk of type 2 diabetes, suggest results from the Women's Health Study, possibly due to the high unsaturated-fat content, which can help regulate blood sugar levels and insulin balance.

- A review of nut studies (mostly involving almonds, peanuts, and walnuts) showed decreases in total cholesterol between 2 and 16 percent and LDL cholesterol between 2 and 19 percent, compared with subjects consuming control diets.

- Some nuts and seeds are potentially important sources of vitamin E, an antioxidant that is hard to find in many foods. Almonds, hazelnuts, and sunflower seeds contribute more than 20 percent of the recommended daily allowance for vitamin E (with a 28.3-gram serving), and Brazil nuts and peanuts provide between 10 and 20 percent.

JUST THE FLAX

If we were to look for an ideal case study to broaden our appreciation for food synergy, we'd need look no further than flax. The synergy inherent in this little seed is drawn from a number of its components, though the specific dynamics remain unclear. For example, many studies have clearly demonstrated that flaxseed offers cancer-protective effects in the body, but researchers aren't sure just which specific component accomplishes that. It could be the plant's lignans, its omega-3s—or the synergistic interactions between these components.

To get the biggest bang for your one buck (that's about what a pound of flaxseed costs), you are probably better off getting everything in the ground seed. For example, lignans are known to help the immune system, but so are the omega-3s, just through different metabolic pathways. Lignans also appear

---

Fast Flax Facts

Recent studies have shown that flaxseed has protective effects against cancer, particularly of the breast, prostate, and colon, with the effect depending on the stage of carcinogenesis. Here's a snapshot of the nutrients in flax responsible for those feats.

✓ Flaxseed contains 75 to 800 times more lignans (a plant-based form of estrogen) than other plant foods do.

✓ Flaxseed contains about 40 percent oil, 57 percent of which is plant-based omega-3 (alpha-linolenic acid).

✓ A small amount of the omega-3s in flaxseed can be metabolized into the same form found in fish (EPA and DHA). Omega-3s, especially those found in fish, may help decrease blood clotting, decrease abnormal heart rhythms, reduce triglycerides, and promote normal blood pressure. There is also some evidence that plant omega-3s lower heart disease risk in their own right.

to offer a measure of protection against some cancers, but so do omega-3s —again through different mechanisms.

Even more interesting, these two components appear to work better together in fighting some diseases than alone. Recent lab studies indicated that the combination of a specific lignan known as SDG and the omega-3–rich oil in flaxseed was more effective in reducing the spread of established tumors than either was alone. SDG and its metabolites (enterodiol and enterolactone) have known antioxidant activity that benefits the body. According to Pennsylvania Hospital (Philadelphia) medical director Paul Kinniry, MD, who just published the results of an animal study with flaxseed boosting lung health, SDG may inhibit the lipid peroxidation process, which helps reduce oxidative stress on the body.

Flaxseed fights cancer. Researchers from the Netherlands found that a high food intake of plant lignans (ground flax is the most concentrated source) could reduce the risk of colorectal cancer by 50 percent. They also found that the breakdown products of dietary lignans may be helpful for people with colorectal adenomas (growths in the colon and rectum that are considered potential precursors for colorectal cancer). The higher the blood level of the lignan breakdown metabolites (enterodiol and enterolactone), the greater the benefit, the researchers noted.

For breast cancer patients, the news on flax also sounds promising. In animal studies, flaxseed increased the effectiveness of the breast cancer drug tamoxifen, but no clinical trials on the flaxseed interaction with tamoxifen, or other breast cancer drugs, have been conducted on breast cancer patients. German research, meanwhile, has linked plant lignan intake and a reduced risk of breast cancer. Studies there have found that premenopausal women eating a high level of lignans experienced a 64 percent reduction in breast cancer risk.

Food sources of lignans besides ground flaxseed include whole grain cereals, berries, vegetables, and fruits in general. At the level of 1 to 2 tablespoons

How to Add In Flax

Here's a helpful handful of nutrition-boosting add-in ingredients and tips. Go forth and boost your health!

- ✓ Add ground flaxseed to smoothies (this is my favorite way to add flaxseed).
- ✓ Add it to hot or cold breakfast cereals.
- ✓ Add it to homemade muffins and breads. Replace no more than ¼ cup of every cup of flour called for with ground flaxseed.
- ✓ Sprinkle it on yogurt or cottage cheese.

a day, flax offers a few other potential benefits beyond cancer and heart disease prevention, including:

- Better regulation of bowel functions (less constipation)
- Possible improvement in glucose control and insulin resistance
- Possible benefits in many "hyperstimulated" immune system diseases, such as rheumatoid arthritis

Flax is not for everyone. Until more studies on humans are completed, Lilian Thompson, PhD, a professor in the department of nutritional sciences at the University of Toronto and one of the pioneers in flaxseed research, recommends that pregnant women do not eat flaxseed in medicinal quantities.

FRUIT AND VEGETABLES: HERE'S TO NINE A DAY!

Recently I was leading a nutrition tour in a supermarket, giving copious advice in various aisles, and when I finally arrived at the produce department,

I found myself simply saying five words: "It's all good—eat more!" So out with the old and in with the new—out goes the magic number five used by the 5 A Day program to educate people about the benefits of eating five servings of fruits and vegetables a day. And in comes the new number—nine! Recent studies suggest that *nine* servings of fruits and vegetables is the amount that should be eaten for optimal health.

The scientific evidence is overwhelming that fruits and vegetables provide a wealth of vitamins, minerals, phytochemicals, antioxidants, and other

Powerhouse Fruits and Vegetables

A diet rich in fruits and vegetables offers a powerful blend of antioxidants and phytochemicals. Together, they are involved in numerous body functions, including stimulating the immune system, offering antibacterial and antiviral activity, regulating detoxification enzymes, decreasing platelet aggregation (sticking together), reducing blood pressure, and altering cholesterol and hormone metabolism. Of course, some have greater antioxidation power than others. A way of measuring this power is called ORAC (oxygen radical absorbance capacity), and a bunch of produce was put to the test. The higher the number, the greater the antioxidant power.

FRUITS AND VEGETABLES WITH HIGH ORAC VALUES

ORAC	FRUITS	VEGETABLES
2,000+	Prunes, raisins, blueberries, blackberries	
900–1,600	Strawberries, raspberries, plums	Kale, spinach, Brussels sprouts, alfalfa sprouts
500–899	Oranges, red grapes, cherries	Broccoli florets, beets, red bell pepper

What fruit can you count on to be fresh and crisp and wonderful through the dead of winter? Apples! While other fruit bins can look sad and dreary that time of year, the apple section comes alive with color and is filled to the brim.

Numerous population studies have linked eating apples with a reduced risk of some cancers, cardiovascular disease, asthma, and diabetes. And in the laboratory, apples have exhibited very strong antioxidant activity to inhibit cell proliferation (the type of rapid multiplication that occurs in tumors), decrease lipid oxidation (when fats in the body combine with oxygen), and lower cholesterol. Here are some more apple research tidbits.

Load up on phytochemicals. Simple phenolics and flavonoids represent the majority of antioxidant activity found in apples, and it's the phenolics in apple peel specifically that account for the majority of the antioxidant and antiproliferating activity. Apples offer a powerful assortment of phytochemicals, including quercetin, catechin, phloridzin, and chlorogenic acid. Procyanidins, also found in high concentrations in red wine, grapes, cocoa, and cranberries, are thought to have a protective effect on the vascular system. Quercetin, also found in onions, red wine, broccoli, tea, and ginkgo biloba, appears to influence some carcinogenic markers.

Savor the skins! In lab studies, researchers at Cornell University in Ithaca, New York, found that apple extract given together with apple skin worked better to prevent

substances that protect against a variety of conditions and chronic diseases, including cancer, coronary heart disease, and cataracts. These nutrients are literally powerhouses of protection. And because there is so much evidence that the real benefit comes from the mix of nutrients you can only get by eating fruits and vegetables in their whole form, these foods are the epitome of food synergy!

A review of 200 studies demonstrated a 50 percent lower cancer risk in

oxidation of free radicals (unstable molecules that damage cells and are believed to contribute to many diseases) than apple extract without the skin. They also found that catechins, when combined with two other phytochemicals in apples, prevented the oxidation of free radicals *five times* greater than expected. The phenolic phytochemicals in apple peel account for the majority of the antioxidant and antiproliferating activity noted in apples.

Eat at least an apple a day to help keep breast cancer away? In a recent lab study at Cornell, researchers found that breast tumor incidence was reduced by 17 percent when rats were fed the human equivalent of one apple a day over 24 weeks and 39 percent when fed the human equivalent of three a day.

ENJOY APPLES AT THEIR BEST

Fruits and vegetables are a great boost to nutrition and can be a valuable ally in the battle to lose or maintain ideal weight. But does it matter how they are processed and prepared? You know the answer to this—a whole apple cut into wedges is more satisfying than pureed apples or fiber-free juice. The same can be said about oranges and orange juice or grapes and grape juice. So remember to choose your fruits and vegetables with this in mind—the less processed the better.

people who ate diets high in fruits and vegetables, compared with people who ate only a few fruits and vegetables. Other research at the University of San Francisco suggests that increasing vegetable and fruit consumption, already recommended for the prevention of several other chronic diseases, may protect against pancreatic cancer as well. The most protective produce included onions and garlic, beans, carrots, yellow vegetables, and dark, leafy vegetables.

Helping to prevent cancer is only one of the many health benefits of produce. Men eating five servings or more of fruits and vegetables a day (and no more than 12 percent calories from saturated fat) were 76 percent less likely to die from coronary heart disease, according to a recent study from the Jean Mayer USDA Human Nutrition Research Center on Aging at Tufts University. And the list goes on.

Aim for 400 grams to fight heart disease. When our fruit and vegetable consumption reaches 400 grams a day, we'll see significant benefits in reducing heart disease, studies show. Don't let that number scare you; it's actually pretty easy to get 400 grams a day. I picked two fruits and two vegetables from the list of high-antioxidant choices below and added up their weight in grams. This is what I got.

1 cup steamed broccoli
2 cups raw spinach leaves (for a salad)
1 cup orange segments (or other citrus fruit)
1 cup blackberries (or other berries)
Total = 592 grams

One way high produce consumption helps your heart is via your blood pressure. As intake rises, systolic and diastolic blood pressure go down, according to a prospective study of more than 40,000 women. Other results suggest that diets higher in fruits and vegetables and lower in animal meats may prevent or delay the development of hypertension.

Unclog arteries with vegetables. In a very exciting study using mice bred to have a high genetic risk for developing artery-clogging plaque, researchers fed one group a diet in which 30 percent of the calories came from vegetables common in the American diet (corn, carrots, green beans, broccoli, and peas) for 4 months. The other group of mice ate a vegetable-free diet.

The researchers found 38 percent less arterial plaque in the veggie-eating mice, along with lower levels of an inflammatory marker in the blood and a slight decrease in LDL cholesterol, and they had lower body weights as well (they gained 7 percent less weight than the vegetable-free mice). The researchers noted that the differences in weight and cholesterol levels didn't totally explain the favorable significant change in arterial plaque. Could be some synergy at work here! Either way, we definitely don't want to develop fatty plaque in our arteries, and eating vegetables is a wonderful way to avoid it!

Lose weight with fruits and vegetables. If you are hoping for a secret weapon to jump-start your weight loss, point yourself in the direction of the nearest produce section. It's not quite as simple as just eating more servings and watching the pounds melt away, but due to their high water and fiber content, fruits and vegetables fill you up without a lot of extra calories (unlike foods that are higher in fat).

If you need more evidence, consider this: A recent study looked at what happens when you feed overweight people prepared meals that are much higher in vegetables and fruits and lower in fat than what they normally eat. They had significant weight loss! In another study, when people ate more vegetables and fruits in meals, they reduced their total calorie consumption by more than 400 per day.

Experts sum up the weight-loss power of produce in two words—*energy density*. Energy density is the relationship of calories to volume of food (the three-dimensional space that a food takes up on your plate and in your stomach). For weight loss, foods that are low in energy density are good to include—they're low in calories for their volume or space. Dried fruits, because they contain less water, tend to have an energy density four times that of their fresh fruit counterparts. Grapes, for example, have an energy density (calories divided by weight in grams) of 0.7, while raisins have an energy density of 3.0. Fat also increases the energy density of food. To lower the energy density of foods like soups, sandwiches, or casseroles, substitute fruits and vegetables when possible for higher energy-density ingredients (like high-fat cheese, cooking fat, or sausage).

WHY MILK MATTERS

It seems that my generation, the baby boomers, grew up without the beverage monopoly we call the soda business in full force like it is today. As kids, many of us drank milk at every meal. Frankly, I don't even remember having soda every day. I think it was reserved for parties or the occasional trip to the golden arches or downtown diner.

What's been happening to dairy consumption lately? While whole milk and butter consumption have gone down, cheese and premium ice cream are rising. Are we trading one high-fat dairy food for another? The good news is that the yogurt aisle has exploded with choices beyond our wildest imaginations, and reduced-fat cheeses have taken their permanent place in the dairy case as well. Never before has it been so easy to work in a few servings of low-fat dairy a day. But here's the question: Why should we? The short answer: because there are important health benefits. Now for the long answer.

Benefits reach beyond calcium. Many researchers agree that dairy foods are the best source of dietary calcium, a mineral that protects against osteoporosis. But the bone benefits of dairy go well beyond its calcium content. Dairy products sport a team of players that are all important for healthy bones (calcium, vitamin D, protein, phosphorus, magnesium, vitamin A, vitamin B_6, and trace elements like zinc). This is our first clue that there's synergy in dairy. Our second clue comes with research showing weight loss and maintenance benefits, too. Most of the health benefits described below suggest there is some synergy involved. It's not just about calcium anymore.

Consider the calcium and protein dynamic. Most dairy foods have pretty impressive levels of two nutritional components many of us are lacking— calcium and protein. Calcium is a key mineral that helps regulate blood pressure and boost bone strength, and protein is the building block for many enzymes and hormones, as well as muscle tissue, in the body. Unfortunately, ice cream falls a bit short on these two nutrients, but low-fat milk, yogurt, cottage cheese, and reduced-fat cheese pack a protein-and-calcium punch in every serving. Just a cup of fat-free yogurt, for example, gets you a third of the way to your daily recommended calcium intake, along with adding 17 percent of your estimated daily protein.

DAIRY PRODUCTS	CALCIUM (MG)	PROTEIN (G)
Low-fat plain yogurt, 1 c	448	13
Fat-free raspberry yogurt, 1 c	350	8
Fat-free milk, 1 c	301	8.5
Low-fat milk (1%), 1 c, A & D added	270	8
Part-skim mozzarella cheese, 1 oz	207	8
Kraft 2% Milk Sharp Cheddar cheese, 1 oz	200	7
Low-fat cottage cheese (2%), 1 c	180	26

Boost your disease-fighting potential with vitamin D. With adequate sunlight, our bodies can make vitamin D, but getting enough is a real problem for

(continued on page 127)

Bet you never thought bacteria would be a good thing! Well, your body actually needs a healthy amount of "good," or beneficial, bacteria in the digestive tract. We can promote the activity of these beneficial bacteria by eating probiotic and prebiotic foods. Probiotic foods contain the good bacteria, while prebiotic foods are the "helpers," providing nutrients that the good bacteria thrive on.

So what does all this have to do with yogurt? Yogurt, which is made using active good bacteria, is considered to be a probiotic. In the United States, generally lactic acid–producing bacteria are used in making yogurt, including *Lactobacillus* and *Streptococcus* species. Most major brands of yogurt contain probiotic bacteria.

Other probiotic foods, according to the American Institute for Cancer Research (AICR), include kefir (fermented milk drink), tempeh (cake made of fermented, cooked soybeans), miso (fermented soybean paste), and sauerkraut. Foods considered to be prebiotic include whole grains (like barley and oatmeal), legumes, many vegetables and fruits (including onions, dark leafy greens, berries, and bananas), ground flaxseed, and foods containing inulin (including some yogurts and nondairy frozen desserts).

Yogurt with active cultures helps stimulate the immune system. A healthy immune system can reduce your risk of various diseases such as cancer, infection, gastrointestinal disorders, and asthma. Increased yogurt consumption may enhance the immune system (particularly in immunocompromised populations, such as the elderly), which would potentially increase resistance to immune-related diseases, such as the ones just listed. According to several recent research reviews on the subject of yogurt and the immune system, while more research needs to be done using well-designed human studies, results from past studies (some of which were animal and human studies) generally support the idea that yogurt helps stimulate the immune system. Researchers from the Nestlé Research Center in Switzerland showed that immune stimulation was maintained in human volunteers as long as the probiotic was being taken. Levels declined 6 weeks after the probiotic was stopped.

Yogurt helps the gut. Yogurt with active cultures may prove helpful for certain gastrointestinal conditions, including lactose intolerance, constipation, diarrheal diseases, colon cancer, inflammatory bowel disease, and *Helicobacter pylori* infection.

Researchers from the Jean Mayer USDA Human Nutrition Research Center on Aging at Tufts University recently concluded, in a review article, that patients with any of the aforementioned conditions might benefit from eating yogurt, thanks to favorable changes in the microflora of the gut, the time food takes to go through the bowel, and enhancement of the immune system.

Take, for example, the results from a recent Taiwanese study that tested the effects of a 4-week pretreatment of *Lactobacillus*- and *Bifidobacterium*-containing yogurt on 138 people with persistent *H. pylori* infection (triple antibiotic therapy had failed). They found that the yogurt decreased *H. pylori* amounts and improved the efficacy of a fourth round of antibiotic therapy, eradicating the bacteria that were left. *H. pylori* bacteria can cause infection in the stomach and upper part of the small intestine, leading to peptic ulcers in some people and increasing the risk of developing stomach cancer.

Should the BRAT diet (bananas, rice, applesauce, and toast) be changed to BRATY? Yogurt with live bacterial cultures appears to help alleviate severe diarrhea in children and adults, but is there enough evidence to tell "toast" to move over? According to the AICR, a recent study of adult hospital patients found that live culture yogurt decreased the incidence and duration of diarrhea brought on by antibiotics. At the very least, yogurt adds another meal or snack option for people with intestinal issues. So keep yogurt in your diet as a preventive measure, and should you fall ill with diarrhea, consider incorporating it into your self-treatment.

Yogurt with active cultures can discourage vaginal yeast infections in women. Candida vaginal, or yeast, infections are a common problem for women with diabetes, and in a small study, seven diabetes patients with chronic Candida vaginitis were randomly assigned to consume 6 ounces of aspartame-sweetened yogurt per day (with or without active cultures like lactobacillus). Even though most of the women had poor glycemic control throughout the study, the vaginal pH (acid level) of the group eating yogurt with active cultures decreased from 6.0 (normal pH is 4.0 to 4.5) to 4.0 and reported a decrease in yeast infections. The other group remained at the pH of 6.0.

(continued)

Yogurt may help you eat less. A new study from the University of Washington in Seattle tested hunger, fullness, and calories eaten at the next meal after 16 men and 16 women, ages 18 to 35, consumed a 200-calorie snack either of semisolid, spoonable yogurt with peach pieces, the same yogurt in a drinkable form, a peach-flavored dairy beverage, or peach juice. Although the yogurt did not lead to fewer calories eaten in the next meal, both forms resulted in lower hunger and higher fullness ratings than the fruit drinks.

ENJOY YOGURT AT ITS BEST

Yogurt can replace many higher-fat ingredients in all sorts of recipes. Plain yogurt will sub for sour cream in a pinch (over baked potatoes or garnishing enchiladas). You can also substitute a complementary flavor of yogurt for some of the fat in a muffin, brownie, or cake recipe. It can replace all of the fat called for on the back of those cake mixes, too!

Where flavored yogurt is concerned, the trick is figuring out whether you want artificial sweeteners (added to many light yogurts) or whether you are okay with most of the calories coming from sugar. If you are sensitive to aftertastes, chances are you will want to avoid the light stuff. If you want to create your own flavored yogurt, start with plain and stir in all sorts of foods and flavors until you get something you enjoy. From my kitchen to yours, here are a few ideas for jazzing up 6 ounces of plain yogurt.

- **Strawberries and cream:** $1/4$ cup chopped strawberries and $1/8$ teaspoon pure vanilla extract

- **Piña colada:** $1/8$ cup canned crushed pineapple and 1 tablespoon flaked or shredded coconut

- **Mochaccino:** 1 tablespoon cool espresso or extra-strong coffee and 1 tablespoon chocolate syrup

- **Orange burst:** $1/4$ cup chopped orange segments or mandarin oranges and 1 tablespoon reduced-sugar orange marmalade

many people who are housebound or live in areas without a lot of sun. In response to that need, many milk products are fortified with vitamin D, and now some yogurt manufacturers are joining in.

Vitamin D has a long-standing reputation as the vitamin that helps the body absorb calcium and build healthy bones, but recent research has revealed that it may play a role in all sorts of health-boosting functions, from reducing the risk of certain cancers to lowering blood pressure. "Activated vitamin D is one of the most potent inhibitors of cancer cell growth," says Michael F. Holick, MD, PhD, who heads the Vitamin D, Skin, and Bone Research Laboratory at Boston University School of Medicine. "It also stimulates your pancreas to make insulin. And it regulates your immune system."

Boost bone density. Getting your calcium from food rather than supplements seems to be best for your bones. A study in Finland compared changes in bone thickness and density in two groups of 10- to 12-year-olds receiving the same amount of calcium. One group consumed calcium and vitamin D in the form of cheese, while the other received supplements. The cheese-eating group appeared to have the larger increase in bone mass.

Lower risk of high blood pressure. Researchers in Spain studied more than 5,000 adults between 20 and 90 years of age and found that the people who consumed the most low-fat dairy (mostly fat-free and reduced-fat milk) were 54 percent less likely to develop high blood pressure over a 2-year period than the people with the lowest intakes. While other studies have credited calcium for having an effect on blood pressure, the researchers examining this body of evidence suspect the results could also have something to do with the proteins (casein and whey) in dairy, which may have an effect similar to blood-pressure-lowering drugs.

Regulate your weight. High-calcium, low-calorie diets have been shown to help reduce body fat and preserve muscle mass, but some experts suspect that other components besides calcium in dairy products aid the effort. In recent clinical trials of people receiving comparable low-fat diets—one with calcium from dairy products and the other from supplements—those taking supplements lost less weight and body fat.

One theory is that two milk proteins, casein and whey, represent the ideal combination of fast and slow proteins. I bet you didn't know protein could be fast or slow, did you? Eighty percent of the protein in milk is casein, which is a "slow" protein because it leaves the stomach slowly. The other 20 percent comes from whey, which is "fast" because it stays soluble in the acidic stomach and rapidly empties into the small intestine.

In a recent review article on several foods (including dairy) and weight control, nutrition researcher Marie-Pierre St-Onge, PhD, from the University of Alabama at Birmingham, noted that although a meta-analysis has not linked overall calcium consumption with greater weight loss, there is increasing evidence that calcium from dairy products may play a role in weight regulation.

Go with low-fat dairy. A study of adults in Bogalusa, Louisiana, found that as the number of dairy servings increased, so did the percentage of calories from saturated fat—which last I checked was definitely not a good thing. But the other side of the story is that the intake of many key nutrients (like protein, calcium, magnesium, folate, B_1, B_2, B_6, B_{12}, and vitamins A, D, and E) also increased.

What's the answer to capitalizing on the beneficial nutrients in dairy while losing the unfavorable components? Low-fat dairy! As you decrease the fat, you also reduce the calories, saturated fat, and cholesterol, while the amounts of protein, calcium, and most other vitamins and minerals remain high. Aim to work in some low-fat dairy each day, whether it's with fat-free or low-fat milk, low-fat yogurt or cottage cheese, reduced-fat cheese, or a combination.

COMPARISON OF CHOLESTEROL AND SATURATED FAT IN DAIRY FOODS

DAIRY PRODUCTS	CALORIES	FAT (G)	SATURATED FAT (G)	CHOLESTEROL (MG)
Whole milk, 1 c	150	8.2	5.1	33
2% milk, 1 c	121	4.7	2.9	18
Fat-free milk, 1 c	85	0.4	0.2	4
Cheddar or Jack cheese, 1 oz	114	9.4	6	30
Reduced-fat Cheddar or Jack cheese, 1 oz	80	6	3	20
Cream cheese, 1 oz	99	9.9	6.2	31
Light cream cheese, 1 oz	62	4.4	3.1	13
Sour cream, ¼ c	123	12	7.5	26
Light sour cream, ¼ c	80	5	4	20
Fat-free sour cream, ¼ c	62	0	0	0

Choose cheese carefully. Not a day goes by that I don't enjoy a morsel or two of cheese. Maybe it's my Dutch heritage kicking in (Holland is a big cheese producer); maybe it's my body craving calcium because I'm not a big milk drinker. Whatever the case, I always have several types of cheese in my refrigerator, including reduced-fat brands of both Jack and Cheddar because I make Mexican meals often. I also find it handy to have preshredded part-skim mozzarella and Parmesan cheese on hand because I cook quick Italian cuisine even more often.

It's important to keep in mind that cheese does carry a potentially hefty

Healthy Cooking with Cheese

What about using cheese in recipes when you are trying to trim down and eat less saturated fat? Well, you've got lots of choices here, folks. Here are six Recipe Doctor cheese tips.

Slash the fat and calories. There are two basic ways to cut the fat and calories when cooking with cheese. Obviously, you can use regular cheese but in smaller amounts. However, you also get only half the beneficial protein and calcium. The other strategy is to switch to a reduced-fat cheese that tastes good and melts well. The calories will usually decrease by 30 percent, the fat grams by about 40 percent, and the saturated fat by a third! But the calcium and protein will still be high.

Choose wisely. Full-fat cheese does have a place in certain situations. Sometimes reduced-fat versions are not available—such as with blue cheese or Brie. If that's the case, I tend to use the real stuff, but maybe less, and cut back on fat in other steps and ingredients of the recipe.

Don't fear flavor. Switch to a high-flavor cheese so you can use less when reduced-fat isn't an option. Some high-flavor cheeses that come to mind are:

✓ Parmesan and Romano

✓ Any smoked cheese

✓ Blue cheese, Gorgonzola, or other pungent-tasting types

nutritional downside—after meat, the milk group is the largest source of fat, cholesterol, and, more important, saturated fat in the American diet. But on the plus side, cheese is a great source of protein and calcium (two nutrients some of us need more of). Just 2 ounces of reduced-fat cheese a day will give you about 40 to 50 percent of the Daily Value for calcium and around 15 grams of protein for an investment of only 160 to 180 calories. By comparison,

✓ Extra-sharp Cheddar

✓ Feta or goat cheese

Sprinkle, don't smother. There's no reason to completely cover your dish with cheese. Often recipes call for a blanket of cheese as the final step in a casserole or mixed dish. A sprinkle can do just as well; say, 1–1½ cups of shredded cheese instead of 3 cups to cover a 13" x 9" baking dish.

Pair with healthy partners. Because cheese is a source of saturated fat, try to pair it with lower-fat and higher-fiber foods such as pears, pasta, whole grains, beans, and even vegetables instead of butter, high-fat crackers or pastries, or high-fat meats like salami or sausage.

Fat-free cheese may not please. I've personally never met a fat-free cheese I liked, so if you are looking to find one, proceed with caution. It just isn't going to melt like real cheese or taste like real cheese. The brands I've tried are more on the order of, well, plastic. I've learned over the years that there is a line that manufacturers can cross, when taking the fat out of food ingredients, where they have gone too far. The fat-free food has very little in common chemically and aesthetically with the original ingredient. Fat-free margarine, anyone?

the same amount of regular cheese gives you just as much calcium and protein, but the calorie and fat price tag is noticeably steeper.

228 calories in full-fat versus 160 to 180 in reduced-fat

19 grams of fat versus 10 to 12 grams

12 grams of saturated fat versus 8

50 to 60 milligrams of cholesterol versus 30 to 40 milligrams

CHEESE COMPARISONS

There are lots of different types of cheese out there in supermarket land. You can even buy cheese made from soy milk or goat's milk. And if your grocery store has a deli cheese section, you'll find all sorts of imported and domestic cheese, from feta and farmer to Gouda and Gruyère. Here are just a few of the more common cheese options. All data are for 1-ounce portions.

	CALORIES	FAT (G)	SATURATED FAT (G)	PROTEIN (G)	CHOLESTEROL (MG)	CALCIUM (% DV)
Reduced Fat						
Kraft 2% Milk Sharp Cheddar	90	6	4	7	20	20
Part-skim mozzarella	80	5	3	8	15	25
Borden 2% Milk American singles	67	4	2.7	5.4	14	40
Regular Fat						
Cheddar	114	9.4	6	7	30	26
Monterey Jack	106	8.6	5.4	7	25	26
Parmesan	111	7.3	4.7	10	19	42
Brie	95	8	5	6	28	7

TEA FOR TWO AND TEA FOR YOU!

In the interest of cutting excess calories, it behooves us all to avoid regular sodas and other sweetened drinks whenever possible. The best way to do this is to drink "no calorie" beverages instead. Some of the more obvious options are flavored mineral waters, seltzer water with a slice of lemon or lime, diet sodas (although some experts advise limiting these because they contain artificial sweeteners), and plain tea and coffee.

Even better, of course, is drinking beverages that contain potentially protective substances! Tea is the latest trend in beverages, and the variety of health benefits associated with tea probably has a lot to do with it.

Green and black tea both contain phytochemicals thought to have a host of health benefits. Although we don't have definite answers about the whats and hows of tea health benefits, we do have some important clues.

Eighty to 90 percent of the total flavonoid (family of phytochemicals) content in tea is catechins, with possible actions ranging from antioxidant to anti-inflammatory to immune system stimulant and weight loss booster. The

Two Easy Ways to Enjoy Iced Tea

There's nothing like a glass of iced tea on a hot summer day. Granted, it takes a bit of a time to boil water, then steep your tea bag in your glass pitcher, but those few minutes are well worth the effort. You can save yourself a few dollars over a restaurant's glass, and if you have a glass of no-calorie iced tea waiting for you, you might pass up another beverage that has sugar or artificial sweeteners.

When it comes to the phytochemicals in tea, freshly brewed is best! Apparently, bottled teas have fewer of these phytochemicals than freshly brewed tea. All that said, I've been on the lookout for some fun and flavorful iced teas, and I've found two to tell you about.

Brand: Republic of Tea (www.republicoftea.com)

Type: Man Kind Tea

Description: Green tea infused with blueberry; available in 2.65-ounce tins (a portion of the profits go to the Prostate Cancer Foundation)

Brand: Peet's Tea (www.peets.com)

Type: Mango Iced Tea

Description: Black tea infused with mango flavor; available in 3.2-ounce boxes

greatest antioxidant activity comes specifically from EGCG (epigallocatechin gallate), which accounts for 50 to 60 percent of tea's total catechins.

Most of the studies suggesting cancer-protective effects of tea have been carried out with green tea, but black tea may also have some protective qualities, just possibly less than green tea. White tea is unprocessed, so experts suspect it offers plenty of phytochemicals as well.

Whether a tea is black, green, or white depends on the way it is processed. Black tea comes from leaves that have been fermented before being heated and dried. Green tea leaves are steamed before drying, but not fermented, producing a greenish-yellow brew that tastes closer to the flavor of a fresh leaf.

Fight heart disease with green tea. Food synergy is most certainly at play with the many cardiovascular benefits linked to green tea. Consider this: Antioxidants make up a third of the weight of dried green tea leaves. And one of these antioxidants is EGCG, which was shown to slow the buildup of artery-clogging plaque in mice in a recent study.

Green tea's abundant antioxidants may also lower total cholesterol levels by increasing intestinal excretion of cholesterol and bile acids (via your stool) and increase HDL cholesterol levels and protect against rising LDL cholesterol. In addition, green tea catechins may help the body recycle the antioxidant alpha-tocopherol (a form of vitamin E) and increase plasma blood levels of alpha-tocopherol. Because it's difficult to get enough vitamin E from food alone, recycling what we do have is a great way to extend its antioxidant protection.

Lower your risk of ovarian cancer. When you drink your tea each day, you kill at least two birds with one stone because one of the flavonoids found in tea, kaempferol, has recently been linked to lowering the risk of ovarian cancer.

Researcher Margaret Gates, a doctoral candidate at Harvard University's School of Public Health, suggests that consuming between 10 and 12 milligrams a day of kaempferol (an amount you can get from 4 cups of tea) offers some protection against ovarian cancer.

Drink your way to weight loss. In the cooler months, it is definitely easier to down a couple of mugs of hot green tea. Here's why you might want to go out of your way to do that year-round. In a recent study, participants who drank a bottle of tea (fortified with green tea extract) every day for 3 months lost more body fat than those who drank a bottle of regular oolong tea. Other than the different teas, their overall diets were similar. The researchers suspect that the catechins (helpful phytochemicals) in green tea may trigger weight loss by stimulating the body to burn calories and mildly decrease body fat.

Chapter 5

Working Together:
Powerful Food Combinations

This book is about how different components within the same food and between different foods work together in the body for maximum health benefit. This chapter in particular focuses on the latter—different foods working together.

For example, no one would argue the inherent health benefits of broccoli. It's rich in vitamins C and A as well as carotenes and fiber; it even contains some plant omega-3s. It's hard to imagine that you can boost its healing powers even further by eating it with another particular produce item, but you can. Likewise, most of us know that when we eat fish, we are getting the incredibly health-promoting fish omega-3s that can help decrease blood clotting, decrease abnormal heart rhythms, reduce triglycerides, and promote normal blood pressure. But did you also know that eating fish omega-3s with plant omega-3s brings even bigger and better results?

New research is revealing that different foods with the same or complementary mechanisms of action in the body can provide greater health benefits when enjoyed together than either single food could alone. That sounds like food synergy to me, folks! Keep reading because, in this chapter, we will talk about the amazing food partnerships that we know or suspect have synergy!

DYNAMIC DUOS: THE EMERGING SCIENCE OF FOOD SYNERGY

As we've discussed, studying the specific health-boosting benefits that different foods can offer one another is a very new approach to the science of nutrition. However, this is only the beginning; emerging research suggests that more studies will follow.

One researcher leading the pack is John W. Erdman, Jr., PhD, professor of food science and human nutrition at the University of Illinois at Urbana-Champaign. He decided to start looking at foods in combination as a way to learn more about real diets eaten by real people. "People don't eat nutrients, they eat food. And they don't eat one food, they eat many foods in combination," he explains.

Studies that examine individual nutrients in isolation are really not designed to tell us anything about the interactions that occur between those substances, much less between foods that each contain their own anti-disease arsenals. Dr. Erdman agrees: "Of course, it's important to analyze how specific food components influence our health, but such findings provide only tools for further study. They should open the debate, not close it down." I'm sure there are many examples of food pairs that have powerful synergy in the body, but while we wait for more research clues, consider the following:

Broccoli with tomatoes fights prostate cancer. Pairing these two powerhouse foods could be a match made not only in Italy but in health heaven. In a study led by Dr. Erdman and published in a recent issue of the *Journal of Nutrition*, prostate tumors grew much less in rats that were fed tomato and broccoli powders than in rats who ate diets containing either just one of those powders or cancer-fighting substances that had been isolated from tomatoes or broccoli.

In an earlier study, Erdman found that rats fed isolated lycopene (a natural substance from tomatoes believed to help fight prostate cancer) didn't have significant protection from prostate cancer, but rats fed freeze-dried-tomato powder (it's easier to feed rats the powder, and it contains the full range of nutrients in tomatoes) had much greater prostate cancer survival. Meanwhile, broccoli contains substances called glucosinolates that break down into compounds that help enzymes flush carcinogens from the body. But just like with lycopene, research has shown that glucosinolates work better when eaten with the other natural substances found in broccoli.

The take-home message: A lycopene supplement may not hurt, but the whole tomato will probably help more. Even better, a tomato eaten with broccoli may help the most. "Separately, these two foods appear to have enormous cancer-fighting potential," says Dr. Erdman. "Together, they bring out the best in each other and maximize the cancer-fighting effect."

Alfalfa sprouts with cherries lowers cholesterol. Can't say I've thought about putting alfalfa sprouts and cherries together in a dish, but maybe I should start! In a preliminary study, researchers in the department of molecular pharmacology and toxicology at the University of Southern California's School of Pharmacy observed a strong antioxidant synergy between alfalfa and acerola cherry extracts that may help reduce oxidation of low-density lipoprotein (LDL) cholesterol. It could be the flavonoids from the sprouts working together with vitamin C from the cherries. If you want to incorporate this combo into your diet, the hardest part is going to be getting your hands on cherries year-round. The answer lies in the frozen-fruit section of your supermarket.

Flaxseed with soybeans fights breast cancer. Previous research has implicated soy as actually having tumor-promoting effects in late-stage breast cancer, but in recent lab studies, flaxseed has been shown to weaken this effect.

After another lab study analyzing the breakdown products from the lignans in flaxseed in combination with the primary isoflavone in soy (called genistein), flaxseed researcher Lilian Thompson, PhD, from the University of Toronto, concluded that for postmenopausal women with low estrogen levels, the combination of soy and flaxseed may be more beneficial than soy alone in controlling breast cancer growth. In this case, the two are better than one!

Tofu with tea tames tumors. People in Asian countries tend to eat soy products and drink tea on a regular basis. Certain types of cancer, including prostate and breast cancer, are significantly lower in the Asian population than in the United States, which begs the question: Is there some anticancer synergy going on between those two Asian staples? Fascinating research with green tea and black tea suggests there is a link.

One Harvard Medical School study that examined estrogen-dependent human breast cancer progression in female mice found that the combination of soy phytochemical concentrate with green tea synergistically reduced breast tumor growth by 72 percent, whereas the concentrate alone reduced tumor growth by 23 percent and tea alone by 56 percent. Green tea proved to be more potent than black in anti–breast tumor activity.

But soy is an equal opportunity synergist! In another study at Harvard, mice inoculated with human prostate cancer cells experienced less cancer growth and spreading to lymph nodes when they received a combination of soy phytochemicals paired with black tea. In a similar experiment, researchers found that the same phytochemicals paired with green tea also inhibited tumor growth and spreading. The researchers assert that this is the first study of its kind to demonstrate that two major components of the Asian diet can synergistically prevent prostate cancer.

Garlic with onions improves heart health. Organosulfur compounds are the primary active phytochemicals in garlic and onions, and several of them may protect the heart by helping to keep arteries flexible and clear of plaque damage. For example, DADS (diallyl disulfide) has been shown to possess the strongest antioxidant activity that can prevent oxidation of LDL cholesterol in the bloodstream; another compound, SEC (sethylcysteine), has demonstrated great antiglycation activity. Glycation occurs when sugar molecules attach to proteins and other structures, rendering them nonfunctional; the entire process eventually damages the internal lining of blood vessels, causing them to stiffen. Having antiglycation properties, therefore, is definitely a great thing, particularly for people with diabetes who tend to form more advanced glycation compounds. Yet another study noted that DADS and another organosulfur compound, DAS (diallyl sulfide), were best at increasing phase II enzymes that work to detoxify carcinogens.

So where are all these awesome organosulfur compounds? If you eat garlic and onions together, will you be more likely to cover your bases and get plenty of DADS and SEC? Scientists are still answering that question, but given what a delicious flavor that is, there's certainly no harm in enjoying them together as often as you can.

JUST THE FATS: THE ROLE OF DIETARY FAT IN FOOD SYNERGY

It's the million-dollar question: Is fat in the diet a health boost or bust? Nutrition researchers have learned a lot about fat and health in recent years, and it seems the answer is both. Let's start with the good news. There are some "smart fats" that, when eaten as part of a healthy, plant-rich diet, actually benefit the body. I find this personally liberating because without some good fats to play with, I would have a tough time creating recipes I think you would love.

I usually try to lower the fat in recipes I make over, if only to slash calories. But I still include some fat, and it's great to be able to use certain smarter fats with confidence. Before we discuss the many ways different fats interact with other nutrients, let's begin with a quick overview of the types of fats our food contains, where we find them, and how much we should be eating.

MONOUNSATURATED FATS

Many experts urge us to make oils that are high in monounsaturated fat our first choice in cooking. Technically speaking, monounsaturated fats contain one double bond in their carbon-carbon structure, and they stay liquid at room temperature.

Monounsaturated fats in the diet, especially if they replace saturated or trans fats, help reduce LDL cholesterol along with the risk of heart disease. They may also increase levels of high-density lipoprotein (HDL, or "good") cholesterol, reduce blood pressure, and improve insulin sensitivity when part of a reduced-carbohydrate diet. Most experts advise aiming for 10 to 15 percent of calories from monounsaturated fats (for a 2,000-calorie diet, 15 percent computes to 33 grams of monounsaturated fat per day).

Common food sources include olive oil (78 percent monounsaturated fat and 14 percent saturated), canola oil (62 percent monounsaturated and 6 percent saturated), peanut oil (48 percent monounsaturated), hazelnut oil (82 percent monounsaturated), almond oil (73 percent monounsaturated), avocados, and nuts such as almonds.

POLYUNSATURATED FATS

At the molecular level, fatty acids contain two or more carbon-carbon double bonds, which means the fatty acid is missing at least two pairs of hydrogen on the chain. There are two main families of polyunsaturated fats—omega-3s and omega-6s—and each includes a fatty acid essential to health.

OMEGA-3 FATTY ACIDS

Omega-3s are a group of fatty acids that all have their first carbon-carbon double bond (unsaturated) starting in the same place, the third carbon atom. ALA is the major omega-3 fatty acid found in plants, while DHA and EPA are in fish. Fish omega-3s help protect you against heart disease and heart attacks by:

- Inhibiting the accumulation of fatty plaque in the artery walls and minimizing inflammation throughout the body, especially in artery walls and joints
- Enhancing a special layer of cells that line certain parts of the body, like the inside of the heart, called the endothelium
- Possibly helping to decrease blood clotting by thinning the blood, decreasing abnormal heart rhythms and blood pressure, and reducing triglyceride and LDL cholesterol levels while increasing HDL cholesterol levels

Scientists also continue to study omega-3 fatty acids and their potential to lower cancer risk. According to the American Institute for Cancer Research, omega-3s have displayed a range of anticancer activities in the laboratory and have been repeatedly associated with lower cancer risk in population studies. "Populations in countries that consume high amounts of omega-3 fatty acids from fish have lower incidences of breast, prostate, and colon cancer than people in countries that consume less omega-3s," explains omega-3 researcher W. Elaine Hardman, PhD, with the Pennington Biomedical Research Center of Louisiana State University in Baton Rouge. Granted, the cancer prevention link is still being investigated, but so far, laboratory research suggests that omega-3s may:

- Break down into molecules that reduce production of cancer-promoting compounds (in partnership with certain enzymes)
- Promote self-destruction of cancer cells
- Hinder growth of the blood vessels that tumors need to survive
- Suppress cancer-promoting activity of omega-6 fatty acids by competing with them for enzymes

Common food sources of omega-3s include fish (especially coldwater fish like salmon, tuna, mackerel, trout, herring, and bluefish), ground flaxseed, canola oil, walnuts, tofu, soy nuts and soybean oil, red kidney beans and soybeans, walnuts and pecans, and broccoli and other green leafy vegetables. Our bodies can actually convert a small amount of the plant omega-3s (ALA) you eat into the omega-3s found in fish (DHA and EPA).

In new guidelines from the American Heart Association, people without heart disease are advised to eat a variety of fish at least twice a week and regularly include oils, nuts, and seeds rich in omega-3s in their diets. Those living with heart disease should consume about 1 gram of fish omega-3s per day from fatty fish when possible. The National Academy of Sciences is still in the process of setting an "adequate intake" recommendation for omega-3s, but some experts advise at least 2 grams of plant omega-3s per day for a 2,000-calorie diet. According to the American Heart Association, a total intake of 1.5–3 grams of plant omega-3s seems beneficial.

OMEGA-6 FATTY ACIDS

Omega-6s are a type of fat with the first carbon-carbon double bond (unsaturated) beginning at the sixth carbon atom. Linoleic acid is the major omega-6

Cooking the High–Omega-3 Way

The simple decision of which fat we choose to cook and bake with can have a huge impact on our health. So which fats are best? The highest in omega-3s is canola oil, then soybean oil. The highest in monounsaturated fat is olive oil, followed by safflower and canola oil. So what do I do?

Canola oil is also pretty high in vitamin E, so I use it for most of my baking and oven frying. I also use olive oil whenever I can for sauces, dressing, sautéing, bread dips, etc.

COMPARISON OF COMMON COOKING FATS

	TYPE OF FAT (1 TBSP)			TYPE OF FATTY ACID	
	SATURATED	MONOUNSATURATED	POLYUNSATURATED	OMEGA-3	OMEGA-6
Canola oil	7%	59%	29%	9%	20%
Soybean oil	15%	23.5%	58%	7%	51%
Olive oil	14%	77%	9%	1%	8%
Butter	62%	29%	4%	1%	3%
Lard	39%	45%	11%	1%	10%
Safflower oil	7%	71%	21%	0%	21%
Grapeseed oil	9.5%	16%	70%	0%	70%
Peanut oil	17%	46%	32%	0%	32%

found in food. Common sources include walnuts, safflower oil, sunflower seeds and oil, soy nuts, corn oil, Brazil nuts, soybean oil, pecans, tofu, peanuts, peanut butter, almonds, and dark-meat chicken.

Studies show that omega-6 fats can reduce total and LDL cholesterol when they replace saturated fat in the diet. But excessive intake of omega-6 fats can cause a few health problems.

What Does It Mean If Our Omega-6s Are Sabotaging Our Omega-3s?

Omega-6 fatty acids do have a place in healthy meals; it's just that in the typical Western diet, we get so many more of them than we do omega-3s that we might be cutting ourselves off from the protective and powerful effects of omega-3s. While omega-3s partner with enzymes to reduce cancer-promoting compounds, omega-6s pair with an enzyme that promotes inflammation, encourages cells to multiply, and decreases cancer cell death.

- Some studies have shown that omega-6s can cause small decreases in HDL cholesterol levels, compared with monounsaturated fats.

- They can spur the production of hormonelike substances called eicosanoids that can lead to inflammation and damage blood vessels, eventually leading to blood clots and constricted arteries.

- Excessive omega-6 fats can interfere with the body's conversion of plant omega-3s to the more powerful omega-3s found in fish.

So what's the bottom line? These are better fats than saturated or trans fats, and some omega-6 fatty acids are actually essential to the body. Plus, they can lower heart disease risk if they replace saturated or trans fats in the diet. But when eaten in excess, they can cause trouble.

SATURATED FATS

Saturated fats are fatty acids that have the maximum number of hydrogen atoms attached to every carbon atom—they are "saturated" with hydrogen. Some saturated fats (like butter or lard) are solid at room temperature, while others (whole milk or cream) are suspended in liquid.

In the body, saturated fats are known to raise total and LDL cholesterol, increasing the risk of heart disease and stroke, and may also increase the risk of certain cancers.

What's the bottom line? These fatty acids should be minimized! Experts with the National Cholesterol Education Program recommend that less than 7 percent of our total calories come from saturated fat—that's 16 grams per day for a person eating 2,000 calories.

TRANS FATS

Trans fatty acids are unsaturated fats that contain at least one double bond in the "trans" configuration. They occur naturally at low levels in meat and dairy products, but most of the trans fats in the American diet are formed during a hydrogenation process that renders vegetable oils solid.

Trans fatty acids inflict damage akin to the effects of saturated fats, except trans fats hit you with a double whammy—in addition to raising LDL levels, trans fats decrease your HDL levels at the same time. This is one reason many researchers consider trans fats to be a bigger bad boy than saturated fats. They suspect that trans fats increase the risk of not only heart disease but also type 2 diabetes, colon cancer, and breast cancer.

Experts advise getting as few trans fats as possible. Some margarines and shortenings contain as much as 20 to 40 percent trans fatty acids, though with new labeling laws now in effect, consumer demand for trans-free products may make unhealthier products harder to find in the future.

FOOD SYNERGY AND THE GOOD FATS

Here are just a few exciting examples of the synergistic partnerships good fats can offer, but I'm sure there are many more we haven't discovered yet.

Boost nutrient absorption with good fat. Eating a little good fat along with your vegetables appears to help your body absorb protective phytochemicals,

The More Nutritious Omega-6 Food Sources

Aside from chicken (without skin), most nuts and seeds offer the best means to incorporate the right amount of omega-6s into your diet. Try to get a serving of nuts or seeds every day not only because of the omega-6s but because they offer valuable phytochemicals, too.

✓ Nuts

✓ Sunflower seeds and sunflower oil

✓ Peanuts and peanut oil

✓ Hazelnuts and hazelnut oil

✓ Peanut butter

✓ Pumpkin seeds

✓ Almonds and almond oil

like lycopene from tomatoes and lutein from dark green vegetables. A recent study at Ohio State University in Columbus measured how well phytochemicals were absorbed after people ate a lettuce, carrot, and spinach salad with or without 2½ tablespoons of avocado. The avocado eaters absorbed 8.3 times more alpha-carotene and 13.6 times more beta-carotene (both help protect against cancer and heart disease) and 4.3 times more lutein (promotes eye health) than the others.

Another study found similar results when seven women ate salads prepared with either fat-free dressing, reduced-fat dressing containing 6 grams of canola oil per serving, or a full-fat version with 28 grams of canola oil. The researchers measured the amount of carotenoids in the women's blood to see how much of the nutrients had been absorbed. The level detected corresponded to the increased oil: Numbers were higher for the reduced-fat dressing than the fat-free dressing and highest for the full-fat. Canola oil, like avocados, is composed of mainly monounsaturated fat (8 grams per tablespoon), with about a third polyunsaturated fat (4 grams per tablespoon), some of which is plant omega-3s.

Control inflammation with the right ratio of omega-3s and -6s. Even though we need to eat more omega-3s and less omega-6s, there is evidence that the two can get along and work together. The researchers at the Harvard School of Public Health and Harvard Medical School concluded, after studying 405 healthy men and 454 healthy women, that omega-6s do not inhibit the desirable anti-inflammatory effects of omega-3 fatty acids. In fact, quite surprisingly, a combination of both was associated with the lowest levels of inflammation.

Lower the risk of heart disease with fish and olive oil. Given that fish oil has been shown to decrease the risk of cardiovascular disease, while olive oil has demonstrated cholesterol-lowering effects, some researchers have tested the two together to determine if any synergy exists. While some trials have shown no effect, others have had favorable results with lowering LDL cholesterol and triglycerides, so the outlook is positive. More research is needed, but meanwhile, consider the following preliminary observations.

- DHA (a type of omega-3 found in fish) and polyunsaturated-fat–rich diets with a reduced omega-6 to omega-3 ratio (perhaps in a meal plan that includes olive oil) have been shown to prevent high blood pressure. DHA seems to have an even stronger effect than the other fish omega-3, EPA. And in some research, adding extra-virgin olive oil to a low-saturated-fat diet reduced blood pressure to the point that participants no longer required medication to treat hypertension.
- In lab studies, avocado oil (rich in monounsaturated fat and oleic acid) incorporated into a cholesterol-rich diet significantly reduced the severity of aortic lesions, compared with coconut oil (high in saturated fat). The avocado oil also raised levels of HDL cholesterol.

Improve cholesterol levels with fish and garlic. Good old garlic and fish omega-3s have been shown to synergistically lower total cholesterol, triglycerides, and the ratio of bad to good cholesterol as well as total to good cholesterol ratios. Together, they've demonstrated more power to improve blood chemistry than they do alone. Pairing garlic with fish for synergistic benefits . . . now, that I can wrap my head around.

One group of researchers from the University of Guelph in Ontario tested the combination of garlic (900 milligrams a day) with fish oil supplements (12 grams) and each alone in 50 men with moderately high blood cholesterol. They concluded that taking in garlic with fish oil favorably lowered triglycerides, total cholesterol, and LDL cholesterol. The researchers suggested that the combination reversed the moderate increase in LDL cholesterol that normally results from fish oil supplements. Synergy at work, perhaps?

THE GOOD FATS YOU SHOULD GET

According to the American Heart Association, an ideal diet includes a variety of fish (preferably fatty fish) at least twice a week. Specifically, aim for an average of 650 milligrams to 1 gram of fish omega-3s daily (preferably from food), and a total intake of 1.5–3 grams of plant omega-3s (amounts you can get by enjoying the following foods) also seems beneficial.

	SERVING SIZE	OMEGA-3S (G)	CALORIES
Sardines, canned in tomato sauce	2 sardines	1.4	135
Coho salmon, steamed	3 oz	1.3	156
Pacific oysters	3 oz	1.2	139
Mackerel, baked	3 oz	1.1	223
Tuna steak (bluefin), baked	3 oz	1.1	156
Rainbow trout, wild, baked	3 oz	1	128
Shark steak, cooked	3 oz	1	153
Albacore tuna (white tuna in water)	½ can	0.8	110
Pickled herring	2 oz	0.8	148

TOP OMEGA-3 PLANT SOURCES

	SERVING SIZE	ALA (G)	CALORIES
Walnut pieces	¼ c	2.7	196
Flaxseed, ground	1 Tbsp	2.2	59
Canola oil	1 Tbsp	1.3	123
Omega-3 eggs (cage-free)	1 egg	0.23	70
Cauliflower, cooked	1 c	0.2	29
Broccoli, cooked	1 c	0.2	44
Pinto beans, cooked	½ c	0.2	103
Pine nuts	¼ c	0.2	192
Green soybeans, blanched, shelled	½ c	0.16	120
Broccoli florets, raw	1 c	0.1	20
Cantaloupe cubes	1 c	0.1	56
Red kidney beans (canned)	½ c	0.1	109
Spinach, raw	2 c	0.1	13

USDA food composition data was used to compute the numbers in the above tables.

WHY WATCHING SATURATED FAT MAKES SENSE

Eating less saturated fat is one of the most important food changes you can make for your health. Saturated fat is often referred to as bad fat because of its relationship to raising LDL cholesterol levels, which raises the risk of developing heart disease. The strongest dietary factor behind high cholesterol levels, in fact, involves the saturated fat and trans fat we eat. (Dietary cholesterol and obesity are also related to LDL levels, but to a lesser extent.) You might be thinking, *Tell me something I don't know!*

Well, how about this: New research suggests that even if your cholesterol isn't high, too much saturated fat may raise the risk of diabetes and some types of cancers, as well as ovarian disorders and other health problems.

(continued on page 154)

Your Top 10 Sources of Saturated Fat and Quick Cooking Tips!

In my opinion, the best way to eat less saturated fat is to take a long, hard look at where it crops up in the average diet. The following list provides just such a breakdown, along with some easy suggestions for cutting back. Here's the best news, though: If we just look at the top three offenders, we will deal with more than 35 percent of the saturated fat we typically take in. So if you are going to make any changes, it makes sense to start with these three categories first.

1. Cheese (12.7 percent of the saturated fat we consume)
   - Choose reduced-fat cheese when possible.
   - Use less, whether cooking with it or eating it.

2. Beef (12.4 percent)
   - Select leaner cuts.
   - Trim off visible fat.
   - Eat smaller, more sensible portion sizes.
   - Eat beef less often; have fish or vegetarian entrées instead.

3. Milk (10.5 percent)
   - Use fat-free, 1%, or 2% milk or fat-free half-and-half in recipes.
   - Drink fat-free, 1%, or 2% milk instead of whole.
   - If you are a big milk drinker, ask yourself if you are drinking enough water.

4. Oils and other fats (6.6 percent)
   - Switch to canola or olive oil in your recipes when possible.
   - Use the least amount of oil possible so food still tastes great.

5. Cakes/cookies/quick breads/doughnuts (5 percent)
   - Bake with canola oil (using less than the recipe calls for) or no-trans-fat margarine with 8 grams of fat per tablespoon.

6. Margarine (4.8 percent)
   - Choose a margarine with less saturated fat and preferably no trans fat.
   - Use less margarine on the table and in recipes.

• Switch from using melted margarine to an oil with smarter fats, such as canola or olive oil, when possible.

7. Butter (4.1 percent)
    • Use less when it's the best choice for a recipe, and buy the whipped butter.
    • Substitute with no-trans margarine with less saturated fat when possible.
    • Replace it with canola oil or olive oil in recipes when you can.
    • Skip it when a recipe calls for dotting a casserole or pie with butter, and don't use it for topping vegetables.

8. Ice cream/sherbet/frozen yogurt (3.8 percent)
    • Seek out great-tasting low-fat and light ice creams and frozen yogurts. (I know they exist because many have spent time in my freezer!) If they are lower in fat, the saturated fat will be lower as well.
    • Read labels to make sure calories and sugar are also lower than in regular versions.
    • Enjoy ½ cup of a light frozen dessert instead of regular ice cream.

9. Salad dressing/mayonnaise (3.7 percent)
    • Make tasty reduced-fat dressings using olive or canola oil.
    • Choose bottled dressings that use canola or olive oil and contain 5 to 7 grams of fat per 2-tablespoon serving.
    • Choose a light mayonnaise and use less of it.
    • Blend light mayo with fat-free sour cream to make a great-tasting but lighter, lower-saturated-fat dressing for potato and pasta salad recipes.

10. Poultry (3.5 percent)
    • Take off the skin before you cook chicken whenever possible.
    • Stick to low-fat poultry recipes and products.
    • Choose canola or olive oil when you need a fat for cooking.

(Note that the increase in cancer risk is associated with mainly very high levels of saturated fat in the diet.) It seems that too much saturated fat in a meal might decrease the pancreas's secretion of insulin, which may then cause an unhealthful chain of events if this takes place meal after meal, day after day.

Looking at the issues from a different perspective, research also confirms that a low-saturated-fat diet coupled with a rich supply of fruits and vegetables improves the longevity of aging men than either factor alone. A study at Tufts University found that men eating more than five servings of fruits and vegetables a day and less than 13 percent calories from saturated fat were 31 percent less likely to die of any cause and 76 percent less likely to die from coronary heart disease, compared with men eating less produce and more saturated fat. But here's the suggestion of synergy: The men consuming either a diet low in saturated fat or high in fruits and vegetables, but not both, did not have a significantly lower risk of total mortality nor did they have as high a risk reduction for heart disease.

When Tufts researchers tested a low-saturated-fat diet (with 26 percent calories from total fat, 4 percent saturated fat) on 19 men and 14 women over age 40 with moderately high cholesterol, they found a more favorable response in the men. The men's total cholesterol decreased 19 percent, compared with 12 percent in women, and the plasma apolipoprotein B (ApoB) concentrations decreased 18 percent in men and 9 percent in women. ApoB levels are a marker for cardiovascular disease risk because ApoB measures small dense LDL particles, which are considered more harmful than normal LDL particles.

It's possible that a low-saturated-fat diet also improves bone mineral density. A high-saturated-fat diet was associated with lower hip-bone mineral density in a recent Pennsylvania State University study that analyzed data from

NHANES III (the Third National Health and Nutrition Examination Survey), including more than 14,000 men and women. The greatest difference was seen in men under 50 years old. Bone mineral density was 4.3 percent lower in men with the highest saturated fat intake, compared with the lowest saturated fat intake.

Fight cancer with fruits and vegetables. A low-fat diet plus plenty of fruits and vegetables equals synergy that potentially slows breast cancer! In 2005, researchers at UCLA examining the findings of a large, population-based study found that women with early-stage breast cancer had significantly less chance of recurrence after 5 years if they ate a low-fat diet with plenty of fruits and vegetables (compared with the typical high-fat American diet).

Then, in another UCLA study, blood samples from 26 postmenopausal women with breast cancer participating in a 13-day program at the Pritikin Longevity Center and Spa that included exercise and a low-fat, high-fiber diet rich in fruits, vegetables, and whole grains revealed a 20 to 30 percent increase in tumor-cell death at the end of the program. More needs to be known and tested along this front, admittedly, but there's no question that this is very exciting! Clearly, women (and men, too, I'm assuming) can make major changes in their diet that, literally within a couple of weeks, can have a positive and dramatic impact on their health.

Chapter 6

Mediterranean Magic and Other Dietary Patterns with Synergy

One day soon I'm going to get to Italy (one of the countries I have been dying to visit even before I discovered the joy of pasta). And when I do, you can bet I'm going to experience Italian cuisine to its fullest—enjoying every dip of my bread in rich, delicious olive oil and savoring every spoonful of slow-cooked marinara.

Of course, before we can begin to appreciate the way another culture approaches food, it helps to take a look at our own habits. Our tendencies to hurry through meals, mindlessly snack as we watch TV, and dine at the dashboard aren't exactly helping Americans eat less and move more. Generally, in other countries, each meal is more of a celebration, the act of eating is honored, and meals are not rushed but savored. And the slower you eat, the less you tend to eat.

In this chapter, we will examine the collective synergy of certain dietary patterns and cultures. We'll start with the traditional Mediterranean diet, and we'll finish with Asian. In between, we'll look at three dietary patterns, studied here in the United States and Canada, proven to have many health benefits—the PortfolioEatingPlan, the DASH diet, and a traditional vegetarian diet. For all of these dietary patterns, the benefits come not just from one specific food or dietary characteristic. The magic, it seems, is in the mix!

MEDITERRANEAN MAGIC

Today, when you hear the words *Mediterranean cuisine*, a mental association with the word *healthy* seems practically automatic. But it was only half a century ago that researcher Ancel Keys, MD, PhD, first pointed out the health benefits of the Mediterranean diet. He studied the way rural villagers ate on the Greek island of Crete, where they enjoyed a plant-rich diet with fish and very little meat and plenty of fruits and green vegetables. The people on Crete also drank wine every day and got more than one-third of their calories from fat, most of it from olive oil, which is rich in monounsaturated fat.

But where was all the pasta, you ask? Interestingly, refined flours were never part of the original Mediterranean way of eating. When Dr. Keys made his initial observations, the farmers and laborers he studied ate whole grains, including a few whole grain pastas, because at that time the white flour options were more expensive.

From the research conducted since then, we know that people who follow traditional Mediterranean diets tend to:

- Eat an abundance of plant foods, including fruits, vegetables, beans, whole grains, and nuts.
- Eat fish often but go lighter on meat.
- Have a low to moderate intake of dairy products, mostly cheese and yogurt.

- Drink alcohol in moderation, usually wine. While many believe that red wine offers health advantages over other forms of alcohol, some researchers say that is still not clear. One drink equals 1.5 ounces of liquor (whiskey, gin, vodka, etc.), 5 ounces of wine, or 12 ounces of beer.

- Enjoy fats that are derived from plants versus animals and not overly refined. First and foremost in most Mediterranean cuisine is olive oil. There's the standard use of olive oil, which studies now suggest may bolster each one of the previously mentioned benefits! Seventy-five

THE MEDITERRANEAN PANTRY

In general, some of the ingredients called for in traditional Mediterranean dishes/meals are:

VEGETABLES	DAIRY	FRUIT	FISH, SEAFOOD, AND POULTRY	BEANS AND GRAINS	NUTS	HERBS AND SPICES	OTHER FLAVORINGS
Artichokes	Cheese	Dates	Red	Chickpeas	Almonds	Basil	Capers
Eggplant	(cow's,	Figs	mullet	Lentils	Pine nuts	Black	Garlic
Fava or	goat's,	Grapes	Sea bass	Navy beans	Pistachios	pepper	Lemons
broad	sheep's,	Melons	Squid	Bulgur	Walnuts	Chervil	and limes
beans	Italian	Olives	Salt cod	Pasta		Chives	Oranges
Fennel	mozzarella,	(Italy,	Tuna	(including		Cilantro	Tomato
Onions	water	France,	Crab	couscous)		Dill	paste
Peppers	buffalo's	and	Mussels	Rice		Marjoram	
Radicchio	milk, cream	Spain	Shrimp			Mint	
Spinach	cheese)	produce	Chicken			Parsley	
Zucchini	Yogurt	some of				Rosemary	
		the best				Sage	
		olive oil)				Tarragon	
		Oranges				Thyme	
		Peaches				Cardamom	
		and				Cinnamon	
		nectarines				Coriander	
		Tomatoes				seeds	
						Cumin	
						seeds	
						Mace	
						Nutmeg	
						Saffron	

percent of the fat in olive oil comes from monounsaturated fat; only 13 percent is from saturated fat.

- Finish meals simply, with some fresh fruit. Sweet pastries, frozen ices, and other treats are usually served at other times with black coffee.

As a result, a population that enjoys the Mediterranean diet, which is low in saturated fats and rich in both omega-3 fats and a wealth of phytonutrients, has a markedly lower incidence of many forms of cancer and heart disease.

THE STUDIES THAT PUT THE MEDITERRANEAN ON THE DIETARY MAP

Decades after Dr. Keys first observed the health and habits of the people in Crete, researchers are still examining the Mediterranean diet, with some of the most recent studies finding that the magic seems to be in the combination of foods rather than one or two particular ingredients (like olive oil or wine). In fact, the Mediterranean-style diet is a perfect example of food synergy because it includes several healthful food patterns (it's rich in plant foods, whole grains, legumes, and fish; low in meat and dairy products; and contains more monounsaturated than saturated fat because of its emphasis on olives, olive oil, and walnuts). A recent study concluded that this way of eating might reduce the prevalence of both metabolic syndrome (a condition that includes excess body fat, high blood fats, and high blood pressure) and the cardiovascular risk that goes along with it. It also doesn't hurt that the Mediterranean diet is associated with a lower body mass index (BMI) and lower levels of obesity.

According to Dimitrios Trichopoulos, MD, PhD, from the Harvard School of Public Health, who recently studied the diets of more than 20,000 Greeks

Aside from being flavorful and delicious, olive oil is rich in monounsaturated fat and offers a wealth of benefits over the higher polyunsaturated vegetable oils. Consider the following:

Olive oil may decrease the risk of cancer. The phytochemicals in olive oil appear to slow the development of some cancer cells and increase the body's ability to speed their removal from the body. Karen Collins, MS, RD, nutrition advisor to the American Institute for Cancer Research, believes that while these benefits have been observed in laboratory studies rather than controlled human intervention trials, they are supported by what is seen in population studies of the Mediterranean diet.

Olive oil may lower inflammation. Although olive oil doesn't boast healthful omega-3s (one type of polyunsaturated fat found in seafood and in plant foods like ground flaxseed and canola oil), it may strengthen the anti-inflammatory effects of omega-3s. How does it do this? It could have something to do with olive oil's 30-plus phytochemicals, many of which have antioxidant and anti-inflammatory properties that help promote heart health and protect against cancer.

ENJOY OLIVE OIL AT ITS BEST

Choose extra-virgin olive oil, the least processed form, to get the highest levels of these protective plant compounds. Light olive oil is lighter in flavor and color and better for baking or recipes where the distinctive olive oil flavor isn't desired. But the process of making the olive oil light removes many of the protective phytochemicals. In these situations, canola oil is probably your best option because it provides mono-unsaturated fat along with some plant omega-3s and a dose of vitamin E as well.

To maximize the phytochemical content of extra-virgin olive oil, store it away from light and heat. You can even store olive oil in the refrigerator; it will thicken slightly and become cloudy, but it will thin and clear up again after about 15 minutes at room temperature.

ages 20 to 86, researchers examining individual components of the Mediterranean diet have found no significant decrease in death associated with any one type of food—even olive oil. But when the Mediterranean diet was examined as a whole, studies showed that people who most closely followed the Mediterranean diet had lower death rates from both heart disease and cancer. The researchers did, however, also note a significant reduction in death rates from a higher overall ratio of monounsaturated fat to saturated fat. "In this case, the total is better than the sum of the parts," says Dr. Trichopoulos. "You can't point to one thing and say that is what does it."

Combat inflammation. A Mediterranean diet rich in olive oil and low in red meat can combat inflammation that raises the risk of heart attack, according to a study from Harokopio University in Athens, Greece. "The Mediterranean diet, independent of any other factor, reduces levels of inflammation related to heart disease risk," says lead researcher Demosthenes Panagiotakos, PhD. He and his colleagues showed that the more closely participants' eating habits matched the Mediterranean diet (2,200 men and women, ages 18 to 89), the lower their levels of C-reactive protein, a marker of general inflammation in the bloodstream.

Lower the risk of Alzheimer's. A recent study of New Yorkers by the Taub Institute for Research on Alzheimer's Disease and the Aging Brain at Columbia University Medical Center found that closely following the patterns of the Mediterranean diet was associated with a lower risk of Alzheimer's disease. More needs to be known about this possible food synergy benefit, but so far this looks like another reason to eat the Mediterranean way!

Reduce levels of oxidized LDL in the circulation. After a 12-week nutritional intervention promoting the Mediterranean food pyramid with 71 healthy women, researchers from Laval University in Quebec reported that the women showed an 11 percent decrease in low-density lipoprotein (LDL) cholesterol. Now, that's what I call instant gratification! Plus, the results revealed that the more closely participants followed the diet, the greater the decrease. Increases in the servings of two food groups in particular were individually associated with decreases in oxidized LDL concentrations—fruits and vegetables!

Improve blood pressure—and more. Want an excuse for visiting the Mediterranean? How about lowering your high blood pressure? There is some evidence that the more closely one follows the traditional Mediterranean diet, the more both blood pressure numbers (systolic and diastolic) go down. A recent Greek study also noted that as intakes of olive oil, vegetables, and fruit went up, blood pressure went down. In contrast, that same research found that as cereals, meat, and alcohol intake went up, blood pressure went up, too.

Lowering both blood pressure numbers is, of course, a welcome feather in the Mediterranean cap, but I'll do you one better. Some new research from the University of Western Ontario tested a Mediterranean diet and exercise program on 38 people with high-normal blood pressure or prediabetes (impaired fasting glucose or impaired glucose tolerance). They noticed a big improvement in the elasticity of subjects' carotid arteries—an increase of about 16 percent (the thicker and less elastic the arteries, the greater the load on the heart). Improving the health of blood vessels might not sound like it would have a big payoff, but boy, does it. It might lower the risk of high blood pressure, diabetes, heart attacks, and stroke, explains the study's lead researcher.

THE PORTFOLIO PROVES THE POINT

Food as medicine? It stands to reason when you look at the mounting evidence about the PortfolioEatingPlan. Developed by researchers in Toronto,

(continued on page 166)

The 10 Steps to Mediterraneanizing American Cuisine

Keep in mind that countries throughout southern Europe have different diets, religions, and cultures, so there really isn't one "Mediterranean diet" that represents the entire region. Each country differs in the amount of total fat its people enjoy, largely because of differences in type of meat and the way they use olive oil; wine intake, dairy consumption, and availability of different fruits and vegetable are also important variables.

The traditional diet of Greece (before 1960) is the one linked to lowered death rates and longer life expectancy. It is characterized by a high intake of fruits, vegetables, nuts, and cereals (mostly in the form of sourdough bread rather than pasta); more olive oil and olives; less milk but more cheese; more fish and less meat; and moderate amounts of wine. Obviously, most of us can't drop everything and start eating the traditional Mediterranean way. But we can embrace the following 10 steps to incorporate as many aspects of traditional Mediterranean cuisine as possible.

STEP 1

Fill your plate with fruits and vegetables, emphasizing green leafy veggies.

STEP 2

Eat more fish and less meat and dairy. When dining out, choose entrées with plenty of vegetables, and avoid those with cream or butter or lots of cheese. For example, enjoy grilled fish served with vegetables, or vegetarian pasta drizzled with olive oil and a little Parmesan.

STEP 3

Go for whole grains and flour whenever possible. According to researcher Ancel Keys, MD, PhD, less-processed whole grain foods provide a more sustained level of energy over a longer period, making them more healthful.

STEP 4

Reach for extra-virgin olive oil instead of another vegetable oil, especially when olive oil will enhance or complement other flavors in a dish.

STEP 5

Snack on nuts almost every day, and feature beans in your entrée or side dish when possible.

STEP 6

Get a little fruity with dessert. End your meal with a treat that provides a serving of fruit. Grapes or baked apples, for example, contribute phytochemicals (in the case of grapes, same as those you'd get from wine).

STEP 7

If you drink wine or other alcoholic beverages, have it only with meals, and don't overdo it.

STEP 8

Enjoy olives (green or black) as accents in entrée dishes or sandwiches and salads, or set them out on the table as appetizers.

STEP 9

Take in dairy as cheese and yogurt; milk is less of a focus in Mediterranean cuisine.

STEP 10

Become a "dipper" instead of a "spreader." Instead of serving sourdough or French bread with butter or margarine, try setting out a small dish of tasty extra-virgin olive oil to dip slices in. You can punch up the flavor of the olive oil with a splash of balsamic vinegar and/or a sprinkle of black pepper, Italian herbs, or salt.

this eating pattern reveals that a predominantly plant-based diet, including small daily investments in certain cholesterol-lowering foods, can improve blood cholesterol levels almost as well as taking cholesterol-lowering statin drugs. The four key foods include soy protein, almonds, plant sterol–enriched margarines (such as Benecol or Take Control), and soluble fiber (from foods like oats, barley, psyllium, and vegetables like okra and eggplant).

HOW CHOLESTEROL-LOWERING FOODS WORK TOGETHER

The Portfolio of four cholesterol-lowering foods has been tested in several different studies at the Clinical Nutrition and Risk Factor Modification Center at St. Michael's Hospital in Toronto and the University of Toronto using people with hyperlipidemia (the scientific name for high cholesterol and high triglyceride levels). Following this plan admittedly requires a bit of diligence, so what did these participants get for their trouble? In one of the most recent studies, more than 30 percent of motivated participants lowered their LDL cholesterol levels more than 20 percent! The exciting point in this headline is that these responses are similar to the amount of improvement usually seen with statin medications. Other studies have shown similar results.

According to David Jenkins, MD, PhD, chair in nutrition and metabolism at the University of Toronto and creator of the Portfolio plan, each of the diet's four featured foods has been found to lower cholesterol by up to 7 percent. Plant sterols, for example, have a noted cholesterol-lowering effect. But when they're combined with soy protein, almonds, and soluble fiber, synergy occurs because the cholesterol-lowering effect is greater than that of plant sterols alone.

But that's not all the good news—if those cholesterol-lowering benefits are the cake, here's the icing. The inflammatory marker C-reactive protein, an important risk factor for heart disease, was also reduced in two Portfolio studies. C-reactive protein levels were lowered 24 percent, an amount also similar to reductions seen with statin drug therapy.

What's the bottom line? An eating plan that includes soy protein, viscous fiber, plant sterol–enriched margarine, and a handful of nuts is a wise choice

The Lowdown on Blood Lipids

Lipid is the scientific term for fats in the blood. At proper levels, lipids perform important functions in your body, but they can cause health problems if they are present in excess. Hyperlipidemia—high lipid levels—includes several conditions, but it usually means that you have high cholesterol and high triglyceride levels. A desired lipid profile, according to the American Heart Association, includes:

1. Low LDL cholesterol levels, ideally with a large LDL particle size
   - Optimal: <100 mg/dL
   - Near optimal: 100–129 mg/dL
   - Borderline high: 130–159 mg/dL
   - High: 160–189 mg/dL
   - Very high: 190+ mg/dL

2. High HDL cholesterol (considered "good" cholesterol)
   - High: > 60 mg/dL
   - Low: < 40 mg/dL

3. Low triglyceride levels
   - Normal: < 150 mg/dL
   - Borderline high: 150–199 mg/dL
   - High: 200–499 mg/dL (may necessitate treatment)
   - Very high: > 500 mg/dL

Using Medication with the Portfolio Plan

What if you are already on cholesterol-lowering medication? The PortfolioEatingPlan may still help by keeping you at a lower dosage. According to its creator, David Jenkins, MD, PhD, the drugs have more side effects at high doses. He suggests that the Portfolio foods may help people get the most out of their medication, without having to increase the dosage. "Emphasizing diet changes in general can boost the success rate of statins, while providing additional health benefits and a possible alternative for those for whom drugs are not a viable option," Dr. Jenkins adds. Most exciting is that these two together show more beneficial LDL cholesterol changes than doubling the dose of the statin medication. Talk with your doctor if you want to follow the plan, as your medication may need to be adjusted.

for anyone concerned about reducing their risk of heart disease. Here's what you need to know.

Power up with plant sterols. Although they sound like they might have been hatched in a laboratory as some kind of Frankenfood experiment, plant sterols are actually quite natural. Sterols are part of the cell membranes in plants, and they are structurally similar to cholesterol. In the body, they go to work during digestion, displacing dietary cholesterol in the cells lining the small intestine (where cholesterol is normally absorbed). The less dietary cholesterol absorbed through the intestines, the less cholesterol enters the bloodstream.

According to a recent scientific review, a diet enriched with plant sterols can, on average, reduce LDL cholesterol by approximately 10 percent. So how much is enough? The review also revealed that the favorable effect on LDL appears to be at its greatest at a dose of 2 grams a day. Taking in more than this amount doesn't seem to offer further benefits. The research that examined the Portfolio plan used plant sterol–enriched margarines, such as Benecol or Take Control, which contribute about 1,700 milligrams (1.7 grams) of plant sterol per tablespoon, as well as other sterol-rich foods such as almonds and soybeans.

In light of this research, the Adult Treatment Panel of the National Cholesterol Education Program recently added its support to the recommendation to add 10 to 25 grams a day of viscous fiber along with 2 grams a day of plant sterols to our daily diet.

Natural Plant Sources of Phytosterols

The average American diet contains around 250 to 500 milligrams of plant sterols per day, but Portfolio research suggests striving for 2 grams (2,000 milligrams) as part of a 2,000-calorie diet. Plant sterols are found in small amounts in many healthful plant foods including grains, fruits, nuts, and vegetables.

PLANT FOOD	PHYSTOSTEROLS (MG)
Avocado, 6 oz (1 small)	132
Soybeans, 1 c	90
Chickpeas, ½ c	35
Almonds, 1 oz (about 23)	34
Olive oil, 1 Tbsp	30

Is there a difference between plant sterol esters and plant stanol esters (both added to various products like margarine)? Plant sterols occur naturally in vegetable oils and are normally found at low levels in the diet, whereas plant stanols are created by chemical hydrogenation of sterols extracted from wood pulp and other sources. They are thought to function similarly in the intestine, and research suggests both help to reduce LDL cholesterol.

Save sterols for mealtime to get bigger results. In observing the effects of plant sterol–enriched low-fat yogurts, researchers found they worked similar to the plant sterol–enriched margarines, and they worked better when taken with meals instead of as snacks. When the yogurts were eaten at mealtime, total cholesterol decreased by about 10 percent, compared with a placebo, and LDL cholesterol dropped 14 percent. Why is mealtime a must? Eating the enriched yogurt with a slow-emptying solid food gives the sterol more time to mix with the intestinal contents (liquids pass through the digestive tract faster than solids). Though the yogurts are not available in supermarkets, the same logic applies to other sterol-rich foods.

Look for viscous fibers. Viscous fiber is the new name to look for when it comes to fiber . . . sort of. Viscosity refers to the thick and sticky consistency some types of fiber assume as they move along the small intestine. This sticky fiber seems to work its magic by preventing bile acid (which contains cholesterol) from being reabsorbed through the intestinal wall. And if these bile acids are not reabsorbed, there's only one place for them to go: outside the body through the normal course of digestion. Increased loss of bile is associated with a reduction in LDL cholesterol (because the body requires blood cholesterol to manufacture more of the bile acid it just lost), which is a very good thing. There is even evidence that the presence of viscous fiber in the intestines may decrease the body's natural production of cholesterol—you're beating cholesterol coming and going, so to speak.

So where do you get these valuable viscous fibers? Basically, many of the foods we know of as being high in the type of fiber formerly known as soluble fiber are high in viscous fiber. The following table provides a detailed list.

VISCOUS FIBER—WATCH IT ADD UP!

The PortfolioEatingPlan suggests taking in 20 grams of viscous fiber per day as part of a 2,000-calorie diet. Here are some examples of foods that contribute some viscous fiber.

FOOD	VISCOUS FIBER (G)
Kidney beans, 1 c, cooked	6
Lima beans, 1 c, cooked	5.2
Oats, 1 c, cooked*	4
Pinto beans, 1 c, cooked	3.8
Strawberries, 1 c	3.4
Broccoli, 1 c, raw or cooked	3.2
Dried prunes, ½ c	3.1
Apple, 1 large	3
Chickpeas, 1 c raw	3
Metamucil wafers, 2	3
Sweet potatoes, 1 c, mashed	2.8
White beans, 1 c, cooked	2.8
Barley, 1 c, cooked	2.6
Metamucil powder, 1 Tbsp	2.4
Grapefruit, 1 medium	2.3

* Oat bran bread and oat bran cereal also contribute viscous fiber.

Stock up on soy protein. Soy proteins derived from soybeans and other soy products appear to reduce serum cholesterol by decreasing the body's urge to make its own. (Remember, the body can make cholesterol, so levels are affected not just by the amount you eat but also by how much your body's cholesterol adds to the mix.) The Portfolio plan suggests 50 grams of soy protein as part of a 2,000-calorie diet. Here are some of the soy products suggested by the plan to meet the 50-gram goal.

SOY PRODUCT	SOY PROTEIN (G)
Lightlife Organic Wild Rice Soy Tempeh, 4 oz	18
Soybeans, 5 oz, cooked	12
Boca Original Chik'n Patty, 1 patty	11
Boca All American Classic Burger, 1 patty	10
Firm tofu, ⅓ c	10
Pacific Foods Ultra Soy beverage, vanilla, 1 c	8
Lifeway Organic SoyTreat beverage, 1 c	6.25
Mori-Nu Silken Tofu, 3 oz	6
Lightlife Smart Deli Roast Turkey Style, 3 slices	5

A recent analysis of various soy studies suggested that soy protein had a modest effect on lowering LDL cholesterol (a 4 percent reduction). But it's possible putting low levels of saturated fat in the diet (9 grams a day) together with soy protein weakens the cholesterol-lowering effect. Certainly, if you look at the populations that typically consume more soy, you see a link between high soy consumption and low coronary heart disease rates.

For almonds and other nuts, a 1-ounce daily dose results in an approximately 4 percent reduction in LDL cholesterol, according to recent studies. The reduction in heart disease risk, though, has been much more impressive. For somewhat modest increases of nut consumption (up to 20 grams a day or a few tablespoons, depending on the nut in question), the reduction in risk has been around 18 to 48 percent.

THE FAB FOUR FOODS IN THE PORTFOLIO PLAN

In addition to eating 5 to 10 serving of fruits and vegetables a day, as well as more plant protein (like beans), the Portfolio plan involves getting the following foods into your diet every day.

1. About 20 grams of soy protein per 1,000 calories as soy milk, soy burgers, and tofu (substitute soy-based foods for meat, and soy milk as a dairy substitute)

2. About 10 grams of viscous, or sticky, fiber per 1,000 calories (including three servings of psyllium as Metamucil as well as oats and barley that replace other grains, and vegetables like eggplant and okra)

3. Plant sterol–enriched margarine in place of butter and margarine, with the aim of taking in about 1 gram of plant sterols per 1,000 calories (It's not hard to reach this range. For example, 1 tablespoon of Take Control [regular] margarine provides 1.7 grams of plant sterol esters from natural soybean extract.)

4. Twenty-three grams of whole almonds per 1,000 calories (about 1½ ounces for a typical 2,000-calorie diet). For a list of 10 ways to eat more almonds, see Chapter 7.

THE DASH DIET DOES THE TRICK

DASH—Dietary Approaches to Stop Hypertension—is a well-studied pattern proven to lower blood pressure as well as blood fat levels in people with either high or normal blood pressure. High blood pressure, a major risk factor for both stroke and coronary heart disease, is also problematic for people with type 2 diabetes, who are twice as likely to get hypertension as people without diabetes. Because they are already at an increased risk of bloodflow problems, people dealing with both diabetes and high blood pressure also face kidney damage and numerous other vascular diseases. As further evidence of the link between these two diseases, high blood pressure

Nuts in general contain a combination of various cholesterol-lowering plant food components. Here's the fact that got my attention, though: In virtually all studies that examined the impact of nuts in our diet, nut consumption has been associated with a reduction in coronary heart disease risk.

Each nut contains its own unique profile of phytochemicals, types of fatty acids, and types and amounts of fiber. It's no accident that the Portfolio study chose to use almonds.

Almonds may improve cholesterol levels. Almonds (and most nuts) contain large amounts of oleic acid (a monounsaturated fatty acid), which may help raise HDL cholesterol and possibly lower LDL cholesterol. Plus, almonds contain a vegetable protein that may also lower LDL. One-quarter cup of roasted almonds contributes around 11 grams of monounsaturated fat and contains almost 8 grams of plant protein.

Almonds offer a fiber benefit. Almonds contain mostly insoluble fiber, which helps keep bowel movements regular and may help reduce the risk of colon problems, hemorrhoids, varicose veins, and obesity (by making us feel full). One-quarter cup of roasted almonds adds just over 4 grams of total fiber—3.6 grams insoluble fiber and 0.5 grams soluble.

is one of several disorders that defines metabolic syndrome, a precursor to diabetes.

The original DASH study followed 459 participants with three dietary patterns for 8 weeks. It was designed to measure the impact of different combinations of fiber, key minerals (calcium, magnesium, and potassium), and macronutrients (protein, fat, saturated fat, polyunsaturated fat, and monounsaturated fat) on participants.

A second round of research used the same diet (if it ain't broke, don't fix it, right?), but salt intake was monitored at three levels: the current US sodium levels of around 3,450 milligrams per day, the upper daily limit of the current recommendations of 2,300 milligrams, and the optimal lower level of 1,150 milligrams. Guess what happened? After 30 days, the biggest drops in blood pressure were seen with the DASH diet at the lowest level of salt intake. Here's the lowdown on why scientists think it works.

Fiber, potassium, magnesium, and calcium create synergy. Scientists attribute the DASH diet success in part to the fiber, potassium, magnesium, and calcium found in this combination of foods. Fruit and vegetables are rich in potassium, while dairy products provide a boost of calcium and magnesium. It makes sense that these minerals could help with blood pressure because a diet low in calcium, potassium, and magnesium and high in sodium is suspected of causing high blood pressure in the first place. But keep in mind that simply adding these minerals as *supplements* to the diet has not been shown to lower blood pressure effectively.

The DASH diet is also rich in phytochemicals, notes Marlene Most, PhD, RD, of the Pennington Biomedical Research Center of Louisiana State University in Baton Rouge, who analyzed the DASH diet specifically for its phytochemical content. According to Dr. Most, lycopene (found in tomatoes and may help fight prostate cancer) is abundant in the DASH diet, along with flavonols (found in fruits, vegetables, tea, and red wine and may protect against heart disease), carotenoids, and flavonoids (which may protect against coronary heart disease and stroke). "It is recognized that plant-based diets are associated with a reduced incidence of chronic diseases," she says. With 8 to 11 servings of fruits and vegetables a day and 6 to 12 servings of whole grains, the DASH diet can be a great ally in the battle against a number of chronic, diet-related diseases.

The Five Elements of the DASH Diet

In a nutshell, the DASH diet is a way of eating that is low in cholesterol, saturated fat, and total fat but rich in low-fat dairy foods, whole grains, fruits, and vegetables. Specifically, the DASH diet calls for the following daily nutrients.

✓ 8 to 10 servings of fruits and vegetables. One serving equals:
   ¾ cup of fruit or vegetable juice
   ½ cup of raw or cooked fruits or vegetables
   1 medium apple or banana
   1 cup of raw, leafy vegetables (like romaine lettuce)

✓ 6 to 12 servings of whole grain products

✓ 2 to 3 servings of low-fat or fat-free dairy products. One serving equals:
   1 cup of milk or yogurt
   1.5 to 2 ounces of reduced-fat cheese
   ½ cup of cottage cheese

✓ No more than two 3-ounce servings of lean meat, poultry, or fish

✓ 2 to 3 tablespoons of added fat and oil, as well as nuts

Controlling sodium, fiber, and fat also creates synergy. While the DASH diet and lower sodium intake have both been proven to reduce blood pressure, employing both strategies at the same time has shown to yield even better results. Adding more physical activity to the mix appears to reduce blood pressure even more.

Think it can't get any better? Consider fiber as part of the equation, too. A low-sodium, low-fat, high-fiber diet has been linked to even larger improvements in blood pressure and body weight. In the DASH research, the diet rich in fruits and veggies provided roughly 24 grams of fiber and 1,600 calories.

The fiber came from the usual suspects—almost half from whole grains, with the rest from fruit and juices, vegetables, nuts, seeds, and legumes. When researchers examined the factors in isolation, they found that each had only a small effect on blood pressure, but when combined, the story changed entirely. The combination of the three diets (high fiber, low sodium, and low fat) produced larger and highly significant decreases in blood pressure and body weight.

THE PART-TIME VEGETARIAN (A HEALTHFUL HAPPY MEDIUM)

I call myself a part-time vegetarian because I like to eat vegetarian meals often, including at restaurants—just to get some new ideas on making meatless dishes. I still eat fish and chicken and lean beef and pork, but I would guess at least half my meals qualify as lacto-ovo-vegetarian. There was a time when all my meals were meatless (can you say "UC Berkeley grad school"?), and, oddly enough, the one thing I totally craved every so often was a good lean cheeseburger—but that was before all these great vegetarian burgers hit restaurants and supermarkets.

Two decades and two kids later, I have definitely evolved into a happy part-time vegetarian. Lucky for me, this has also come with a slew of benefits! Meatless eating often costs less, helps the environment (some would argue), and confers health advantages. "Besides reducing the saturated fat content of your diet because you aren't eating animal fats, there are other benefits to a meatless day or two each week," says Julie Upton, MS, RD, with the *Environmental Nutrition* newsletter. According to Upton, vegetarian diets are lower in total fat, saturated fat, and cholesterol, plus they include more of the beneficial nutrients found in plant foods, like vitamins A and C, potassium, fiber, and phytonutrients like beta-carotene and lycopene.

So what exactly does it take to call oneself a vegetarian? In reality, there are many forms of vegetarianism, each based on varying degrees of dependence on animal products. For the purposes of our discussion, "semi-vegetarian" refers to someone who eats some fish and poultry sometimes, but also eats meals that are meat-free. The other common type of vegetarianism is lacto-ovo-vegetarian, which includes dairy products and eggs but excludes meat, fish, and fowl. The lacto-vegetarian excludes eggs as well.

Vegetarian Options Abound

There's never been a better time to become a part-time vegetarian and eat meatless meals more often. Today's supermarkets have many healthful and creative options for when you fire up the grill and beyond. Look for meatless convenience items to keep in your freezer. They're great fast fixes for action-packed weeknights or microwave lunches.

I love soy and veggie burgers. They usually contain less saturated fat than beef burgers, some feature high-quality soy protein, and most of the veggie/soy options add at least a couple grams of fiber. Here are a few examples.

BOCA Vegan Burger: 110 calories, 2 g fat, 13 g protein, 5 g fiber

Gardenburger Flame Grilled Soy Burger: 120 calories, 4 g fat, 14 g protein, 4 g fiber

Gardenburger Portabella Burger: 100 calories, 2.5 g fat, 9 g protein, 4 g fiber

Morningstar Farms Grillers Original: 140 calories, 6 g fat, 15 g protein, 2 g fiber

Amy's Kitchen All American Veggie Burger: 120 calories, 3 g fat, 10 g protein, 3 g fiber

Whole Foods 365 Organic Classic Veggie Burger: 100 calories, 2.7 g fat, 14 g protein, 4 g fiber

A vegetarian diet is linked to weight loss. What's this? A recent scientific review compiling data from 87 observational and clinical studies on vegetarian diets noted weight loss of up to a pound a week, and it didn't appear to depend on exercise or calorie count? Sign me up!

What's behind this? Well, vegetarians typically consume more than 50 percent of energy from carbohydrate-rich plant foods known for having some nutritional synergy (fruits, vegetables, legumes and nuts, and whole grain breads and cereals). Vegetarian diets also tend to be higher in fiber and lower in calories, protein, total fat, cholesterol, and saturated fat, compared with your average meat-eater's diet.

"There is evidence that a vegetarian diet causes an increased calorie burn after meals, meaning plant-based foods are being used more efficiently as fuel for the body, as opposed to being stored as fat," notes one of the reviewers, Neal Barnard, MD, of the Physicians Committee for Responsible Medicine, a nonprofit organization based in Washington, DC. The reviewers also reported that vegetarians experienced increased insulin sensitivity, meaning their cells absorbed nutrients more easily.

Part-time vegetarians reap health benefits. There's not a great deal of research on part-time vegetarians, but in my opinion, eating vegetarian more often and being carnivorous less often offers a number of distinct benefits. In one Swedish study, healthy semivegetarian or lacto-vegetarian women had a lower risk of overweight and obesity than did omnivorous women. There's one of the most prized benefits right there! The researchers concluded that the advice to consume more plant foods and fewer animal products might help individuals control their weight.

Further, research has demonstrated time and again that eating a diet both high in fruits and vegetables and low in saturated fat is more protective against mortality than either factor alone. What's one of the easiest ways to

(continued on page 182)

Beans offer an amazing package of nutrients—every piece is important—but the beauty is in the balance. This plant food is uniquely high in protein and bursting with beneficial phytochemicals. You get some good-quality carbohydrates that interact with lots of fiber to be digested slowly. Beans have been shown to result in relatively small increases in blood glucose levels following meals in people with and without diabetes.

Beans help fight cancer. Beans (also known as legumes) and soy (considered a bean) are two of 11 plant foods that the AICR recently named as "foods that fight cancer." The active ingredients in beans that seem to play a protective role include three distinguished phytochemicals: saponins, protease inhibitors, and phytic acid. According to the AICR, they protect cells from the type of genetic damage that can lead to cancer. Laboratory studies have shown saponins' ability to inhibit the reproduction of cancer cells and slow the growth of tumors in several types of tissues. Protease inhibitors seem to slow the division of cancer cells and help prevent tumors from releasing substances called proteases that destroy nearby cells. Slowing down the progression of tumors is phytic acid's contribution. In one recent case-control study involving 3,237 men, the men who ate the most beans had a 38 percent lower risk of prostate cancer than subjects who ate the least.

The other big anticancer benefit is all the fiber, both insoluble and soluble, you get in a ½-cup serving of beans. Diets high in fiber have been repeatedly linked to lower risk of colorectal, pancreatic, and breast cancers.

Beans are tops in antioxidant power. Ronald Prior, PhD, with the USDA Agricultural Research Service, performed an antioxidant study and found beans to be supreme, with ½ cup—a mere 100 calories—of red beans yielding 13,727 antioxidants; red kidney beans, 13,259; pinto beans, 11,864; and black beans, 4,191. Beans are also full of B vitamins, potassium, and fiber, which promote digestive health and relieve constipation. Eating beans may also help prevent colon cancer and reduce blood cholesterol, a leading cause of heart disease.

Beans may help reduce the risk for cardiovascular disease. In terms of possible heart protection, start with the antioxidants and phytochemicals in beans, then add in the fact that beans are one of the highest-fiber plant foods on the planet, with ½ cup generally contributing 7 grams of fiber. Fiber is one of many nutritional factors that may lessen your risk of atherosclerotic cardiovascular disease, and, generally, the more fiber in your diet, the lower your risk.

Beans may lead to better blood sugar control. According to a recent scientific review, the use of beans (along with whole grains) is associated with better blood sugar control in diabetic and insulin-resistant people. High in soluble fiber, beans release carbohydrates slowly and steadily, preventing that rapid rise in blood sugar that follows the wrong kind of meals. Enjoy a bowl of zesty black bean soup, or slather your sandwich with a delicious layer of hummus, and you may benefit from better-controlled blood sugar.

ENJOY BEANS AT THEIR BEST

The general recommendation is to eat beans several times a week, possibly taking the place of red meat (which lowers intake of saturated fat and cholesterol) and also serving as a source of folic acid (in lentils and pinto beans), fiber, and assorted phyto-chemicals (in soybeans and soybean products). Here are a few bean tips to get you started.

Canned beans save the day! Just open a can, rinse, and go. Otherwise, you'll probably be stuck soaking dry beans in water overnight and then boiling until tender. Kidney beans and black beans seem to fare the best in most recipes including salads and soups.

Frozen beans are lifesavers, too. In my opinion, having frozen beans on hand is a great idea because leftovers are easy to store—you take only what you need and put the rest of the bag back in the freezer. My favorite frozen item is edamame (shelled), and one of my daughter's favorite quick snacks is microwaved shelled edamame.

Beat gas. If beans bother your digestive system, try canned beans. Rinse them well in a colander to remove any gas-producing substances. The over-the-counter product Beano contains an enzyme supplement that breaks down problematic substances.

accomplish both? Eat vegetarian more often. Substituting dishes with plant protein for meals with ample animal protein will typically bring down the overall amount of saturated fat while boosting the fruit and vegetable totals!

MEATLESS MEALS FOR THE CHRONICALLY CARNIVOROUS

Curious to see what vegetarian meals can do for you? The following tips can help you work more meatless meals into your week. Start with a "meatless Monday," and add more vegetarian meals each week as you find new dishes you like. It might be easier than you think.

- Substitute a soy "meat" product for the meat ingredient in casseroles, stews, tacos, chili, etc.
- Break out a can of beans. There's such a wide variety, and beans make great meat-replacers because they are supersatisfying, with high amounts of protein and fiber. You might not notice the meat's missing in a nice chili or vegetable stew bursting with beans.
- Try a veggie potpie featuring potatoes, peas, mushrooms, and any other vegetables with vegetarian gravy and pie crust (if desired).
- Make Mexican dishes (burritos, nachos, enchiladas, etc.) featuring beans and veggies instead of beef and chicken.
- Stir-fry Chinese cuisine with veggies and tofu and serve over rice or noodles.
- Stuff bell peppers with a mixture of rice with spices and vegetables plus vegetarian sausage, tofu, or beans to make the dish more satisfying.
- Layer lasagna with veggies instead of meat. Lasagna has so much going for it—sauce, cheese, noodles, and herbs—that you won't even

miss the meat. Same goes for other pasta dishes: Macaroni and cheese doesn't need meat to pass muster, and neither does fettuccine Alfredo, cheese tortellini with pesto, or marinara sauce.

- Substitute hearty vegetables that have a substantial texture and rich, satisfying flavor (eggplant, spinach, portobello mushrooms, zucchini, etc.) for the meat in favorite dishes. Thick slices of broiled eggplant take the place of chicken in eggplant Parmesan, and spinach replaces ground beef in spinach lasagna. Tofu can take the place of beef in chili, and a grilled portobello mushroom can stand in for a burger on a bun.

DOES ASIAN CUISINE REIGN SUPREME?

Talk about a cuisine and culture that's different from our own—where to begin with the Asian diet? Well, for starters, we could discuss portion size. While Americans tend to see meat as an entrée, and the mantra is usually "bigger is better," Asian cuisine tends to use shavings of meat as a garnish or flavoring. Most traditional Asian meals include a lot of vegetables that are "spiced" with the flavor of meat. One-third pound of meat (5 ounces) will often be used to feed four to six people. In the United States, we'll order a ⅓-pound burger just for one! The traditional Chinese diet, in fact, is composed of only 20 percent animal foods, and all those vegetables provide a slew of disease-fighting antioxidants and phytochemicals. Perhaps the Chinese were the original vegetarians and part-time vegetarians—the traditional Chinese diet is primarily vegetarian, featuring lots of vegetables, rice, and soybeans.

It's a no-brainer that the typical Asian diet is markedly different from the standard American one, but you may still be wondering how much is really known about its health benefits. For that information, we turn to the Cornell-China-Oxford Project on Nutrition, Health, and Environment, a long-term study comparing the diets of rural China with average American ones. Since the early 1980s, T. Colin Campbell, PhD, director of the project, has been tracking the eating habits of people living in 100 Chinese rural villages. What has he discovered so far? In rural China, the rates of major chronic diseases, including breast, colon, and rectal cancer, are mere fractions of those reported in the United States. "There are some regions in China in which breast cancer and heart disease are almost unknown," Campbell says. Type 2 diabetes and bone-weakening osteoporosis are much less prevalent, even though the Chinese consume far fewer dairy products than we do in the United States, according to Campbell.

Does soy offer breast cancer benefits? Eating lots of soy-based food may protect older women against breast cancer, suggests a study of Chinese Singaporeans. Researchers, including Anna H. Wu, PhD, from the University of Southern California, analyzed the diets of 144 healthy postmenopausal Chinese women in Singapore. Until recently, women in Japan and China had a sixfold lower risk of breast cancer than Western women. And we know it's not entirely genetic because as Asian women adopt Western lifestyles and diets, this protection disappears.

Wu's study found that women whose diets put them in the highest 25 percent of soy consumption (the equivalent of more than three servings of tofu a day) had 15 percent lower blood levels of an important form of estrogen. Women who ate average amounts of soy, however, showed no drop in estrogen.

So is it the soy? In my opinion, soy is one big piece of the Asian cuisine puzzle. Certainly the smaller servings of red meat and ample servings of vegetables don't hurt, either.

Is miso a must? If you've eaten at a Japanese restaurant, you may have met up with a bowl of miso soup, a thin stock made from a paste of fermented soybeans. Doesn't sound too appetizing? Trust me, it's tastier than you might think. But if my endorsement alone doesn't convince you, consider this: A group of Japanese researchers conducted a large study on Japanese women between ages 40 and 59, looking at soy, isoflavones (a plant estrogen found in soy), and breast cancer. After a decade of collecting data, the researchers found some magic in that miso!

First of all, for the women in the study, miso soup was a part of daily life. Seventy-five percent ate it almost every day, and most had two or more cups a day. The researchers also found that women, especially postmenopausal women, with the most isoflavones in their diet had the lowest risk of breast cancer. Strangely, though, the researchers also found that eating soy foods in general did not seem to lower the risk of breast cancer.

Think beyond soy. The same study also found that other traditional Asian eating habits, such as eating more rice, pickles, vegetables, and fish, were also linked with lower breast cancer risk, suggesting to me that there are many health-promoting aspects to the traditional Asian cuisine, probably a result of synergy within their food patterns. Favorite Chinese vegetables, which likely have some phytochemical synergy going on themselves, include bok choy, kale, Swiss chard, sweet potatoes, bean sprouts, spinach, and eggplant. Four out of seven are nutrient-packed dark green leafy vegetables. Coincidence? I think not.

Make the tea connection. As we discussed in Chapter 4, there's an amazing amount of food synergy in green tea (and black and white tea, too). In fact, the American Institute for Cancer Research advises that people concerned about lowering their cancer risk consider adding green tea to a diet rich in various plant foods and low in fat and salt. That sounds like synergy in motion to me! Yes, there is certainly more to know about the potential benefits and ideal amounts of tea, but adding a couple cups of green tea to a healthy diet just seems smart.

But which is best: white, green, or black? The less processed the tea, such as in green and white, the higher the concentration of its beneficial compounds. White tea is very unprocessed, whereas green tea is steamed a little more but still has loads of phytochemicals. Black tea is the most processed, and while it still contributes helpful compounds, there are fewer reported benefits compared to green or white tea.

The half-life of the phytochemicals in tea is a few hours in humans, which suggests that drinking tea throughout the day rather than at one particular time would give the biggest nutritional bang for your buck.

TRADITIONAL ASIAN CUISINE

Want to explore the health benefits traditional Asian cuisine has to offer? If you're not a fan of the standard take-out options, which are actually often high in sodium and fat, take heart. You don't necessarily have to eat Asian dishes to reap the rewards. There are plenty of ways to benefit from an Asian diet without drastically changing the way you eat. Just keep the following points in mind.

- Meals consist mainly of plant foods with small amounts of fish and poultry and only occasionally red meat.
- Vitamin-packed vegetables often used in Chinese dishes include bok choy, kale, Swiss chard, sweet potatoes, bean sprouts, spinach, and eggplant.
- Fresh fruit is considered a treat or dessert in Chinese and other Asian cuisines. So skip that slice of cheesecake, and instead enjoy fresh slices of mango drizzled with honey and lime juice.

- Green tea (black tea, too) is a mainstay beverage. Try replacing a few cups of coffee with tea.
- Soy is a common protein source, coming from tofu, miso, edamame (green soybeans), etc. Try mixing soft silken tofu into a smoothie instead of yogurt. Or dice some extra-firm tofu, toss with barbecue sauce, and bake until heated through for a delicious alternative to meat-based fare.

Chapter 7

Putting Food Synergy into Action

If you've read the book this far, is your head now swimming with all sorts of food synergy examples? Was it flaxseed that you are supposed to eat with soy–or was it citrus? And what were the fruits and vegetables that seemed to have the most food synergy going for them? Was it broccoli and tomatoes or citrus and blueberries?

Don't worry; I'll try to tie up this whole food synergy thing for you with a nice, pretty (and practical) bow. Previous chapters contain actionable how-to tips and tables, but this is the chapter that pulls as much of the information as possible back into the disease categories, so you can see which food synergy possibilities might help protect against heart disease and which relate to cancer prevention, stroke and blood pressure, and diabetes. I even have a list of food synergy examples that help with weight loss! But don't flip ahead to that part yet.

First, I'm going to highlight the foods and diet themes that kept popping up all over the book. When these came up, as you were reading, you would say, "Didn't we just talk about this food?" These are what I like to call Synergy Super Foods because they have several things going for them. These are the foods that research suggests you should try to eat as frequently as possible, if you do nothing else after reading this book.

While we're on the subject of research . . . You might have wondered as you read the other chapters why I used so many "soft" words when reporting on the food synergy science—terms like *may, might, possibly, seems to, is thought to, appears to, is believed to,* etc. This is because what we know for sure about many of these food synergy relationships is not set in stone. There are still more studies to be conducted, more journal abstracts to be written. Some of the studies were done in laboratories, and human studies are necessary before we can report with confidence the exact implications for people.

That said, you'll also notice that these "clues" seem to be leading us down a certain path, one I feel completely comfortable recommending to you. It's a path that points toward more plant foods and away from processed foods; a path that seeks balance within broad dietary patterns instead of focusing on one or two particular miracle foods or ingredients. It's a path that leads us beyond "low-fat" or "low-carb." It's about making smart choices most of the time. It's about slowing down to enjoy each meal as a celebration; it's about savoring each bite. When we nourish our bodies with the best foods that nature has to offer, our bodies spontaneously respond in kind.

ACHIEVING FOOD SYNERGY: 12 RULES TO LIVE BY

Certainly the recipes in this book are one way to immerse yourself in the power of food synergy, but I want you to be able to translate this information to your own kitchen and consider your personal food preferences. So the following rules are designed to help you do just that. Circle the ones that interest you most, then go back and create your Personalized Food Synergy Action Plan by including all the foods mentioned that you liked and are willing to include.

1. EAT MORE WHOLE FOODS

Quite simply, in terms of your health, whole foods are the best options, compared with processed or refined foods and products. Food in its whole form means beans, fruits and vegetables, whole grains, nuts and seeds, chicken (feel free to take off the skin), and unprocessed lean meats.

Remember all that you learned about the different phytochemicals in foods? Many are powerful antioxidants, and some are thought to wield more power than vitamins C and E! Well, the only way to make sure we are receiving all the phytochemicals possible (even the ones we don't know about yet) is to eat plant foods in the least processed form possible.

For example, you're more likely to get the maximum amount of the 30-plus phytochemicals in olive oil from oils that are the least processed—that's why buying extra-virgin oil is best. And you are more likely to get the phytochemicals in grains when you use whole grains or buy products that use mostly whole and unprocessed grains. So have I convinced you yet? Are you ready to eat a mostly whole foods diet? See "10 Tips for Enjoying a Whole Foods Diet" on page 192 for suggestions to get you started.

2. SWITCH TO WHOLE GRAINS EVERYWHERE YOU CAN!

You probably already know that we should all be eating more whole grains for all sorts of health reasons. But how do we go about doing that in our white-bread world? Listen, I grew up on that balloon bread that got stuck between your teeth. But switching to 100 percent whole wheat or whole grain bread is one of the easiest things I've done. It took trying a few different brands, but I finally found one my two teenage girls like.

I look for opportunities to switch to whole grain everywhere possible. While you may not be ready to switch to whole grains entirely, everyone can add a serving here and there. And that can be enough to make a difference in your health.

10 Tips for Enjoying a Whole Foods Diet

1. Check labels carefully to make sure they contain the nutrients that are suggested by advertising claims. Many foods like breads and bread products, cereals and cereal bars, crackers, whole grain–blend pastas, and even some frozen entrées advertise that they use "whole grains," but some contain such a small amount that it hardly makes a difference in the overall quality of the food.

2. Choose 100 percent whole grain products as much as possible.

3. Use half whole wheat flour in your baking and half the amount of sweetener when you can.

4. Eat lots of fresh vegetables and fruits; try to include them in almost every meal and snack.

5. Have beans more often; they're a great source of plant protein, fiber, phyto-chemicals, and other nutrients.

6. Eat processed food less often; it's often loaded with added fats, sugar, salt, and additives.

7. Choose beverages wisely and have plenty of nonsugary options available, like water, mineral water, green tea (iced or hot), and fat-free or soy milk.

8. Make your own frozen entrées (instead of buying them) by freezing homemade leftovers. Consider making double batches of family favorites like meat loaf, spaghetti sauce, and soups.

9. Look for recipes that call for mostly "whole foods" and are easy to fix (because then you're more likely to actually try them).

10. Eat in more often. Do the fast-food thing less often. And when you do need to get food out, go to the chains with more whole foods, like fresh Mexican food (Baja Fresh, Chipotle), fresh sandwiches (with whole wheat buns, real chicken breast and sliced roast beef), and fresh pasta and Italian foods (some restaurants offer whole wheat pasta). If you go to a Chinese restaurant, choose traditional dishes that are not deep-fried, and aim for less meat and more vegetables.

Your goal should be to eat at least three 1-ounce servings per day of whole grain foods—preferably in place of refined grains, according to the latest dietary guidelines. And with the new and improved whole grain–blend pastas available and the emphasis on whole grains in the cereal aisle, I'm at my "three a day" goal by lunch!

3. BECOME VORACIOUS FOR VEGGIES

How many times do we have to hear about how amazing vegetables are for us before we really take it to heart? You knew they were nutritious before you read this book, I'm sure, but now you know more about all the powerful phytochemicals they pump into our bodies along with the vitamins and minerals we need more of. Whether it's the two vegetables high in viscous fiber (like eggplant and okra) or the cruciferous vegetables (like kale and broccoli) with all those anticancer organosulfur compounds or the carotenoid family (carrots, sweet potatoes, spinach, etc.) that offers a rich mix of phytochemicals, the message is simple: The more the merrier! Get as many vegetables as you can as often as you can.

Get your daily dark greens. Try to enjoy a dark green veggie almost every day. The dark green veggies ended up on many of the lists in this book—for vegetables high in vitamin C; with multiple carotenoids; and tops in potassium, calcium, magnesium, and vitamin E. My favorite way to get a daily dose of dark green veggies can be summed up in two words: *raw spinach*. Buy a bag of triple-washed, ready-to-go spinach leaves, and a quick salad can be yours at a moment's notice. Every time I make scrambled eggs or an omelet (with omega-3 eggs), I toss in a bunch of raw spinach. It's easy! If you aren't ready to go 100 percent spinach salad, mix some spinach greens with whatever lettuce you prefer. You'll be halfway there!

Don't fear frozen veggies. It's easier to be inspired to eat more vegetables in the middle of summer when the zucchini is firm and the corn is fresh. But

The Quickest Way to Three Servings a Day

One serving can be:

✓ 1 slice of whole wheat or other whole grain bread

✓ 1 small muffin made with a whole grain

✓ 1 cup of ready-to-eat whole grain cereal

✓ ½ cup of hot whole grain cereal

✓ ½ cup of cooked brown rice or whole wheat pasta

It's actually pretty easy to hit the "three servings a day" mark. It's a matter of substituting whole grains for refined ones in foods that we already know and love. Here are examples of some whole grain choices you could make through the day. Have just one at each meal, and you've hit your goal.

BREAKFAST

✓ Hot oatmeal or a cold whole grain cereal

✓ Pancakes, cinnamon rolls, muffins, crepes, or waffles made with part whole wheat flour, part oats, or oat bran

✓ Whole wheat or whole grain toast

what can we do during the most veggie-challenging season of all—winter? The answer is in your grocery freezer case.

Imagine the following scenario. You're running around your kitchen, trying to throw dinner together on a busy weeknight, coordinating what's simmering on the stove with washing the fruit and when to pick up the kids from soccer practice, when you suddenly realize you forgot about the vegetables.

LUNCH

✓ Sandwich on whole wheat or other whole grain bread

✓ Soup made with barley, whole wheat pasta, or bulgur

✓ Burrito or quesadilla made with a whole wheat tortilla

✓ Cold pasta salad made with whole wheat pasta

✓ Fruit-and-cheese plate with 100 percent whole grain crackers

DINNER

✓ Entrée served with cooked brown rice, barley, millet, quinoa, bulgur, or whole wheat or whole wheat–blend pasta

✓ Dinner roll made with part whole wheat flour

✓ Soup or stew made with barley, bulgur, whole wheat pasta, brown rice, etc.

DESSERT

✓ Favorite recipe made with part whole wheat flour

✓ Dessert featuring oats (oatmeal raisin cookies, fruit crisp, etc.)

✓ Rice pudding made with brown rice

No worries; you just pop open your freezer and see what goes best with tonight's entrée. Six minutes later, your ever so lightly microsteamed veggies take their proud place on the dinner table.

That exact scene happens more often than I want to admit at my house. The truth is, frozen veggies come in handy year-round, but I especially rely on them during the months when it's slim pickings in the produce section.

My Personal Picks

Let's face it—certain vegetables manage the stress of being frozen and then heated and eaten better than others. Take peas. I'm not a "pea" person (my mom forced me to eat them, and I think I will be forever influenced by this dinner trauma), but even I have them around to toss in soups, fried rice, and casseroles. And what would I do without frozen chopped spinach for some of my all-time favorite dishes, like spinach garlic dip and spinach lasagna?

Of the 20 most frequently eaten raw veggies, half are available frozen, so you do have lots of options year-round! Those available frozen are followed by an F (for "frozen") in the list below.

20 MOST FREQUENTLY CONSUMED RAW VEGETABLES

Asparagus	F
Bell pepper	F (some stores)
Broccoli	F
Carrots	F
Cauliflower	F
Celery	
Cucumber	
Green cabbage	
Green onions	
Green snap beans	F
Iceberg lettuce	
Leaf lettuce	
Mushrooms	F (some stores)
Onions	F (some stores)
Potatoes	F
Radishes	
Summer squash	
Sweet corn	F
Sweet potatoes	
Tomato	

Source: Federal Register, March 20, 2002

Industry statistics show frozen vegetable sales peak between November and April, but highest sales are during the three holidays that fall within these months—Thanksgiving, Christmas, and Easter.

Sometimes in winter, it isn't the quality of the produce that scares us off as much as it is the price. Frozen vegetables, though, are fairly reasonable throughout the year. And it's tough to beat the convenience of having several bags of vegetables sitting in the freezer, not a worry in the world about having to use them up before they turn brown.

Nutritionally speaking, frozen veggies are similar to and sometimes better than fresh. They're usually picked at the peak of the season and flash-frozen (which suspends the "aging" and nutrient losses) immediately after harvest. I ran a nutritional comparison on the vitamins in a cup of fresh and frozen broccoli florets (uncooked), and the frozen broccoli contained a bit more of vitamins A, B_2, and C, and folic acid. A recent government study found no change in the amounts of folic acid after 12 months of freezing. So don't let nutrition concerns stop you from buying frozen.

4. HAVE A HANDFUL OF NUTS EVERY DAY

Did you notice that nuts were mentioned in almost every chapter? In general, nuts contain mostly monounsaturated fat, and most contribute phytosterols, which in sufficient amounts help lower blood cholesterol, enhance the immune system, and decrease the risk of some cancers. Pistachios and sunflower seeds have the most phytosterols, followed by Brazil nuts and English walnuts. Nuts also contribute some vitamins and minerals we tend to lack, such as vitamin E, potassium, and magnesium. Two forms of vitamin E work best together (alpha- and gamma-tocopherol), and you'll find them in almonds, cashews, and walnuts. Walnuts also contain some plant omega-3s.

One nut in particular, however, takes the cake—*A* is for almond. Almonds were the preferred nuts in the PortfolioEatingPlan, and they were mentioned

10 Ways to Eat More Almonds

1. Sprinkle them over hot or cold cereal.

2. Top a green salad with a couple tablespoons of toasted slivered or sliced almonds.

3. Stir 1 cup of chopped almonds into muffin batter, or sprinkle 1½ tablespoons of chopped almonds over the tops of unbaked muffins. The nuts will toast while the muffins bake.

4. Stir chopped almonds into pancake or waffle batter.

5. Sprinkle a heaping tablespoon of toasted sliced or slivered almonds on top of a serving of fish or chicken.

6. Keep a can of roasted almonds in your car or desk for a quick snack.

7. Carry a bag or two of almonds in your purse or briefcase to tide you over when you have to postpone a meal.

8. Stir some toasted almonds into your daily yogurt.

9. Make trail mix by tossing your favorite dried fruits with some toasted almonds. It makes a great energy-boosting snack because it has a nice blend of carbohydrates, protein, fat, and fiber!

10. Set out small bowls of roasted almonds on the kitchen counter and the coffee table in your family room (like you would a bowl of candy), inviting everyone to nibble on almonds.

in a few different synergy examples, too. They are probably the most studied nut, which is why we know they have phytochemicals that can help lower cholesterol, vegetable protein that may also lower low-density lipoprotein (LDL, or "bad") cholesterol, and monounsaturated fat that may increase high-density lipoprotein (HDL, or "good") cholesterol while lowering LDL.

And they're rich in antioxidants, thanks to flavonoids (catechin, epicatechin, and kaempferol).

For me, 2006 was the year of the nut. I started eating a handful almost every day. You could say I'm a bit nutty. I've never met a nut I didn't like. I have all sorts in my pantry, and I like to buy some of the more exotic trail mixes from Trader Joe's and mix things up a bit with cashews, pistachios, almonds, and walnuts.

Adding something like almonds on an almost daily basis just takes changing some old eating habits or adding some new ones. FYI: I've found that adding tends to be a lot easier than changing. For me, munching on some trail mix in the afternoon when I want a snack before I work out seems to do the trick. I keep trail mix in my car and in my kitchen so I can't miss. In "10 Ways to Eat More Almonds," you'll find lots of different ways to add almonds (or other nuts); see which ones work for you!

5. DRINK TEA (ESPECIALLY GREEN TEA)

Believe it or not, drinking green tea every day was my New Year's resolution. I like the way it tastes, but just thinking about all the health benefits gives me extra incentive. With each sip, I get two potent flavonoids—anthocyanin and proanthocyanidin—as well as a healthy dose of catechin, which may enhance the antioxidant activity of alpha-tocopherol (a form of vitamin E) and trigger weight loss by stimulating my body to burn calories and decrease body fat.

All that's great, but I'm probably most excited about this research breakthrough: Green and black tea contain antioxidant polyphenols thought to block cell damage that can lead to cancer. Green tea happens to be loaded with a certain polyphenol catechin called EGCG (epigallocatechin gallate), which has a knack for binding to a certain procancer protein, interfering with its ability to activate cancer cells, possibly stopping cancer before it starts!

So I started this year armed with an arsenal of exciting flavored green tea options (I take my New Year's resolutions seriously). Since it was winter, drinking a hot cup of green tea in the morning and at night was a cinch. Then came summer. It took me a couple weeks to transition, but I was sipping iced green tea in no time. The flavored green teas, like the mango or blueberry types I'm drinking right now, just keep it interesting.

A few things to keep in mind as you embark on this beverage adventure:

- The phytochemicals in tea have a half-life of a few hours, so have 1 cup now, another later to get the biggest bang for your tea bag.
- Tea components may have synergy with nut components, so it's a great idea to enjoy your morning or afternoon tea as a snack with a handful of nuts. This can work out well at the office; just keep some tea bags and a can of nuts in your desk!
- If you are sensitive to small amounts of caffeine, look for the decaf options; you still get all the good stuff from the tea.
- When selecting which teas to buy, remember that your nose always knows! If a tea bag smells delicious, that's how it will usually taste when brewed.
- Drink 2 to 3 cups of green tea a day, but feel free to have black and white tea at times, too; each has its own anticancer benefits.

6. BECOME AN OLIVE OIL AFICIONADO

If you haven't already, you can learn to appreciate and taste olive oil like many people do with wine. If you truly enjoy the flavor of your olive oil, you will be more likely to use it for cooking and as a dip for bread (instead of butter). If a dish I'm making doesn't require high heat and the flavor of olive oil complements the other ingredients, then I'm all over it! I make sure I am using reasonable amounts, though—I drizzle, not drench. It is still oil, after all, and each tablespoon adds more than 100 calories.

Eating olives as an appetizer, garnish, or entrée embellishment is always an option, too. Those 30-plus precious phytochemicals in olive oil, many of which have antioxidant and anti-inflammatory action in the body, helping to promote heart health and protect against cancer, are also in the olives themselves.

7. PUT PLANT STEROL–ENRICHED MARGARINE TO WORK

Sometimes you need a spreadable fat option for waffles or toast or for a nonoil fat when baking. You might as well reach for a great-tasting margarine with a dose of plant sterols and a healthier fatty-acid profile. These margarines have reduced LDL by up to 14 percent and total cholesterol levels by 10 percent (with 2 grams of plant sterols a day for the maximum LDL-lowering effect).

The truth is, some brands taste better than others. I did a taste test with three major brands a few years back, and at that time, Take Control was the clear winner. I've been buying it ever since. Try to enjoy the margarine at mealtimes because this is when the plant sterols will be most effective. When comparing margarine labels, look for one with:

- Plant sterol or stanols added
- The least saturated fat
- No trans fats
- A high amount of monounsaturated fat
- Possibly some plant omega-3s as part of the polyunsaturated fat total
- Around 8 grams of fat per tablespoon (so it works in recipes calling for butter or regular margarine but has a third less fat and one-quarter fewer calories than regular butter or stick margarine)
- Great flavor!

8. EAT FISH SEVERAL TIMES A WEEK

Fish offers powerful omega-3s, along with a dose of potassium. It's also a rare natural food source of vitamin D. Fish omega-3s have some synergy with plant omega-3s, so serve seafood with a side dish like spinach salad topped with wal-

Fast Fish Tips

Shop for your fish at a busy fish counter; the fish is more likely to be fresh. If your purchase was previously frozen and is now thawed, it should be used the same day—don't refreeze it. In fact, it's preferable to cook any fish the day you buy it. If you have to keep it longer, make sure to store it well sealed and in the coldest part of your refrigerator. Discard any fish that has a strong fishy smell or appears discolored. Remember, fresh fish has a sweet, briny scent (like the ocean it came from).

Although I relish the crispy crumb and moist interior of fried fish fillets just as much as the next person, it pains me to see something so innately healthful transformed within minutes into high-calorie, high-fat fare. I'm here to help you think outside the deep-fryer box.

GRILLING

In my opinion, grilling is the tastiest way to cook fish. The first key is to keep most of the moisture of the fish inside it as it cooks. Coating the fish lightly with oil will help seal in some of this moisture. If you choose a smart oil like canola or olive, with high amounts of the preferred monounsaturated fats and desirable plant omega-3s (canola oil), and you don't drench the fish with it, this will add around 1.1 grams of fat and 10 calories per serving (about ¼ teaspoon of oil per 4- or 5-ounce raw fillet).

The second key to grilling fish is to watch it carefully because it's very vulnerable to drying out. Remember, most fish on the grill takes only a few minutes per side. Flip the fillets over the second you cut into the fish and see that it's cooked halfway through. Continue to watch the fish closely and remove it as soon as it is cooked throughout—

nuts and a canola-oil dressing or a salad with red kidney beans and a canola-oil dressing, or finish the meal with a shot of fruit juice mixed with a tablespoon of ground flaxseed. And don't overlook other types of seafood: Crab in particular has all three B vitamins with synergy (folic acid, B_6, and B_{12}).

preferably, slightly before because the fish will continue to cook after you remove it from the heat.

Another method that's especially good for more delicate types of whitefish is to wrap each serving in foil and place it on the grill. The fish will marinate in its own moisture as it cooks. You can add seasonings like fresh garlic, fresh rosemary or basil, freshly ground pepper, garden tomatoes, white wine, orange, or lemon peel to create a subtly flavored dish.

BROILING

Broiling is basically grilling in the oven. You are still cooking your fish at a high temperature using a direct heat source. You can use a sauce or marinade, but this time the sauce won't fall through the grill and hit the coals below. My favorite way to broil fish is to thickly line a shallow baking pan with foil and coat it with canola-oil cooking spray before adding my fish or sauce. Cleanup is a snap this way.

BAKING

This is the antithesis to grilling, where you need to lovingly watch your fish carefully for the 10 or so minutes it's over the hot grill. Baking fish is more of a toss-and-go setup. Prepare the cooking sauce or coating (because you don't want to bake your fish dry) while you preheat the oven. Then pop the fish dish into the oven, following the recipe instructions for cooking times (so you don't overcook it). It's only tricky if your fish isn't the same size or thickness called for in your recipe; a thin fish fillet will cook more quickly, and a thicker one will generally take longer.

9. SEEK OUT TOMATOES

Here's to the high-powered fruit that acts like a vegetable! I'll take tomatoes any way I can: as cherry or grape tomatoes in salads, tucked in a two-slice sandwich or topping an open-faced one, chopped and added to an egg dish or vegetable sauté, or cooked into marinara or pizza sauce (check out the recipe in Chapter 8). Bottom line, tomatoes are loaded with food synergy potential because they contain:

- All four major carotenoids, which have synergy as a group (alpha- and beta-carotene, lutein, and lycopene). Few fruits and vegetables can say that.
- Three high-powered antioxidants also thought to have synergy together (beta-carotene, vitamin E, vitamin C)
- Great amounts of lycopene (thought to have the highest antioxidant activity of all the carotenoids), which has synergy with vitamin E and other food components
- Rich amounts of potassium, a mineral we need more of and that has synergy with other nutrients and food components

10. GO CRAZY FOR CITRUS

The whole citrus family is loaded with synergy because it boasts awesome amounts of the phytochemical subgroup flavones, which are believed to have antioxidant, anti-inflammatory, antithrombotic, and antiatherogenic action in the body. Oranges offer two carotenoids: lutein and zeaxanthin. Citrus also contains vitamin C, which was named in several synergistic partnerships in this book, plus potassium. Orange juice contains around 124 milligrams of vitamin C and 484 milligrams of potassium per cup, and grapefruit juice contains around 94 milligrams of vitamin C and

388 milligrams of potassium. Speaking of grapefruit, red grapefruit has been shown to have antioxidant synergy, and it's also rich in the high antioxidant lycopene.

Citrus fruits are suspected of some synergy with soy because vitamin C and phytoestrogens may help inhibit LDL cholesterol oxidation. If you like making smoothies, you could blend orange juice or oranges with soy yogurt or soft tofu as two of your ingredients.

Having some citrus juice every day as a beverage or in a smoothie is something many of us can do. I spend the extra money and buy freshly squeezed OJ (in plastic bottles) because the difference in flavor is amazing; once I tried it, it was darn hard to go back. If you prefer fruits to juice, make sure you always have some on hand. Cut oranges into wedges and chill them in the refrigerator for a great table snack. Buy grapefruit segments or mandarin oranges in jars so all you have to do is spoon them out onto your spinach salad or into your blender for a smoothie. Here are some ways to spruce up your juice so you won't get bored with it.

- Make a spritzer by adding seltzer water, club soda, or sparkling mineral water to your citrus juice.
- Make a sunrise drink by pouring ⅓ cup cranberry juice into your glass with ⅔ cup orange juice.
- Blend orange juice and grapefruit juices for a citrus blend.
- Make a citrus freeze by popping juice and crushed ice into a blender.

11. STIR IN A SPOONFUL OF GROUND FLAXSEED

Ground flaxseed seems to have synergy within itself on many levels, through fiber, lignans (plant estrogens), and plant omega-3s. But the seed may have synergy with several other foods (like fish omega-3s and soy), and these are just the ones we know about. Keep in mind, too, that small amounts of plant omega-3s are converted by the body into the long-chain omega-3s (normally found in fish).

It's ground flaxseed, not whole, you want to add a spoon of here and there because all those wonderful components aren't absorbed and available until the seed is ground. Keep your ground flax in the freezer to preserve its freshness, and add a tablespoon a day, if you can, by stirring it into your yogurt, cereal, smoothie, or stew.

When baking, you can usually replace ¼ cup of every 1 cup of flour in recipes with ground flaxseed. This means that instead of 1 cup of flour, you could use ¼ cup flaxseed and ¾ cup flour.

12. LEARN TO LOVE LOW-FAT DAIRY

Dairy foods deliver a team of players that are all important for healthy bones (calcium, vitamin D, protein, phosphorus, magnesium, vitamins A and B_6), some of which have synergy together. There's no better way to consume your calcium (a cup of yogurt contains 448 milligrams and a cup of fat-free milk, 300). Calcium combined with vitamin D may possibly reduce the risk of colon cancer. Low-fat dairy foods are packed with potassium, too (573 milligrams potassium per cup of yogurt; 407 per cup of fat-free milk). Including a couple low-fat dairy servings a day is also part of the DASH diet to lower hypertension. And if PMS is a problem, calcium and vitamin D together may ease symptoms (as part of a low-fat diet).

I'm not a milk drinker (just don't like it) or a cottage-cheese eater (don't care for the texture), but I have no problem ordering an iced or hot fat-free latte at a coffee bar. I also enjoy a nice serving of cheese almost every day and snack on yogurt a few times a week. I've worked out my plan; see if you can come up with some low-fat dairy options you'll enjoy, too.

SYNERGY AND MATTERS OF THE HEART

As this book has shown, there are many ways that food synergy can help reduce your risk of heart disease. Overall, eating lots of fruits and vegetables while keeping saturated fat intake on the low side (all the features of a traditional Mediterranean diet) can reduce your risk of dying from heart disease. If you know which facets of heart disease you're prone to, refer to the following list of foods and food combinations that may help the most.

To Reduce Effects of LDL Cholesterol:

- Garlic + onions, which contain organosulfur phytochemicals
- Oat phytochemicals + vitamin C
- Almond skin + vitamins C and E
- Vitamin C and E + beta-carotene
- Citrus extracts + vitamin C in citrus
- Soy protein
- Soy (phytoestrogens) + vitamin C in citrus
- Ground flaxseed (highest food source for lignans)
- Red wine (polyphenols)
- Grapefruit (part of a low-fat heart-healthy diet)
- Green tea

To Reduce LDL Blood Levels:

- The Portfolio plan (may reduce LDL by 30 percent)
- Nuts
- Ground flaxseed

(continued on page 210)

Putting Synergy Super Foods to the Test!

What happens if we have most of these Synergy Super Foods every day? Specifically, what do we get nutritionally if we do *all* of the following in a day? In putting my advice to the test, I calculated a daily menu plan incorporating the following:

✓ A few servings of whole grains (I included ½ cup of oats and two slices of 100 percent whole wheat bread in our analysis)

✓ A dark green vegetable (such as 1 cup of raw broccoli florets)

✓ A handful of nuts (3 tablespoons of almonds, for example)

✓ Green and/or black tea (as much as you want—tea is calorie free!)

✓ Olives or a little olive oil (I included 2 teaspoons of olive oil)

✓ 1 tablespoon of plant sterol–enriched margarine

✓ Fish (recommended several times a week; I included half a serving)

✓ Tomatoes (I included ½ cup of canned crushed tomato)

✓ Citrus (I included one orange)

✓ 1 tablespoon of ground flaxseed

✓ An antioxidant-rich fruit (I included ½ cup of mango and ½ cup of blueberries)

✓ A couple servings of low-fat dairy (in this case, 1 cup of fat-free milk and 1 cup of low-fat plain yogurt)

If you got every single Synergy Super Food listed above in one day, what's the calorie cost? What do you gain altogether nutritionally? It's probably fewer calories than you think. The grand total: 1,340 calories.

And here's the part that got me jumping up and down: Notice how you meet almost all of your nutritional needs—fiber, protein, vitamins, and minerals—by having these Synergy Super Foods! They delivered more nutritionally than I ever dreamed; it's amazing! Even the omega-6 to omega-3 ratio was an ideal 2 to 1 (6.6 grams omega-6 to 3.7 grams omega-3).

DAILY TOTAL

Calories	1,340
Protein	68 g
Carbohydrate	163 g
Fiber	27 g
Fat	49 g
Cholesterol	60 mg
Saturated fat	7.4 g
Monounsaturated fat	23 g
Polyunsaturated fat	14 g
Omega-3 fatty acids	3.7 g
Omega-6 fatty acids	6.6 g
Sodium	645 mg

PERCENTAGE DAILY VALUE (WOMEN 31–50 YEARS) FOR:

Vitamin A	139
Vitamin C	277
Vitamin E	82
Vitamin B_1	121
Vitamin B_2	213
Vitamin B_3	138
Vitamin B_6	153
Vitamin B_{12}	254
Folate (folic acid)	105
Calcium	110
Vitamin D	165
Magnesium	104
Potassium	97
Selenium	71
Zinc	154

To Lower Triglyceride Levels in the Blood:

- Red grapefruit as part of a low-fat heart-healthy diet
- Garlic + fish omega-3s
- Red wine (polyphenols) + soy protein
- Ground flaxseed

To Lower Total Cholesterol Levels:

- Garlic + fish omega-3s
- Whole grains
- Oats
- Fiber-rich foods
- Green tea
- The Portfolio plan (linked to lower cholesterol levels)

To Protect against Inflammation:

- Fish + plant omega-3s
- Red wine (polyphenols)
- Grapes (resveratrol)
- The Portfolio plan (reduces C-reactive protein, a marker of inflammation)

To Fight Plaque Buildup in Arteries:

- Blueberries + grapes (especially Gamay or Pinot Noir)
- Carotenoid-rich foods
- Soy isoflavones (phytoestrogens)
- Pomegranate juice
- Citrus extracts + vitamin C in citrus
- Green tea (may slow buildup of artery-clogging plaque)

USE FOOD SYNERGY TO PREVENT STROKES

Overall, one of the best ways to reduce the risk of stroke, particularly for women, is to eat plenty of whole grains. Other foods that play a significant role in stroke prevention are ground flaxseed, which may lower the risk of blood clots, and soy foods, which can help relax blood vessels.

To Prevent and Improve High Blood Pressure:

- Soy in general and perhaps soy protein in particular
- DHA (one of the fish omega-3s)
- Whole grains
- Oats
- Ground flaxseed
- Fruits and vegetables
- Low-fat dairy
- The traditional Mediterranean diet
- Olive oil
- The Portfolio plan

USE FOOD SYNERGY TO FIGHT CANCER

Overall, the Mediterranean diet, with its emphasis on fruits and vegetables, has been linked to 50 percent lower cancer risk. To fight specific aspects of the disease, the following combinations may prove helpful.

To Slow Development of Cancer Cells:

- Olive oil
- Tomatoes + broccoli (prostate tumors grew slower in rats)
- Soy + green tea (reduced breast tumor growth by 72 percent in mice)

Fight Cancer with Color

Certain fruits and vegetables may target specific cancers. Of course, we aren't playing Russian roulette, where we guess which cancer we need to prevent. We want to prevent them all! To benefit from the most cancer-fighting substances in produce, like carotenoids, isothiocyanates, limonene, vitamin C, and folic acid, just think of the three Cs.

- ✓ **C**olor (the deeper the better)
- ✓ **C**ruciferous vegetables (cabbage family of broccoli, cauliflower, Brussels sprouts, kale, etc.)
- ✓ **C**itrus fruits and juice (oranges, grapefruit, tangerines, etc.)

The vegetables thought to have the highest anticancer effect:

- ✓ Soybeans
- ✓ Cabbage
- ✓ Carrots
- ✓ Celery
- ✓ Parsnips

Other fruits and vegetables with an anticancer effect:

- ✓ Citrus
- ✓ Broccoli
- ✓ Brussels sprouts
- ✓ Cauliflower
- ✓ Onions
- ✓ Tomatoes
- ✓ Sweet bell peppers
- ✓ Cucumber
- ✓ Cantaloupe
- ✓ Berries

Herbs with anticancer effects:

- ✓ Garlic
- ✓ Ginger
- ✓ Coriander
- ✓ Parsley
- ✓ Licorice root

- Green tea (reduced breast tumor growth by 56 percent in mice)
- Soy
- Ground flaxseed
- Pomegranate juice
- Limonoids (phytochemicals) in citrus peel

To Reduce Risk of Certain Types of Cancer:

- Organosulfur compounds (found in garlic, onions, leeks, scallions, chives, broccoli, and other cruciferous veggies)
- Plant lignans (may cut colorectal cancer risk in half)
- Plant lignans from soy and ground flaxseed (may reduce breast cancer risk)
- Oranges (lutein may help reduce colon cancer risk)

To Prevent Damage from Free Radicals:

- Vitamin E + selenium
- Carotenoids working together (lutein + zeaxanthin)
- Broccoli, garlic, Brussels sprouts (contain a form of selenium that the body easily converts to an anticancer agent)

USE FOOD SYNERGY TO HELP PREVENT TYPE 2 DIABETES

Everything listed previously in "Synergy and Matters of the Heart" would help anyone who already has type 2 diabetes because when you develop diabetes, your risk of heart disease quadruples. But let's say you don't have diabetes, but your doctor told you that you are "prediabetic." Or perhaps you are at risk for diabetes and are interested in doing everything within your power to avoid it. These are the possible foods or food partnerships with the type of synergy that might help reduce your risk of this disease that has fast become an epidemic, striking children as well as adults.

To Improve Blood Sugar (Glucose) Control:

- Fiber
- Whole grains
- Soluble fiber in oats
- Beans (and possibly soy protein)
- Ground flaxseed
- The Portfolio plan

To Keep Insulin Levels Steady:

- Whole grains
- Oats (soluble fiber)
- Soy protein
- Ground flaxseed
- The Portfolio plan

To Reduce Risk of Kidney Disease Associated with Diabetes:

- Plant protein (like beans) when it replaces animal protein
- Soy protein

USE FOOD SYNERGY TO WORK TOWARD WEIGHT LOSS

I don't know about you, but I am so sick of hearing how overweight Americans are, I could scream. How could a country so obsessed with plastic surgery and being thin, spending billions a year on fad diets and dieting products, get itself in this mess?

Well, I've got my theories. First of all, when it comes to food variety and taste, the United States has it made. Both of these factors stimulate food intake. We may have started as the land of opportunity, but we are now the land of huge portions. Our extralarge servings and the fact that we eat out more often than ever are two more factors that encourage overeating in America.

As a country, we definitely don't exercise like people in other countries do, and our day-to-day lives appear to be more harried and stressful than in other cultures—more factors that encourage obesity.

Add in the fact that there is a fast-food restaurant on practically every

The Hormones Behind the Headlines

Leptin is a hormone that sends messages to the brain to say when we can stop eating—simply put, it calls a halt to hunger pangs. But a new study suggests that something quite common in the typical American diet actually gets in the way of leptin doing its job properly: high triglycerides.

According to some compelling research on obese mice, high levels of triglycerides in the blood block this much-welcome "stop eating" signal before it gets to the brain. The researchers believe these findings may hold some important clues to our understanding of obesity.

In particular, they found that the more triglycerides the mice ate, the less leptin reached the rodents' brains. But here's an important distinction: These results occurred only when the triglycerides were from animal fats. Triglycerides from vegetable fats did not block leptin as the animal triglycerides had done.

What do the researchers think is the solution? Theoretically, if you lower triglycerides, you should help the body's own leptin work better, which may help you lose weight. Eating a low-fat diet, they say, is a natural way to reduce triglycerides.

corner, and all the junk and snack food that seems to feed the masses, not to mention our apparent love affair with high-calorie sweetened beverages like soda, fancy coffee drinks, and bottled teas (from 150 to 400 calories a pop), and you've got yourself an obesity epidemic.

The icing on the obesity cake, so to speak, is our practice of dieting, losing weight fast, and gaining it back. Many chronic dieters have lost the ability to eat when they are truly hungry and to stop eating when they're comfortable.

Years of dieting have taught us to follow a certain plan to the letter and deprive ourselves until we can't stand it anymore. We are born with the ability to eat when hungry and stop when comfortable, but this is an easy thing to lose in an environment of fad dieting, with tempting food everywhere you go.

We have our work cut out for us, but it can be done. We have to start focusing on eating and exercising for the health of it and letting the pounds fall where they may. Our obsession with being thin is partly what got us into this mess, after all.

We have to stop the fad diets immediately and make changes in our eating and exercise habits that will serve us well for the rest of our lives. It's not a sexy message, I know, but it's the truth.

Go for whole grains. More whole grains may lead to less VAT fat (visceral adipose tissue). This is the type of abdominal fat that's most dangerous to health, even in teens. Within the whole grains category, some research on oats has shown they slow the emptying of the stomach into the small intestine and may help you feel fuller longer.

Load up on fruits and vegetables. More vegetables equate to lower energy density (food that's low in calories for its volume or space)—meaning it's more satisfying and can decrease the total calories you take in!

Include dairy. A healthful diet that includes a couple servings of low-fat dairy a day might have a connection to losing weight, perhaps even in the dreaded midsection.

Drink green tea. Green tea research indicates this tasty beverage may trigger weight loss by stimulating the body to burn calories and mildly decrease body fat, possibly through catechins.

Consider a vegetarian diet. A review of vegetarian-diet studies noted that weight loss did not appear to depend on exercise or calorie count and could occur at a rate of 1 pound per week. Semivegetarian or lacto-vegetarian women had a lower risk of overweight and obesity, compared with omnivorous women, according to a Swedish study.

MORE MENUS THAN YOU'LL KNOW WHAT TO DO WITH

This section could be retitled "More Food Synergy Than You'll Know What to Do With." We've learned about so many different food components that work together for maximum health benefit, it can be mind-blowing to think about how to put it all together to fit our lifestyles.

If you want to see what a more "whole foods" eating plan looks like, from meal to meal and day to day, incorporating as many Synergy Super Foods and partnerships as practically possible, this next section is just for you.

Following are 2 weeks (5 days each) of possible meals adding up to around 1,500 calories a day (give or take 100) because that's about as low as an active adult should go. The first thing you'll notice when you glance at the menus is that we are talking about a lot of food here! When you start choosing mostly whole foods and deemphasizing junk and processed foods, it takes quite a bit of volume to get to 1,500 calories.

I included a few meals each week that can be found in select fast-food places and restaurants; for many of us, that's a reality of life. I tried to include only one meat-centered meal a day, plus a couple low-fat dairy products, several fruits and vegetables, and at least three whole grain servings.

At the end of the sample menu section, I list a few high-synergy snacks that provide some of the Synergy Super Foods the menu may lack on some days.

Note: Include noncaloric beverages where needed, such as green or black tea (iced or hot), mineral water, or regular water (with slices of lime or lemon for flavor).

WEEK 1 | DAY 1

Breakfast

2 slices 100 percent whole wheat or whole grain bread with 1 tablespoon natural peanut butter and 1 tablespoon light fruit preserves

8 ounces low-fat milk (vitamin D fortified) as a beverage or in a café latte

*Synergy of high fiber and protein from milk controls appetite.

*Synergy of vitamin D with calcium in milk decreases PMS symptoms and boosts bone health.

Lunch

2 cups tomato or clear broth–based soup like minestrone (with beans)

Spinach and avocado salad: 2 cups spinach leaves; 5 cherry tomatoes; ¼ avocado, sliced or diced; 2 chopped hard-cooked egg whites; 2 tablespoons light salad dressing with canola or olive oil

4 whole wheat crackers

*Good fat from avocado and dressing increases absorption of phytochemicals from vegetables.

*Vitamin C from spinach works with phytoestrogens in plant foods like beans to inhibit oxidation of LDL.

*Synergy of protein from egg whites and fiber from beans and veggies controls appetite.

Dinner

Chicken, black bean, and vegetable quesadilla: 1 whole wheat tortilla; ¼ cup canned black beans; 2 ounces reduced-fat cheese; 2 ounces boneless, skinless roasted chicken breast; ½ cup veggies of your choice; 1 tablespoon green onions; and 1 tablespoon salsa

*Synergy between protein and fiber in quesadilla controls appetite.

*Link between whole grains and vegetables protects against heart disease.

*Synergy within whole grains prevents heart disease.

Snack

6 ounces low-fat fruit yogurt (vitamin D fortified)

*Synergy between calcium and vitamin D decreases PMS symptoms and boosts bone health.

DAILY TOTAL

CALORIES	PROTEIN	CARB	FIBER	CHOLEST	TOTAL FAT	SAT FAT	MONO FAT	POLY FAT	OMEGA-3	OMEGA-6	SODIUM
1,497	82 g	189 g	20 g	119 mg	50 g	16 g	10 g	6 g	2.1 g	2.6 g	2,828 mg

% DAILY VALUE (WOMEN 31–50 YEARS) FOR:

VITAMIN A	VITAMIN C	FOLATE	CALCIUM
180%	153%	61%	115%

DAY 2

Breakfast

1 cup cooked oatmeal made with 1 cup low-fat milk (vitamin D fortified) and ½ cup fresh or frozen fruit, such as blueberries, diced apple, or peaches

1 cup orange juice

*Synergy of oat components protects heart health.

*Synergy with calcium and vitamin D in milk decreases PMS symptoms.

*Synergy with fruits and whole grains protects against heart disease.

Lunch

Tuna sandwich: 2 slices 100 percent whole wheat or whole grain bread and tuna salad made with ½ cup tuna packed in water, 1 tablespoon light bottled vinaigrette (with canola or olive oil), tomato slices, and spinach or romaine lettuce leaves

½ cup baby carrots

1 cup grapes

*Synergy between protein and fiber in whole wheat bread and tuna controls appetite.

*Good fat from dressing increases absorption of phytochemicals from veggies.

*Synergy exists between fish omega-3s in tuna and plant omega-3s in oil from dressing and spinach leaves.

*Synergy between fruits and vegetables and whole grains protects against heart disease.

Dinner

Baked potato bar: 1 baked potato split open and topped with ¼ cup shredded reduced-fat Cheddar, ¼ cup fat-free sour cream, ½ cup broccoli, and 1 tablespoon chives or green onions

1 cup cantaloupe cubes

*Synergy of three B vitamins (from broccoli-cheese potato) helps protect artery linings.

*Synergy exists between various phytochemicals in fruits and vegetables.

Snack

12-ounce café latte made with espresso and 1 cup fat-free or low-fat milk (vitamin D fortified)

*Synergy with calcium and vitamin D in milk decreases PMS symptoms.

DAILY TOTAL

CALORIES	PROTEIN	CARB	FIBER	CHOLEST	TOTAL FAT	SAT FAT	MONO FAT	POLY FAT	OMEGA-3	OMEGA-6	SODIUM
1,374	77 g	218 g	20 g	78 mg	22 g	9 g	10.5 g	4.5 g	0.6 g	1.7 g	1,644 mg

% DAILY VALUE (WOMEN 31–50 YEARS) FOR:

VITAMIN A	VITAMIN C	FOLATE	CALCIUM
491%	311%	79%	14%

DAY 3

Breakfast

Smoothie: ½ banana, ½ cup frozen blueberries, ½ cup light vanilla ice cream, ½ cup vanilla soy milk, 1 tablespoon ground flaxseed

1 slice whole wheat toast with 1½ teaspoons light plant sterol–enriched margarine

*Synergy with soy protein, viscous fiber, and plant sterols lowers blood lipid levels.

Lunch

Turkey and avocado sandwich: 2 slices 100 percent whole wheat or whole grain bread; 2 teaspoons mustard; 3 ounces roasted turkey breast; ¼ avocado, sliced; sliced onion, tomato, and lettuce

Orange wedges

¼ cup bean salad made with light Italian dressing

¼ cup almonds

*Synergy with protein and fiber controls appetite.

*Synergy of three Bs (in meat and orange wedges) helps protect artery linings.

*Synergy with skin of almonds with vitamins C and E decreases oxidation of LDL.

Dinner

Spaghetti: 1 cup cooked whole wheat–blend pasta topped with ¾ cup meat sauce made with super-lean ground sirloin and marinara sauce

1 cup steamed or microsteamed broccoli or zucchini

*Synergy between protein from beef and fiber from pasta and broccoli controls appetite.

*Synergy between three Bs (in pasta and meat) helps protect artery linings.

*Synergy between broccoli and tomatoes protects against cancer.

Snack

Fruit and veggie plate: 1 cup apple slices (with skin), 2 stalks celery, 1 tablespoon natural peanut butter

1 cup green tea (hot or iced)

*Synergy between quercetin (apples) and catechin (green tea) helps keep platelets from clumping.

*Synergy between components in apple skin and flesh prevents oxidation of free radicals.

DAILY TOTAL

CALORIES	PROTEIN	CARB	FIBER	CHOLEST	TOTAL FAT	SAT FAT	MONO FAT	POLY FAT	OMEGA-3	OMEGA-6	SODIUM
1,458	73 g	220 g	39 g	110 mg	38 g	8 g	9 g	6 g	2 g	2.4 g	2,810 mg

% DAILY VALUE (WOMEN 31–50 YEARS) FOR:

VITAMIN A	VITAMIN C	FOLATE	CALCIUM
50%	193%	81%	61%

DAY 4

Breakfast

1 medium whole wheat bagel with 1 ounce light cream cheese and 1 ounce lox

8 ounces fresh orange juice (fortified with calcium and vitamin D)

*Synergy of the Bs (fish and orange juice) helps protect artery linings.

*Synergy between calcium and vitamin D decreases PMS symptoms.

*Synergy between whole grains and fruits protects against heart disease.

Lunch

1 barbecue chicken breast sandwich with barbecue sauce on whole grain bun (similar to Carl's Jr. menu item)

Side spinach salad topped with 2 tablespoons light ranch dressing

*Synergy of three Bs (from spinach and chicken) helps protect artery linings.

*Synergy between whole grains and vegetables protects against heart disease.

*Synergy between protein (chicken) and fiber (whole grain bun and spinach) controls appetite.

Dinner

Vegetarian stir-fry: ½ cup tofu, ½ cup snow peas, ½ cup julienned carrots, 2 teaspoons garlic stir-fried with 1 tablespoon canola oil and spices served over 1 cup cooked brown rice

1 pear, sliced or poached, sprinkled with cinnamon

Black or green tea (hot or iced)

*Synergy of good fat (from canola oil) increases absorption of the phytochemicals in veggies.

*Synergy between soy and tea prevents prostate cancer growth and spread to lymph nodes.

*Synergy of fruits and vegetables and whole grains protects against heart disease.

DAILY TOTAL

CALORIES	PROTEIN	CARB	FIBER	CHOLEST	TOTAL FAT	SAT FAT	MONO FAT	POLY FAT	OMEGA-3	OMEGA-6	SODIUM
1,440	74 g	171 g	27 g	85 mg	34 g	6 g	10 g	10.5 g	2 g	8 g	1,798 mg

% DAILY VALUE (WOMEN 31–50 YEARS) FOR:

VITAMIN A	VITAMIN C	FOLATE	CALCIUM
400%	232%	62%	52%

DAY 5

Breakfast

2 buttermilk wheat pancakes (or waffles) made with canola oil and omega-3 egg
  topped with 1 cup strawberry slices (or other berries) and ¼ cup fat-free frozen
  whipped topping

1 cup fat-free or low-fat milk (vitamin D fortified) as beverage or in latte

  *Synergy of fruits and whole grains protects against heart disease.

  *Synergy between calcium and vitamin D decreases PMS symptoms.

Lunch

Small/medium bean burrito at fast-food restaurant (such as Taco Bell)

2 cups melon in season

  *Synergy from protein and fiber in beans controls appetite.

Dinner

3 ounces broiled salmon (use spice rub or nonfat marinade)

1 cup steamed or microsteamed broccoli florets with ¼ cup marinara sauce

Garlic cheese bread: 2½" whole wheat roll halved and drizzled with 1 teaspoon
  olive oil blended with minced garlic (or pesto made with olive oil) and 1 ounce
  shredded low-fat mozzarella cheese

  *Synergy of three Bs (from salmon and broccoli) helps protect artery linings.

  *Synergy between broccoli and tomato decreases prostate tumor growth.

  *Good fat from olive oil and fish increases absorption of phytochemicals
   from vegetables.

  *Synergy from whole grains and vegetables helps protect against heart disease.

  *Synergy from vitamin D (from salmon) and calcium (from cheese) decreases
   PMS symptoms.

Snack

Veggies and dip: 1 cup assorted raw vegetables (such as sugar snap peas, jicama,
  carrot coins) served with 1 tablespoon light ranch dressing as dip

DAILY TOTAL

CALORIES	PROTEIN	CARB	FIBER	CHOLEST	TOTAL FAT	SAT FAT	MONO FAT	POLY FAT	OMEGA-3	OMEGA-6	SODIUM
1,455	73 g	186 g	33 g	108 mg	50 g	12.6 g	15 g	8 g	3.1 g	4.5 g	2,585 mg

% DAILY VALUE (WOMEN 31–50 YEARS) FOR:

VITAMIN A	VITAMIN C	FOLATE	CALCIUM
334%	357%	63%	114%

WEEK 2 | DAY 1

For this second week, I'm including the analysis per meal so you can feel free to mix and match or only use the meal ideas that appeal to you.

Breakfast

Cold cereal and fruit: 1 cup raisin bran with ½ cup vanilla soy milk and 1 sliced banana

Midmorning snack

1 cup light fruit-flavored yogurt with 1 tablespoon ground flaxseed

*Synergy of fruits and whole grains protects against heart disease.

*Synergy between calcium and vitamin D decreases PMS symptoms.

*Synergy with fiber and protein decreases postmeal appetite.

MEAL TOTAL

CALORIES	PROTEIN	CARB	FIBER	CHOLEST	TOTAL FAT	SAT FAT	MONO FAT	POLY FAT	OMEGA-3	OMEGA-6	SODIUM
542	22 g	103 g	16 g	3 mg	9 g	6 g	2 g	4 g	2.1 g	1.6 g	558 mg

% DAILY VALUE (WOMEN 31–50 YEARS) FOR:

VITAMIN A	VITAMIN C	FOLATE	CALCIUM	VITAMIN D	MAGNESIUM	POTASSIUM
49%	90%	92%	60%	51%	76%	63%

Lunch

Fruit and cheese plate: 2 ounces reduced-fat cheese (your choice) and 2 ounces low-fat whole wheat crackers

Fruit salad: 1 cup cantaloupe cubes and ½ cup blueberries

¼ cup nuts (analyzed with almonds)

1 cup green tea (unsweetened iced or hot)

*Synergy from protein and fiber controls appetite.

*Synergy exists between nuts and green tea phytochemicals (catechins in tea enhance antioxidant activity of vitamin E in nuts).

*Synergy exists between carotenoids in carotene-rich cantaloupe.

MEAL TOTAL

CALORIES	PROTEIN	CARB	FIBER	CHOLEST	TOTAL FAT	SAT FAT	MONO FAT	POLY FAT	OMEGA-3	OMEGA-6	SODIUM
587	27 g	54 g	12 g	40 mg	30 g	9 g	12 g	5 g	0.2 g	4.2 g	658 mg

% DAILY VALUE (WOMEN 31–50 YEARS) FOR:

VITAMIN A	VITAMIN C	FOLATE	CALCIUM	MAGNESIUM	POTASSIUM
119%	105%	12%	42%	6%	18%

Dinner

> Shrimp kebab: 4 ounces grilled shrimp on a kebab with 6 large mushrooms, ½ cup pineapple chunks, and 1 tablespoon teriyaki sauce served over ¾ cup cooked brown rice
>
> Spinach salad: 2 cups spinach leaves, ½ cup grated carrot, ½ cup sliced cucumber dressed with 2 tablespoons low-fat sesame ginger or light ranch dressing
>
> > *Synergy exists between fish omega-3s and plant omega-3s from spinach and dressing (if it contains canola oil).
> >
> > *Synergy exists with two antioxidants, carotenes (vitamin A) and vitamin C, from spinach and carrots.
> >
> > *Good fat from canola oil and fish increases absorption of phytochemicals from vegetables.
> >
> > *Synergy from whole grains and vegetables helps protect against heart disease.
> >
> > *Synergy with high-protein, high-fiber meal decreases postmeal appetite.

MEAL TOTAL

CALORIES	PROTEIN	CARB	FIBER	CHOLEST	TOTAL FAT	SAT FAT	MONO FAT	POLY FAT	OMEGA-3	OMEGA-6	SODIUM
485	36 g	65 g	10 g	229 mg	10.5 g	2 g	3 g	4 g	1.5 g	2.5 g	1,426 mg

% DAILY VALUE (WOMEN 31–50 YEARS) FOR:

DAILY TOTAL

VITAMIN A	VITAMIN C	FOLATE	CALCIUM	VITAMIN D	MAGNESIUM	POTASSIUM
303%	77%	18%	17%	134%	61%	39%

CALORIES
1,614

DAY 2

Breakfast

> Veggie scramble: 1 omega-3 egg and ¼ cup egg substitute or 2 egg whites scrambled with ½ cup broccoli florets, 1 medium tomato, ¼ cup reduced-fat sharp Cheddar cheese, and herbs and spices as desired
>
> 2 slices whole wheat bread with 2 teaspoons plant sterol–enriched margarine
>
> > *Synergy between broccoli and tomato helps reduce risk of cancer.
> >
> > *Synergy between calcium and vitamin D decreases PMS symptoms.
> >
> > *Synergy with fiber and protein decreases postmeal appetite.

MEAL TOTAL

CALORIES	PROTEIN	CARB	FIBER	CHOLEST	TOTAL FAT	SAT FAT	MONO FAT	POLY FAT	OMEGA-3	OMEGA-6	SODIUM
403	27 g	36 g	8 g	210 mg	17.5 g	6.7 g	4.1 g	4 g	0.4 g	3 g	743 mg

% DAILY VALUE (WOMEN 31–50 YEARS) FOR:

VITAMIN A	VITAMIN C	FOLATE	CALCIUM	VITAMIN D	MAGNESIUM	POTASSIUM
71%%	71%	33%	39%	46%	25%	19%

Lunch

Chicken stew: 1 cup broth; ½ cup diced potato; ½ cup boneless, skinless chicken breast; ½ cup sliced carrots; ¼ cup peas

1 sliced pear with 1 ounce reduced-fat cheese

Midafternoon snack/beverage

Iced or hot latte made with 1 cup fat-free milk

*Synergy from protein and fiber controls appetite.

*Synergy exists with mixture of carotenes in carrots.

*Synergy between minerals calcium, magnesium, and potassium lowers blood pressure.

*Synergy exists between calcium and vitamin D and from low-fat dairy.

MEAL TOTAL

CALORIES	PROTEIN	CARB	FIBER	CHOLEST	TOTAL FAT	SAT FAT	MONO FAT	POLY FAT	OMEGA-3	OMEGA-6	SODIUM
550	44 g	76 g	16 g	84 mg	9.5 g	4.7 g	1 g	1 g	0.2 g	0.7 g	1,075 mg

% DAILY VALUE (WOMEN 31–50 YEARS) FOR:

VITAMIN A	VITAMIN C	FOLATE	CALCIUM	VITAMIN D	MAGNESIUM	POTASSIUM
324%	41%	15%	58%	53%	23%	44%

Dinner

Fish tacos: 2 soft corn tortillas with ¼ cup green bell pepper and onions sautéed with 1 teaspoon canola oil, 4 ounces broiled halibut, 1 cup shredded cabbage, and 3 tablespoons salsa

1 cup grapefruit segments

*Synergy exists between fish omega-3s and plant omega-3s from canola oil.

*Synergy exists with citrus extracts and vitamin C in grapefruit.

*Good fat from canola oil and fish increases absorption of phytochemicals from the vegetables.

*Synergy with high-protein, high-fiber meal decreases postmeal appetite.

*Synergy exists with phytochemicals in cabbage-family vegetables.

MEAL TOTAL

CALORIES	PROTEIN	CARB	FIBER	CHOLEST	TOTAL FAT	SAT FAT	MONO FAT	POLY FAT	OMEGA-3	OMEGA-6	SODIUM
531 calories	38 g	64 g	10 g	46 mg	15.5 g	2 g	8 g	4 g	1.5 g	2.5 g	201 mg

% DAILY VALUE (WOMEN 31–50 YEARS) FOR:

VITAMIN A	VITAMIN C	FOLATE	CALCIUM	VITAMIN D	MAGNESIUM	POTASSIUM
19%	195%	44%	26%	23%	70%	51%

DAILY TOTAL

CALORIES
1,484

DAY 3

Breakfast

Three-grain waffle: 1 Three-Grain Buttermilk Waffle (page 259) served with
2 teaspoons plant sterol–enriched margarine and 1 tablespoon powdered sugar

8 ounces fresh orange juice

*Synergy between calcium and vitamin D decreases PMS symptoms.

*Synergy with fiber and protein decreases postmeal appetite.

*Synergy Super Foods include whole grains (whole wheat and oats), plant sterol–
enriched margarine, ground flaxseed, and citrus.

*Synergy exists with vitamin C and citrus extracts in juice.

MEAL TOTAL

CALORIES	PROTEIN	CARB	FIBER	CHOLEST	TOTAL FAT	SAT FAT	MONO FAT	POLY FAT	OMEGA-3	OMEGA-6	SODIUM
427	13 g	67 g	6 g	58 mg	12 g	1.7 g	4.5 g	5 g	1.5 g	1.6 g	500 mg

% DAILY VALUE (WOMEN 31–50 YEARS) FOR:

VITAMIN A	VITAMIN C	FOLATE	CALCIUM	VITAMIN D	MAGNESIUM	POTASSIUM
30%	170%	45%	15%	26%	30%	30%

Lunch

Potato salad: 1 cup whole wheat pasta tossed with ½ cup broccoli florets,
1 medium tomato, 5 green olives, and 2 tablespoons commercial pesto

1 large apple, sliced

*Synergy from protein and fiber controls appetite.

*Synergy with the mixture of phytochemicals in broccoli and tomato helps reduce
risk of cancer.

*Synergy between minerals calcium, magnesium, and potassium lowers blood pressure.

*Synergy exists with phytochemicals in apple flesh and peel.

*Synergy with smart fat in olives and pesto increases absorption of nutrients
in vegetables.

*Synergy exists from whole grains.

MEAL TOTAL

CALORIES	PROTEIN	CARB	FIBER	CHOLEST	TOTAL FAT	SAT FAT	MONO FAT	POLY FAT	OMEGA-3	OMEGA-6	SODIUM
452	13 g	79 g	13 g	5 mg	10 g	2.2 g	4 g	1.8 g	0.2 g	1.3 g	624 mg

% DAILY VALUE (WOMEN 31–50 YEARS) FOR:

VITAMIN A	VITAMIN C	FOLATE	CALCIUM	MAGNESIUM	POTASSIUM
49%	95%	14%	15%	25%	20%

Dinner

Turkey dinner: 2 ounces roasted turkey breast; ¾ cup mashed potatoes or mashed sweet potatoes topped with 1½ teaspoons plant sterol–enriched margarine; 1 cup steamed green beans

1 cup red grapes

1 cup fat-free milk (by itself or in a coffee drink)

*Synergy exists with the phytochemical in grapes–resveratrol.

*Synergy exists with low-fat dairy and with calcium and vitamin D in milk.

*Good fat from margarine and fish increases absorption of phytochemicals from vegetables.

*Synergy with high-protein, high-fiber meal decreases postmeal appetite.

MEAL TOTAL (INCLUDING MASHED WHITE POTATOES)

CALORIES	PROTEIN	CARB	FIBER	CHOLEST	TOTAL FAT	SAT FAT	MONO FAT	POLY FAT	OMEGA-3	OMEGA-6	SODIUM
559	40 g	78 g	9 g	73 mg	11.5 g	3.2 g	4 g	4 g	0.3 g	2 g	680 mg

% DAILY VALUE (WOMEN 31–50 YEARS) FOR:

VITAMIN A	VITAMIN C	FOLATE	CALCIUM	VITAMIN D	MAGNESIUM	POTASSIUM
33%	48%	6%	43%	78%	19%	49%

DAILY TOTAL

CALORIES
1,438

DAY 4

Breakfast

Muffin morning: 2 Apple Oat Muffins (page 244) and 2 teaspoons plant sterol–enriched margarine

Latte made with 1 cup fat-free or low-fat milk

*Synergy exists with phytochemicals in apple flesh and peel.

*Synergy exists with phytochemicals in oats.

*Synergy between calcium and vitamin D decreases PMS symptoms.

*Synergy with fiber and protein decreases postmeal appetite.

*Synergy Super Foods include whole grains, plant sterol–enriched margarine, and low-fat dairy.

MEAL TOTAL

CALORIES	PROTEIN	CARB	FIBER	CHOLEST	TOTAL FAT	SAT FAT	MONO FAT	POLY FAT	OMEGA-3	OMEGA-6	SODIUM
430	14 g	70 g	5 g	48 mg	11 g	3 g	3.3 g	4.5 g	0.3 g	3 g	484 mg

% DAILY VALUE (WOMEN 31–50 YEARS) FOR:

VITAMIN A	VITAMIN C	FOLATE	CALCIUM	VITAMIN D	MAGNESIUM	POTASSIUM
59%	9%	11%	36%	98%	19%	17%

Lunch

Deli roast beef sandwich: Arby's Junior Roast Beef Sandwich

Side salad: 2 cups romaine lettuce, ½ cup cherry tomatoes, ⅓ cup sliced cucumbers, 1 tablespoon olive oil vinaigrette

1 orange

¼ cup almonds

*Synergy exists with components in almonds.

*Synergy with protein in roast beef and fiber from salad, fruit, and nuts decreases the postmeal appetite.

*Synergy with smart fat from olive oil vinaigrette increases absorption of plant nutrients and phytochemicals.

MEAL TOTAL

CALORIES	PROTEIN	CARB	FIBER	CHOLEST	TOTAL FAT	SAT FAT	MONO FAT	POLY FAT	OMEGA-3	OMEGA-6	SODIUM
417	20 g	58 g	8 g	40 mg	15 g	5.4 g	5 g	2.6 g	0.2 g	1.6 g	842 mg

% DAILY VALUE (WOMEN 31–50 YEARS) FOR:

VITAMIN A	VITAMIN C	FOLATE	CALCIUM	MAGNESIUM	POTASSIUM
54%	127%	57%	16%	14%	30%

Dinner

Eggplant Parmesan: Grilled or broiled eggplant slices brushed with 2 teaspoons olive oil and layered with ½ cup marinara sauce, 1 ounce part-skim mozzarella cheese, and 2 tablespoons Parmesan cheese

1 cup broccoli florets, steamed or microcooked

1 whole wheat dinner roll

2 kiwifruit

10 stuffed olives (as appetizer)

*Synergy with tomatoes and broccoli helps reduce cancer risk.

*Good fat from canola oil and fish increases absorption of phytochemicals from vegetables.

*Synergy Super Foods include viscous fiber–rich eggplant, whole wheat roll, tomatoes, low-fat dairy, fruits, and dark green vegetables.

MEAL TOTAL

CALORIES	PROTEIN	CARB	FIBER	CHOLEST	TOTAL FAT	SAT FAT	MONO FAT	POLY FAT	OMEGA-3	OMEGA-6	SODIUM
550	21.5 g	68 g	17 g	22 mg	23 g	7 g	13 g	3 g	04 g	2.5 g	1,600 mg

% DAILY VALUE (WOMEN 31–50 YEARS) FOR:

VITAMIN A	VITAMIN C	FOLATE	CALCIUM	VITAMIN D	MAGNESIUM	POTASSIUM
61%	283%	24%	54%	2%	42%	36%

DAILY TOTAL

CALORIES
1,397

DAY 5

Breakfast

Strawberry French toast: 2 slices 100 percent whole grain bread dipped in 3 tablespoons omega-3 egg and 3 tablespoons egg substitute beaten with ground cinnamon, pure vanilla extract, and ¼ cup fat-free half-and-half; topped with 2 teaspoons plant sterol–enriched margarine, 2 teaspoons powdered sugar, and ⅔ cup sliced strawberries

*Synergy between calcium and vitamin D decreases PMS symptoms.

*Synergy with fiber and protein decreases postmeal appetite.

*Synergy exists between the beta-carotene and vitamin C from strawberries.

*Synergy Super Foods include whole grains, plant sterol–enriched margarine, and high-antioxidant strawberries.

MEAL TOTAL

CALORIES	PROTEIN	CARB	FIBER	CHOLEST	TOTAL FAT	SAT FAT	MONO FAT	POLY FAT	OMEGA-3	OMEGA-6	SODIUM
351	20 g	47 g	7 g	162 mg	10 g	2.2 g	3.5 g	3.3 g	0.4 g	2 g	743 mg

% DAILY VALUE (WOMEN 31–50 YEARS) FOR:

VITAMIN A	VITAMIN C	FOLATE	CALCIUM	VITAMIN D	MAGNESIUM	POTASSIUM
45%	85%	22%	28%	67%	25%	19%

Lunch

Peanut butter and jelly bag lunch: 1 (4½") whole grain bagel filled with 2 tablespoons natural peanut butter and 1 tablespoon reduced-sugar jam or jelly

Fruit salad: ¾ cup mango and ¾ cup watermelon

Midafternoon snack/beverage

Iced or hot latte made with 1 cup fat-free milk

*Synergy from protein and fiber controls appetite.

*Synergy exists with mixture of carotenes in mango and phytochemicals in watermelon.

*Synergy exists between calcium and vitamin D and synergy from low-fat dairy.

*Synergy exists with fiber and phytochemicals in nuts.

*Synergy Super Foods include whole grains, nuts, mango, and fat-free dairy.

MEAL TOTAL

CALORIES	PROTEIN	CARB	FIBER	CHOLEST	TOTAL FAT	SAT FAT	MONO FAT	POLY FAT	OMEGA-3	OMEGA-6	SODIUM
744	30.5 g	121 g	16 g	5 mg	15.5 g	3 g	6 g	3 g	0.3 g	2.3 g	871 mg

% DAILY VALUE (WOMEN 31–50 YEARS) FOR:

VITAMIN A	VITAMIN C	FOLATE	CALCIUM	MAGNESIUM	POTASSIUM
89%	71%	22%	36%	45%	36%

Dinner

Time for chili: Chunky chili made with 1 cup chunky canned tomatoes, ½ cup kidney beans, 3 ounces cooked extra-lean ground beef, ¼ cup onion, and 2 teaspoons garlic sautéed in 1 teaspoon olive or canola oil

1 cup steamed or microcooked zucchini

*Synergy between plant omega-3s from oil and beans increases absorption of nutrients in tomatoes and vegetables.

*Synergy with high-protein, high-fiber meal decreases postmeal appetite.

*Synergy with phytochemicals in garlic and onions helps prevent LDL oxidation.

MEAL TOTAL

CALORIES	PROTEIN	CARB	FIBER	CHOLEST	TOTAL FAT	SAT FAT	MONO FAT	POLY FAT	OMEGA-3	OMEGA-6	SODIUM
508	38 g	58 g	19 g	41 mg	15.5 g	4.8 g	8.1 g	1.5 g	0.4 g	0.8 g	1,430 mg

% DAILY VALUE (WOMEN 31–50 YEARS) FOR:

VITAMIN A	VITAMIN C	FOLATE	CALCIUM	VITAMIN D	MAGNESIUM	POTASSIUM
23%	52%	37%	10%	7%	39%	27%

DAILY TOTAL:

CALORIES
1,603

HIGH-SYNERGY SNACK OPTIONS

Snack 1

¼ cup each almonds (roasted whole natural) and dried apricots

SNACK TOTAL

CALORIES	PROTEIN	CARB	FIBER	CHOLEST	TOTAL FAT	SAT FAT	MONO FAT	POLY FAT	OMEGA-3	OMEGA-6	SODIUM
319	9 g	32 g	6.5 g	0 mg	18 g	1.2 g	11 g	4 g	0 g	4 g	1 mg

% DAILY VALUE (WOMEN 31–50 YEARS) FOR:

VITAMIN A	VITAMIN C	FOLATE	CALCIUM	MAGNESIUM	POTASSIUM
4%	9%	4%	11%	31%	22%

Snack 2

20 small stuffed green olives

SNACK TOTAL

CALORIES	PROTEIN	CARB	FIBER	CHOLEST	TOTAL FAT	SAT FAT	MONO FAT	POLY FAT	OMEGA-3	OMEGA-6	SODIUM
82	1 g	2 g	1 g	0 mg	8.8 g	1.2 g	6.4 g	0.8 g	0.1 g	0.7 g	1,600 mg

% DAILY VALUE (WOMEN 31–50 YEARS) FOR:

VITAMIN A	VITAMIN C	CALCIUM	MAGNESIUM	POTASSIUM
8%	12%	4%	4%	2%

Snack 3

1 cup light fruit-flavored yogurt with 1 tablespoon ground flaxseed and ¼ cup frozen unsweetened berries (or fresh)

MEAL TOTAL

CALORIES	PROTEIN	CARB	FIBER	CHOLEST	TOTAL FAT	SAT FAT	MONO FAT	POLY FAT	OMEGA-3	OMEGA-6	SODIUM
217	14 g	30 g	6.2 g	3 mg	5.5 g	0.2 g	1.1 g	3.1 g	2.1 g	1 g	151 mg

% DAILY VALUE (WOMEN 31–50 YEARS) FOR:

VITAMIN A	VITAMIN C	FOLATE	CALCIUM	VITAMIN D	MAGNESIUM	POTASSIUM
9%	81%	59%	42%	1% (if yogurt not fortified with vitamin D)	38%	37%

Snack 4

Veggie bowl: ½ cup shelled edamame (green soybeans), ½ cup cauliflower florets, 1½ teaspoons plant sterol–enriched margarine

SNACK TOTAL

CALORIES	PROTEIN	CARB	FIBER	CHOLEST	TOTAL FAT	SAT FAT	MONO FAT	POLY FAT	OMEGA-3	OMEGA-6	SODIUM
163	12 g	12 g	5 g	0 mg	8.4 g	1 g	1.9 g	4.2 g	0.5 g	2.5 g	237 mg

% DAILY VALUE (WOMEN 31–50 YEARS) FOR:

VITAMIN A	VITAMIN C	FOLATE	CALCIUM	VITAMIN D	MAGNESIUM	POTASSIUM
15%	36%	25%	13%	17%	17%	14%

Snack 5

Got fat-free milk? 1 cup fat-free milk (as is or in a latte, iced or hot)

SNACK TOTAL

CALORIES	PROTEIN	CARB	FIBER	CHOLEST	TOTAL FAT	SAT FAT	MONO FAT	POLY FAT	OMEGA-3	OMEGA-6	SODIUM
100	10 g	15 g	0 g	5 mg	0 g	0 g	0 g	0 g	0 g	0 g	150 mg

% DAILY VALUE (WOMEN 31–50 YEARS) FOR:

VITAMIN A	CALCIUM	VITAMIN D	POTASSIUM
14%	30%	49% (if milk fortified with vitamin D)	13%

Chapter 8

Food Synergy Recipes

This collection of recipes incorporates many of the food combinations we've discussed in earlier chapters. Look for the synergy notes to see what benefits each dish provides. But, as if great nutrition were not enough, I guarantee your family will become hooked on these dishes from the first bite. Enjoy!

Breakfasts, Baked Goods, and Sweet Treats

EDAMAME-SPINACH SCRAMBLE

Don't let the list of ingredients scare you—this is easy to whip up and very filling. If you're cooking for two, just double the ingredients and use a large frying pan.

FOOD SYNERGY NOTES | *You'll find three whole foods with synergy: soy edamame, vegetables, and dairy, along with the phytochemicals in garlic and onions. There's also synergy between the smart fat from the olive oil and the nutrients in the vegetables.*

Makes 1 main-dish or 2 side-dish servings

1	large egg (omega-3, if available)
2	egg whites or ¼ cup egg substitute
1	tablespoon fat-free half-and-half or any type of milk
1	teaspoon olive or canola oil
1½	cups fresh raw spinach leaves, loosely packed
⅓	cup shelled edamame, frozen or thawed
⅛	cup finely chopped red bell pepper
⅛	cup finely chopped sweet or yellow onion
1	teaspoon minced garlic
	Salt and pepper
⅓	cup shredded grated cheese of choice, such as Cheddar or Swiss
1	medium tomato or 1½ roma tomatoes, chopped
2	teaspoons fresh herbs, such as chopped parsley or basil (optional)

PER SERVING (MAIN DISH):

CALORIES	FAT CAL	PROTEIN	CARB	FIBER	CHOLEST	TOTAL FAT	SAT FAT	MONO FAT	POLY FAT	OMEGA-3	OMEGA-6	SODIUM
389	41%	34 g	23 g	6.5 g	215 mg	17 g	6.8 g	6.5 g	3.2 g	0.5 g	2.6 g	469 mg

In a large measuring cup, combine the egg and egg whites or substitute and half-and-half or milk and whisk until smooth. Set aside.

Add the oil to a medium nonstick skillet with a lid and heat over medium-high heat. Add the spinach, edamame, bell pepper, onion, and garlic and cook, stirring constantly, for 2 to 3 minutes or until the spinach shrinks down and onion is lightly brown. Season to taste with salt and pepper.

Pour in the reserved egg mixture and reduce the heat to medium. Continue to gently stir and cook until the eggs are soft and cooked throughout.

Turn off the heat and sprinkle the cheese over the top. Top with the tomato and cover the pan. Let sit for a couple of minutes to melt the cheese. Sprinkle the herbs over the top, if desired.

% DAILY VALUE FOR:

VIT A	VIT C	VIT E	VIT B$_1$	VIT B$_2$	VIT B$_3$	VIT B$_6$	VIT B$_{12}$	FOLATE	CAL	MAG	POT	SELEN	ZINC
102%	113%	23%	30%	124%	15%	40%	48%	59%	47%	30%	32%	33%	27%

BREAKFAST PANINI WITH ROASTED RED PEPPER SPREAD

If you can find whole grain ciabatta rolls, they are the perfect bread for this recipe.

FOOD SYNERGY NOTES | *Red pepper and spinach are both rich in carotenoids (and antioxidant vitamins), and this sandwich has plenty of them. Using whole grain bread will also provide whole grain synergy. And using omega-3 eggs will add to the smart fat (omega-3s) also in spinach.*

Makes 2 servings

½ cup light cream cheese

¾ cup roasted red peppers

½ teaspoon minced fresh garlic

1 teaspoon balsamic vinegar

Pinch ground red pepper

2 ciabatta rolls or 4 slices whole wheat bread

2 large eggs (omega-3, if available)

½ cup egg substitute

1 tablespoon fat-free half-and-half

2 cups fresh spinach leaves, loosely packed and rinsed

Pinch or two of seasoning blend (any desired flavor)

½ cup shredded reduced-fat Swiss cheese or ¼ cup regular Swiss

2–3 strips turkey bacon, cooked until crisp and broken into bits

PER SERVING:

CALORIES	FAT CAL	PROTEIN	CARB	FIBER	CHOLEST	TOTAL FAT	SAT FAT	MONO FAT	POLY FAT	OMEGA-3	OMEGA-6	SODIUM
420	32%	31 g	31 g	6 g	239 mg	15 g	5.5 g	5 g	2 g	0.2 g	1.8 g	896 mg

Place the cream cheese, roasted peppers, garlic, vinegar, and ground red pepper in a small food processor and pulse until completely blended. (If you only have a large food processor, it will work better if you double the recipe for the spread.) Spread the bottom part of each roll or the bottom slice of each sandwich with 1½ tablespoons of the roasted red pepper spread.

In a mixing bowl, combine the eggs, egg substitute, and half-and-half and beat or whisk until nicely blended.

Heat a large nonstick skillet over medium heat, coat generously with canola-oil cooking spray, and add the spinach. Cook, stirring often, for 1 minute, or until the leaves soften nicely. Add a pinch or two of the seasoning blend, if desired.

Pour in the egg mixture and continue to cook and gently stir until the eggs are cooked throughout. Turn off the heat, sprinkle the cheese over the top, and cover with a lid. Let sit for 1 minute.

Sprinkle the turkey bacon over the top of the egg mixture. Remove half of the egg mixture and position it on top of the red pepper spread on the roll half or bread. Top with the remaining roll or bread and serve. Leftover spread can be kept in the refrigerator in a covered dish and used as a dip for veggies or as a spread for other sandwiches.

% DAILY VALUE FOR:

VIT A	VIT C	VIT E	VIT B₁	VIT B₂	VIT B₃	VIT B₆	VIT B₁₂	FOLATE	CAL	MAG	POT	SELEN	ZINC
120%	53%	17%	20%	127%	17%	34%	46%	22%	44%	25%	14%	66%	50%

BREAKFAST SAUSAGE CASSEROLE

Serve this lacto-ovo-vegetarian dish with fresh fruit to bring down the percentage of calories from fat for the meal. Almost every breakfast food group is represented in this recipe. The only thing missing is that fruit plus a cup of coffee.

FOOD SYNERGY NOTES | *A great vegetarian option to a traditional high-fat sausage breakfast, this dish offers some soy and whole grain synergy along with low-fat dairy servings and omega-3s (from the eggs).*

Makes 6 servings

12	ounces soy sausage
4½	cups whole wheat or whole grain bread cubes (toast 6 large slices and cut into ¾" squares)
2	cups (8 ounces) shredded reduced-fat sharp Cheddar or soy Cheddar cheese
1	teaspoon poultry seasoning
1	teaspoon mustard powder
½	teaspoon salt (optional)
2	large eggs (omega-3, if available)
½	cup egg substitute or 4 egg whites
2	cups fat-free half-and-half or low-fat milk

Coat a 13" × 9" baking dish with canola-oil cooking spray and set aside.

In a medium nonstick skillet, cook the sausage over medium heat until nicely brown. Transfer to a large bowl and add the bread cubes, cheese, poultry seasoning, and mustard powder, and salt, if desired.

PER SERVING:

CALORIES	FAT CAL	PROTEIN	CARB	FIBER	CHOLEST	TOTAL FAT	SAT FAT	MONO FAT	POLY FAT	OMEGA-3	OMEGA-6	SODIUM
379	40%	29 g	30 g	9 g	31 mg	14 g	7 g	3 g	4 g	1 g	3 g	464 mg

In a mixing bowl, combine the eggs and egg substitute or egg whites and half-and-half or milk and beat on medium-low speed until smooth and completely blended. Drizzle over the sausage-and-bread mixture and stir to blend. Pour into the prepared baking dish, spread evenly, cover with foil, and chill in the refrigerator for 8 hours or overnight.

Preheat the oven to 350°F.

Bake, covered in foil, for 45 minutes. Remove the foil. Reduce the temperature to 325°F and bake for about 20 minutes more (or until set).

% DAILY VALUE FOR:

VIT A	VIT C	VIT E	VIT B$_1$	VIT B$_2$	VIT B$_3$	VIT B$_6$	VIT B$_{12}$	FOLATE	CAL	MAG	POT	SELEN	ZINC
36%	1%	8%	93%	90%	37%	31%	25%	9%	57%	12%	14%	18%	41%

VEGETARIAN SAUSAGE-AND-SAGE GRAVY

Use this gravy for all sorts of recipes, from a vegetarian shepherd's pie to a vegetarian casserole or potpie.

FOOD SYNERGY NOTES | *Who said gravy can't be nutritious? This particular gravy features the synergy in soy plus the plant omega-3s from canola oil.*

Makes 4 servings (1¼ cups)

4 vegetarian sausage links or patties (about 3 ounces)	¼ teaspoon salt (optional)
	Freshly ground black pepper to taste
1 tablespoon canola oil	
2 tablespoons Wondra quick-mixing flour or all-purpose flour	¼–½ teaspoon dried ground sage
1 cup vegetable broth	

In a large nonstick skillet, fry the sausage in the oil until done, crumbling it into small pieces as it cooks.

In a small nonstick saucepan, mix together the flour and ¼ cup of the broth to make a paste. Slowly whisk in the remaining ¾ cup broth.

Whisk in the salt (if desired), pepper, sage, and cooked sausage. Bring to a simmer and stir for 2 minutes, or until the mixture thickens.

PER SERVING:

CALORIES	FAT CAL	PROTEIN	CARB	FIBER	CHOLEST	TOTAL FAT	SAT FAT	MONO FAT	POLY FAT	OMEGA-3	OMEGA-6	SODIUM
93	48%	5 g	6 g	2 g	0 mg	5 g	0.5 g	2 g	3 g	0.6 g	2.4 g	410 mg

% DAILY VALUE FOR:

VIT A	VIT E	VIT B₁	VIT B₂	VIT B₃	VIT B₆	FOLATE	CAL	MAG	POT	SELEN	ZINC
11%	8%	47%	9%	18%	14%	3%	2%	2%	1%	3%	4%

EASY SWEET POTATO HARVEST ROLLS

Two 16-ounce cans of sweet potatoes will give you what you need in this recipe. These rolls taste great up to 2 days later, warmed up or cut in half and toasted.

These moist and irresistible rolls feature the synergy between whole grains and antioxidant-rich foods by using whole wheat flour along with the antioxidant powerhouse—sweet potatoes.

FOOD SYNERGY NOTES

Makes 18

1½ cups mashed sweet potatoes	¼ cup egg substitute
½ cup fat-free half-and-half or low-fat milk	1¾ cups unbleached all-purpose flour
2 tablespoons canola oil	1½ cups whole wheat flour
2 tablespoons reduced-calorie pancake syrup	1 teaspoon salt
1 large egg (omega-3, if available), lightly beaten	¼–½ teaspoon pumpkin pie spice
	2¼ teaspoons active dry or bread machine yeast

Place the ingredients in the order listed here into a bread machine pan, making a well in the center of the flours to put the yeast. Set the bread machine to the dough cycle (about 1 hour 40 minutes) and press start.

Lightly coat two jelly-roll pans with canola-oil cooking spray. When the dough is ready, turn it out onto a lightly floured surface. Cut into 6 equal pieces, then cut each of these pieces into 3 pieces. Place (shape into balls if desired) on the prepared pans. Cover and let rise about 1 hour, or until the pieces double in size. About midway through the rising, preheat the oven to 375°F.

Bake for 12 to 18 minutes, or until golden brown. Serve warm.

PER ROLL:

CALORIES	FAT CAL	PROTEIN	CARB	FIBER	CHOLEST	TOTAL FAT	SAT FAT	MONO FAT	POLY FAT	OMEGA-3	OMEGA-6	SODIUM
131	16%	5 g	24 g	2 g	12 mg	2.3 g	0.3 g	1.1 g	0.7 g	0.2 g	0.5 g	167 mg

% DAILY VALUE FOR:

VIT A	VIT C	VIT E	VIT B₁	VIT B₂	VIT B₃	VIT B₆	VIT B₁₂	FOLATE	CAL	MAG	POT	SELEN	ZINC
48%	2%	3%	10%	16%	11%	8%	3%	6%	3%	7%	4%	17%	7%

LEMON-ROSEMARY ROLLS

This recipe was inspired by a recent trip to my local farmer's market, where I bought rosemary bread from a baker and lemon-flavored olive oil from another vendor. After I returned home, my whole family starting tearing the bread into pieces and dipping them in the olive oil. My taste buds were singing the "Hallelujah Chorus." That's the exact moment I realized lemon and rosemary are a match made in heaven.

FOOD SYNERGY NOTES *There is synergy within the components in flaxseed and within the whole wheat flour and olive oil.*

Makes 10

1	large egg (omega-3, if available), lightly beaten	1½	cups unbleached all-purpose flour
1	cup + 1 tablespoon low-fat buttermilk	1½	teaspoons salt
1	tablespoon olive oil	1½	tablespoons finely chopped lemon peel
¼	cup honey	1½	tablespoons finely chopped fresh rosemary
1½	cup whole wheat flour	3	teaspoons rapid-rise yeast or bread-machine yeast
¼	cup ground flaxseed		

Add all the ingredients to a bread machine pan in the order recommended by the manufacturer. (Usually, the yeast is added last.)

Set the bread machine to the dough cycle (usually 1 hour 40 minutes) and press start.

Coat a jelly-roll pan with canola-oil cooking spray.

When the cycle is over, remove the dough from the bread machine and divide it in half. Form each half into 5 rolls and place them on the prepared pan. Cover with plastic wrap coated with canola-oil cooking spray so it doesn't

PER ROLL:

CALORIES	FAT CAL	PROTEIN	CARB	FIBER	CHOLEST	TOTAL FAT	SAT FAT	MONO FAT	POLY FAT	OMEGA-3	OMEGA-6	SODIUM
184	19%	7 g	32 g	4 g	22 mg	3.8 g	0.7 g	1.7 g	1.1 g	0.6 g	0.5 g	386 mg

stick to the dough. Place in the refrigerator to rise overnight, or let rise in a warm place until doubled in size.

Preheat the oven to 350°F.

Bake the rolls for 20 to 25 minutes, or until golden brown.

IF YOU DON'T HAVE A BREAD MACHINE:

Place ¼ cup of the buttermilk in a small microwaveable bowl and heat in the microwave so it's warm to the touch but not too hot.

Using a fork, stir in 1 tablespoon of the honey and the yeast and set aside for 10 minutes in a warm place to proof (get bubbly).

In a mixing bowl, by hand or with an electric mixer, combine the egg, oil, remaining honey and buttermilk, and the reserved yeast mixture. Stir in the lemon peel and rosemary.

In a medium bowl, stir together the flours, flaxseed, and salt. Slowly beat or stir into the buttermilk mixture until completely combined. On a lightly floured flat surface, knead the dough for 10 minutes, or until elastic. Place in a lightly oiled bowl, cover with plastic wrap, and let rise in a warm place for 1 hour, or until doubled in size.

Coat a jelly-roll pan with canola-oil cooking spray.

Punch down the dough and divide it in half. Form 5 rolls out of each half and place them on the prepared pan. Cover with plastic wrap coated with canola-oil cooking spray so it doesn't stick to the dough. Place in the refrigerator to rise overnight, or let rise in a warm place until doubled in size.

Preheat the oven to 350°F.

Bake the rolls for 20 to 25 minutes, or until golden brown.

% DAILY VALUE FOR:

VIT A	VIT C	VIT E	VIT B$_1$	VIT B$_2$	VIT B$_3$	VIT B$_6$	VIT B$_{12}$	FOLATE	CAL	VIT D	MAG	POT	SELEN	ZINC
4%	16%	3%	24%	45%	42%	32%	52%	37%	6%	1%	20%	13%	38%	40%

APPLE OAT MUFFINS

FOOD SYNERGY NOTES *In this delicious muffin, you get two of the items from the PortfolioEatingPlan (plant sterol–enriched margarine and oats). You also get plenty of two whole foods with synergy: apples with skin and whole wheat flour.*

Makes 12

TOPPING

¼	cup brown sugar
¼	cup unbleached all-purpose flour
	Pinch of salt
⅛	teaspoon ground cinnamon

2	tablespoons light plant sterol–enriched margarine
2–3	tablespoons oats

MUFFINS

2	tablespoons light plant sterol–enriched margarine
½	cup sugar or sugar blend with Splenda or Equal
2	teaspoons pure vanilla extract
1	large egg (omega-3, if available)
½	cup unbleached all-purpose flour
½	cup whole wheat flour
½	teaspoon baking powder

½	teaspoon baking soda
½	teaspoon salt
¼	cup fat-free sour cream
2	tablespoons buttermilk (or stir ¼ teaspoon vinegar into 2 tablespoons fat-free half-and-half and let stand)
2	apples, cored and diced (about 1½ cups)

Preheat the oven to 375°F. Line the cups of a muffin pan with paper or foil liners.

To make the topping: In a large mixing bowl fitted with the paddle attachment, combine the sugar, flour, salt, and cinnamon and beat briefly to blend. Add the margarine and beat on low until a crumb mixture forms. Work the oats in with your hands, pour into a small bowl, and set aside.

PER SERVING:

CALORIES	FAT CAL	PROTEIN	CARB	FIBER	CHOLEST	TOTAL FAT	SAT FAT	MONO FAT	POLY FAT	OMEGA-3	OMEGA-6	SODIUM
148	15%	6 g	29 g	2.5 g	19 mg	2.5 g	0.4 g	0.8 g	1.2 g	0.2 g	1 g	180 mg

To make the muffins: Return the mixing bowl to the mixer and add the margarine, sugar or sugar blend, and vanilla extract and beat until light and fluffy. Add the egg and beat to combine, scraping the sides of the bowl.

In a large measuring cup, combine the flours, baking powder, baking soda, and salt and whisk to blend. Add all at once to the mixing bowl along with the sour cream and buttermilk. Beat on low speed just until blended, scraping down the sides of the bowl after 5 seconds. Stir in the apples.

Spoon a slightly heaping ⅛ cup of batter into each muffin cup. Sprinkle the reserved topping evenly over the top of each muffin. Bake for 20 minutes, or until the muffins are lightly browned and the tops spring back after being pushed.

% DAILY VALUE FOR:

VIT A	VIT C	VIT E	VIT B$_1$	VIT B$_2$	VIT B$_3$	VIT B$_6$	VIT B$_{12}$	FOLATE	CAL	MAG	POT	SELEN	ZINC
11%	3%	4%	7%	7%	5%	3%	3%	4%	3%	4%	3%	9%	3%

STRAWBERRY-ORANGE SPREAD

This spread tastes so fresh and amazing! I love it on whole wheat toast or toasted whole grain bagels.

FOOD SYNERGY NOTES | *This spread contributes a little bit of synergy from the strawberries and citrus.*

Makes 6 servings (1½ cups)

8 ounces (1 block) light cream cheese	½ teaspoon pure vanilla extract
2 tablespoons sugar	⅔ cup diced strawberries
2 tablespoons Splenda (optional)	1½ teaspoons orange peel

In a food processor, place the cream cheese, sugar, Splenda (if using), vanilla extract, strawberries, and orange zest and pulse to combine. Scrape down the sides of the bowl and break up any chunks of cream cheese. Pulse again for 5 seconds, or until smooth.

Cover and store in the refrigerator until needed. Serve within 24 hours.

PER SERVING:

CALORIES	FAT CAL	PROTEIN	CARB	FIBER	CHOLEST	TOTAL FAT	SAT FAT	MONO FAT	POLY FAT	OMEGA-3	OMEGA-6	SODIUM
107	45%	4 g	8.5 g	1 g	18 mg	5.5 g	4 g	0.8 g	0.7 g	0 g	0 g	177 mg

% DAILY VALUE FOR:

VIT A	VIT C	VIT B₁	VIT B₂	VIT B₆	FOLATE	CAL	MAG	POT
14%	20%	1%	5%	1%	1%	5%	1%	3%

VANILLA-CHERRY-ALMOND GRANOLA

This granola may be more satisfying than your typical breakfast cereal because it's got some fat (mostly from the nuts), dried fruit, and a nice fiber boost from the oats and ground flaxseed. Enjoy this granola as a cold cereal with low-fat milk or as a topping for fruit salad, yogurt, or fruit parfaits.

This recipe maximizes the synergy power of whole grains along with beneficial fats by pairing oats with not one but two types of seeds and one of the most nutritious nuts to boot—almonds!

FOOD SYNERGY NOTES

Makes 18 servings (9 cups)

4½	cups uncooked old-fashioned oats
1½	cups almonds
1	cup unsalted sunflower seeds (optional)
1	cup ground flaxseed
1	teaspoon ground cinnamon
¾	teaspoon ground nutmeg

¾	teaspoon ground allspice
4	tablespoons molasses
4	tablespoons canola oil
3	tablespoons honey
2	tablespoons apple juice
5	teaspoons pure vanilla extract
2	cups dried cherries

Preheat the oven to 300°F.

In a medium roasting pan or 13" × 9" baking pan, combine the oats, almonds, sunflower seeds (if using), flaxseed, cinnamon, nutmeg, and allspice. In a 2-cup measuring cup, combine the molasses, oil, honey, apple juice, and vanilla extract and stir together well. Drizzle over the dry mixture in the pan and stir to coat the dry mixture evenly with the honey mixture.

Bake for 40 minutes, stirring occasionally. When completely cooled, stir in the dried cherries. Store in a large zip-top bag or sealed container.

PER ½ CUP:

CALORIES	FAT CAL	PROTEIN	CARB	FIBER	CHOLEST	TOTAL FAT	SAT FAT	MONO FAT	POLY FAT	OMEGA-3	OMEGA-6	SODIUM
250	39%	9 g	32 g	6 g	0 mg	11 g	1.2 g	6 g	6.3 g	2 g	4 g	4 mg

% DAILY VALUE FOR:

VIT A	VIT E	VIT B₁	VIT B₂	VIT B₃	VIT B₆	VIT B₁₂	FOLATE	CAL	MAG	POT	SELEN	ZINC
1%	42%	15%	17%	11%	11%	1%	6%	10%	29%	10%	22%	17%

ORANGE-CRANBERRY OATMEAL

FOOD
SYNERGY
NOTES *Oats help lower blood sugar, blood pressure, and serum cholesterol. It's hard to argue with that! This dish also offers the synergy of citrus (vitamin C plus citrus extracts), some low-fat dairy (calcium and vitamin D), and a hint of nuts.*

Makes 2 servings

1½	cups orange juice	2	tablespoons dried cranberries
¼	teaspoon ground cinnamon	2	tablespoons toasted pecan pieces
⅛	teaspoon salt (optional)		
¾	cups quick oats (uncooked)	¼	cup fat-free half-and-half or low-fat milk (optional)

In a small nonstick saucepan, bring the orange juice, cinnamon, and salt (if using) to a boil. Stir in the oats and cranberries.

Return to a boil, then reduce the heat to medium. Cook, stirring occasionally, for 1 minute longer, or until most of the juice is absorbed.

Spoon into two bowls and sprinkle each serving with 1 tablespoon of the nuts and a couple tablespoons of the half-and-half or milk, if desired.

PER SERVING:

CALORIES	FAT CAL	PROTEIN	CARB	FIBER	CHOLEST	TOTAL FAT	SAT FAT	MONO FAT	POLY FAT	OMEGA-3	OMEGA-6	SODIUM
275	24%	7 g	45 g	4.5 g	0 mg	7 g	0.8 g	4 g	2 g	0.1 g	1.5 g	3 mg

% DAILY VALUE FOR:

VIT A	VIT C	VIT E	VIT B₁	VIT B₂	VIT B₃	VIT B₆	FOLATE	CAL	MAG	POT	ZINC
6%	124%	2%	30%	9%	7%	8%	16%	4%	19%	14%	13%

BLUEBERRY-VANILLA-WALNUT ALMOST-INSTANT OATMEAL

I know how convenient it is to have those instant oatmeal packets around, so here's a recipe that transforms a packet of instant oatmeal into blueberry bliss.

Oats help lower blood sugar, blood pressure, and serum cholesterol. With every serving you also get the synergy of soy, and a scoop of blueberries gives you some berry synergy. If you want to have the synergy of flaxseed and soy, just stir in a tablespoon of ground flaxseed.

FOOD SYNERGY NOTES

Makes 1 serving

1	packet plain instant oatmeal or any compatible flavor, such as Quaker Instant Oatmeal Nutrition for Women Vanilla Cinnamon
¼	teaspoon pure vanilla extract
⅔	cup vanilla soy milk or low-fat milk

¼	cup frozen blueberries or 2 tablespoons dried
1	tablespoon toasted walnut pieces

Empty the oatmeal packet into a microwave-safe breakfast bowl. In a small bowl, combine the vanilla extract and milk, then add to the oatmeal and stir. (If using vanilla-flavored oatmeal, add the milk only.) Microwave on high for 1 to 2 minutes. Gently stir in the blueberries and top with a sprinkling of the walnuts.

PER SERVING:

CALORIES	FAT CAL	PROTEIN	CARB	FIBER	CHOLEST	TOTAL FAT	SAT FAT	MONO FAT	POLY FAT	OMEGA-3	OMEGA-6	SODIUM
238	32%	11 g	30 g	5 g	0 mg	8.5 g	0.6 g	2 g	3.7 g	0.4 g	3.3 g	349 mg

% DAILY VALUE FOR:

VIT A	VIT C	VIT E	VIT B₁	VIT B₂	VIT B₃	VIT B₆	VIT B₁₂	FOLATE	CAL	MAG	POT	SELEN	ZINC
75%	2%	5%	51%	59%	41%	62%	84%	30%	37%	19%	10%	29%	20%

LEMON-BLUEBERRY BUTTERMILK PANCAKES

FOOD SYNERGY NOTES | *This recipe features the synergy between vitamin C and a phytoestrogen in whole grains, working together to inhibit the oxidation of LDL cholesterol.*

Makes 6 servings

1	cup whole wheat flour
1	cup unbleached all-purpose flour
2	teaspoons baking powder
1	teaspoon baking soda
½	teaspoon salt
2	tablespoons sugar
1	large egg (omega-3, if available), lightly beaten
¼	cup egg substitute
2	cups buttermilk
2	tablespoons canola oil
¼	cup reduced-calorie pancake syrup
1	teaspoon pure vanilla extract or vanilla powder
1	tablespoon finely grated lemon peel
1½	cups small blueberries, fresh or frozen
12	tablespoons light whipped topping or light whipping cream (optional)

In a medium bowl, place the flours, baking powder, baking soda, salt, and sugar and blend with a whisk.

In a mixing bowl, place the egg, egg substitute, buttermilk, oil, syrup, vanilla extract or powder, and lemon peel and beat on medium speed until smooth. Add the flour mixture and beat on medium-low speed just until smooth (scrape the sides after a few seconds). Do not overmix. Let the batter rest for 10 minutes.

PER SERVING (NOT INCLUDING LIGHT WHIPPING CREAM):

CALORIES	FAT CAL	PROTEIN	CARB	FIBER	CHOLEST	TOTAL FAT	SAT FAT	MONO FAT	POLY FAT	OMEGA-3	OMEGA-6	SODIUM
285	22%	10 g	48 g	4.2 g	38 mg	6.5 g	1 g	3.3 g	1.8 g	0.5 g	1.2 g	520 mg

Preheat a nonstick skillet or griddle over medium heat until water skittles. Gently stir in the blueberries.

Pour the batter by ¼-cupfuls onto the hot griddle. Cook over medium heat for 30 to 60 seconds, or until bubbles form on top of the pancakes. Turn over with a spatula and cook another 30 to 60 seconds, or until the pancakes are golden brown. Repeat this step until all the batter is used.

To serve, top each pancake with a dollop of whipped topping or cream.

% DAILY VALUE FOR:

VIT A	VIT C	VIT E	VIT D	VIT B$_1$	VIT B$_2$	VIT B$_3$	VIT B$_6$	VIT B$_{12}$	FOLATE	CAL	MAG	POT	SELEN	ZINC
4%	6%	12%	4%	17%	27%	16%	8%	8%	5%	19%	9%	15%	31%	10%

BEST SWEDISH PANCAKES

I've lightened up this traditional recipe by tossing out half the egg yolks (the fluffiness comes from the whites), replacing half the flour with whole wheat flour, and using fat-free sour cream and low-fat milk. They're delicious with fresh fruit and powdered sugar.

FOOD SYNERGY NOTES | *The ample protein and fiber from whole wheat flour means these pancakes may help you feel more satisfied while you enjoy them; and that feeling of fullness may even last longer after you leave the table!*

Makes 40 (10 per serving)

4	large eggs (omega-3, if available), separated, 2 yolks discarded
¼	cup egg substitute
2	tablespoons granulated sugar
3	tablespoons fat-free sour cream
½	cup whole wheat pastry flour or whole wheat flour
½	cup unbleached all-purpose flour
½	teaspoon salt
½	teaspoon ground cinnamon
1	cup 1% milk
¼	teaspoon pure vanilla extract (optional)

Place the egg whites in a mixing bowl and beat with an electric mixer until soft peaks form. Spoon into another bowl and set aside.

In the mixing bowl (the one used to beat the whites), add 2 egg yolks and the egg substitute and beat until thick and creamy, then beat in the sugar and sour cream.

In a 2-cup measuring cup, using a fork, stir together the flours, salt, and cinnamon.

PER SERVING:

CALORIES	FAT CAL	PROTEIN	CARB	FIBER	CHOLEST	TOTAL FAT	SAT FAT	MONO FAT	POLY FAT	OMEGA-3	OMEGA-6	SODIUM
230	16%	14 g	35 g	3 g	131 mg	4 g	1.4 g	1.4 g	1 g	0.2 g	0.8 g	397 mg

Add half the flour mixture and ½ cup of the milk to the egg yolk mixture, beating on low until combined. Then beat in the remaining flour mixture, ½ cup milk, and vanilla (if desired). Fold in the reserved egg whites.

Heat a nonstick skillet or griddle over medium-high heat. Coat a small area of the skillet or griddle with canola-oil cooking spray and spoon a full tablespoon of batter on that spot. To spread the batter into a circle, tap the measuring spoon against the skillet a few times in the center of the pancake. Repeat coating and dropping batter until you fill the griddle, leaving some space between the pancakes. When the bottoms have nicely browned and bubbles appear on the tops, about 1 to 2 minutes, flip the pancakes over to brown the other side. Remove to a serving plate. Repeat the process until you've used all the batter.

% DAILY VALUE FOR:

VIT A	VIT E	VIT B$_1$	VIT B$_2$	VIT B$_3$	VIT B$_6$	VIT B$_{12}$	FOLATE	CAL	VIT D	MAG	POT	SELEN	ZINC
15%	4%	19%	50%	14%	9%	20%	13%	11%	21%	9%	8%	48%	12%

HOT APPLE-BLUEBERRY COBBLER WITH WALNUT-BUTTER STREUSEL

This fruit-packed dessert gives you all the taste but just half the sugar and less margarine (or butter) than used in traditional versions. When buying plant sterol–enriched margarine, look for brands that have about 8 grams of fat per tablespoon. If you like to bake with Splenda, equal parts Splenda and sugar can replace the sugar.

FOOD SYNERGY NOTES | *A serving of this dessert boasts the synergy of quercetin and catechin (two powerful phytochemicals) and the synergy of unpeeled apples.*

Makes 6 servings

FILLING

1½	cups frozen or fresh blueberries		¼	cup unbleached all-purpose flour
6½	cups thin apple slices		1	teaspoon ground cinnamon
½	cup sugar		1	tablespoon lemon juice

TOPPING

½	cup whole wheat flour		4	tablespoons plant sterol–enriched margarine
½	cup unbleached all-purpose flour			
½	cup toasted walnut or pecan pieces		½	cup fat-free half-and-half
2	tablespoons light pancake syrup		2	teaspoons sugar (optional)
2	teaspoons baking powder		⅛–¼	cup light vanilla ice cream per serving (optional)
½	teaspoon salt			

PER SERVING:

CALORIES	FAT CAL	PROTEIN	CARB	FIBER	CHOLEST	TOTAL FAT	SAT FAT	MONO FAT	POLY FAT	OMEGA-3	OMEGA-6	SODIUM
280	26%	6 g	49 g	4 g	1 mg	8 g	2.8 g	2.1 g	2.4 g	0.4 g	2 g	320 mg

Preheat the oven to 400°F.

To make the filling: In a large bowl, place the blueberries, apples, sugar, flour, cinnamon, and lemon juice and toss gently to blend well. Transfer to a deep 9" × 9" baking dish coated with canola-oil cooking spray. Bake for 20 minutes, or until the fruit is tender and the juices bubble thickly.

To make the topping: Meanwhile, in a food processor, combine the flours, nuts, syrup, baking powder, salt, and margarine and pulse briefly until the mixture resembles coarse meal. Pour into a medium bowl and gradually add the half-and-half, mixing with a fork until moist clumps form.

Drop the topping by small spoonfuls to mostly cover the hot filling. Sprinkle with the sugar, if desired. Bake for 30 minutes more, or until the top is golden brown. Spoon into deep serving bowls and top each with a small scoop of the ice cream, if desired.

% DAILY VALUE FOR:

VIT A	VIT C	VIT E	VIT D	VIT B$_1$	VIT B$_2$	VIT B$_3$	VIT B$_6$	VIT B$_{12}$	FOLATE	CAL	MAG	POT	SELEN	ZINC
15%	17%	9%	9%	21%	17%	13%	11%	2%	8%	16%	13%	10%	19%	14%

LIGHT AND LUSCIOUS BERRY GRUNT

If you want to use margarine, look for plant sterol–enriched types like Take Control and Benecol. They have less fat than many brands of stick margarine. If you prefer not to bake with liqueur, use water instead.

FOOD SYNERGY NOTES | *Each serving provides almost a full cup of berries—bursting with vitamins, minerals, and phytochemicals—so you get a whole lot of berry synergy along with a little bit of whole grain synergy .*

Makes 8 servings

¾	cup sugar
¾	teaspoon ground cinnamon
¼	cup + 3 tablespoons unbleached all-purpose flour
⅓	cup whole wheat flour
¾	teaspoon baking powder
	Pinch of salt
¼	teaspoon ground ginger
⅓	cup fat-free half-and-half or low-fat milk
2	tablespoons plant sterol-enriched margarine, melted

4	cups raspberries
3	cups blackberries
2	tablespoons berry liqueur (such as Chambord)
2	tablespoons lemon or lime juice
2	tablespoons Wondra quick-mixing flour
¼	cup Splenda (optional)
	Light vanilla ice cream (optional)

In a small bowl, stir together 2 tablespoons of the sugar and ½ teaspoon of the cinnamon and set aside.

In a medium bowl, place the white and whole wheat flours, baking powder, salt, ginger, and 2 tablespoons sugar and blend well with a whisk.

PER SERVING:

CALORIES	FAT CAL	PROTEIN	CARB	FIBER	CHOLEST	TOTAL FAT	SAT FAT	MONO FAT	POLY FAT	OMEGA-3	OMEGA-6	SODIUM
217	10%	4 g	47 g	8 g	0 mg	2.3 g	0.3 g	0.8 g	0.8 g	0.2 g	0.6 g	78 mg

In a 1-cup measuring cup, combine the half-and-half or milk and pour into the flour mixture. Stir together with a fork or spoon and set aside.

In a large bowl, place the berries, liqueur, lemon or lime juice, Wondra, Splenda (if using), the remaining sugar, and the remaining ¼ teaspoon cinnamon and gently toss together. Transfer to a large straight-sided skillet, cover, bring to a gentle boil over medium-high heat, and cook, stirring occasionally, for 3 minutes.

Drop heaping tablespoonfuls of the reserved batter evenly on top of the gently boiling berry mixture. Sprinkle the reserved cinnamon-sugar mixture over the dollops of batter. Cover the skillet again and reduce the heat to medium-low. Cook until the biscuits are cooked through and the juices are bubbling, about 15 minutes.

If you wish, top each serving with a cookie-size scoop of ice cream.

% DAILY VALUE FOR:

VIT A	VIT C	VIT E	VIT B$_1$	VIT B$_2$	VIT B$_3$	VIT B$_6$	VIT B$_{12}$	FOLATE	CAL	MAG	POT	SELEN	ZINC
8%	38%	5%	9%	13%	10%	7%	1%	9%	9%	10%	8%	8%	8%

BERRY EASY TOPPING

This creamy, flavorful topping works well for pound cake, shortcake, coffee cake, waffles, or pancakes! Yes, this calls for a very un-"whole" food—nondairy whipped topping—but sometimes you just really need a topping like this. And at least half of it is a fresh "whole" fruit! Blackberries are also a delicious substitute for raspberries.

1 cup raspberries, fresh or frozen and thawed	¼ teaspoon pure vanilla extract
1 cup fat-free or light nondairy whipped topping, thawed in refrigerator	Pinch of cinnamon

In a medium bowl, place the raspberries, topping, vanilla extract, and cinnamon (or more to taste) and stir well with a spoon. Cover and refrigerate until ready to serve or up to 8 hours; after that, moisture from the berries may leak into the mixture.

PER SERVING (USING FAT-FREE TOPPING):

CALORIES	FAT CAL	PROTEIN	CARB	FIBER	CHOLEST	TOTAL FAT	SAT FAT	MONO FAT	POLY FAT	OMEGA-3	OMEGA-6	SODIUM
45	4%	0.3 g	10 g	2 g	0 mg	0.2 g	0 g	0.1 g	0.1 g	0.04 g	0.06 g	0 mg

% DAILY VALUE FOR:

VIT A	VIT C	VIT E	VIT B$_1$	VIT B$_2$	VIT B$_3$	VIT B$_6$	FOLATE	CAL	MAG	POT	ZINC
1%	10%	1%	1%	3%	2%	1%	2%	1%	2%	1%	2%

THREE-GRAIN BUTTERMILK WAFFLES

Get ready for this: Each waffle gives you three delicious grains with whole wheat flour, some oats, and some ground flaxseed (okay, technically that's two grains and one seed).

Each waffle packs the synergy power of whole grains plus some plant omega-3s from the flaxseed, canola oil, and omega-3 egg.

FOOD SYNERGY NOTES

Makes 4 (depending on your waffle maker)

½ cup whole wheat pastry flour	1¼ cups buttermilk
½ cup unbleached all-purpose flour	2 tablespoons light pancake syrup
¼ cup rolled oats	1 large egg (omega-3, if available), lightly beaten
2 tablespoons ground flaxseed	
1 teaspoon baking soda	1 tablespoon canola oil
Pinch of salt	1 teaspoon pure vanilla extract

Heat your waffle iron.

In a mixing bowl, place the flours, oats, flaxseed, baking soda, and salt and beat on low speed until well mixed. Add in the buttermilk, syrup, egg, oil, and vanilla extract all at once and beat on low speed until nicely blended. Let stand 5 minutes or so to thicken. Add extra buttermilk, if desired, to thin the batter slightly.

Coat your waffle iron with canola-oil cooking spray and use the appropriate amount of batter for your waffle iron. Cook to your desired degree of browning and crispness. Remove waffle to a serving plate. Repeat with more batter until all the batter is used. Serve with assorted berries or any other fruit of choice.

PER SERVING:

CALORIES	FAT CAL	PROTEIN	CARB	FIBER	CHOLEST	TOTAL FAT	SAT FAT	MONO FAT	POLY FAT	OMEGA-3	OMEGA-6	SODIUM
264	27%	11 g	36 g	5 g	58 mg	8 g	1.2 g	3.3 g	2.9 g	1.4 g	1.5 g	429 mg

% DAILY VALUE FOR:

VIT A	VIT C	VIT E	VIT D	VIT B$_1$	VIT B$_2$	VIT B$_3$	VIT B$_6$	VIT B$_{12}$	FOLATE	CAL	MAG	POT	SELEN	ZINC
7%	20%	6%	3%	14%	44%	40%	36%	68%	28%	12%	22%	17%	29%	47%

FRUIT AND CREAM CRISP

This warm microwave dessert is just what the doctor ordered on a cold winter's night.

FOOD SYNERGY NOTES *This quick dessert contains the synergy in fruit with a little whole grain synergy thrown in from the granola.*

Makes 1 serving

2 tablespoons light cream cheese	Pinch or 2 of ground cinnamon
1 teaspoon sugar	⅓ cup low-fat granola
⅛ teaspoon pure vanilla extract	⅛ cup light vanilla ice cream or fat-free frozen yogurt (optional)
⅔ cup sliced or diced fresh fruit (blackberries, peaches, or cherry halves)	

In a medium or large microwave-safe dessert cup (such as a Pyrex custard cup), place the cream cheese, sugar, and vanilla extract and stir with a fork to blend. Spread evenly on the bottom of the cup, then top with the fruit. Sprinkle cinnamon over the top, then cover with the granola. Cover and microwave on high for 1½ to 2 minutes, or until the fruit and cream cheese are lightly bubbling. Serve as is or slightly cooled. Top with a small scoop of ice cream or frozen yogurt, if desired.

PER SERVING (WITH ICE CREAM):

CALORIES	FAT CAL	PROTEIN	CARB	FIBER	CHOLEST	TOTAL FAT	SAT FAT	MONO FAT	POLY FAT	OMEGA-3	OMEGA-6	SODIUM
257	24%	7 g	44 g	7 g	15 mg	7 g	3.9 g	0.7 g	0.6 g	0.2 g	0.4 g	223 mg

% DAILY VALUE FOR:

VIT A	VIT C	VIT E	VIT B₁	VIT B₂	VIT B₃	VIT B₆	FOLATE	CAL	MAG	POT	SELEN	ZINC
13%	4%	6%	10%	10%	12%	8%	10%	9%	14%	8%	1%	10%

10-MINUTE SPICED APPLE WEDGES WITH CARAMEL SAUCE

This recipe features apples with skin, a whole food with synergy. If you decide to top this dessert with sliced almonds, you'll be adding the synergy in nuts as well.

FOOD
SYNERGY
NOTES

Makes 6 servings

4	large apples, cored and each cut into 16 wedges
2	tablespoons brown sugar, firmly packed
¼	cup apple cider or apple juice
1	teaspoon pumpkin pie spice

3	cups light vanilla ice cream
4	tablespoons caramel topping
	Toasted sliced almonds for garnish (optional)

In a medium microwave-safe bowl with a lid, place the apples, brown sugar, cider or juice, and spice. Toss to coat the apples well. Cover and microwave on high for 10 minutes, or until the apples are nice and tender.

Add a scoop of the ice cream to six serving bowls. Spoon a serving of the apple mixture around or over each scoop and drizzle each with 2 teaspoons of caramel topping. Sprinkle a heaping teaspoon of the almonds in the middle of each, if desired. Serve and enjoy immediately.

PER SERVING:

CALORIES	FAT CAL	PROTEIN	CARB	FIBER	CHOLEST	TOTAL FAT	SAT FAT	MONO FAT	POLY FAT	OMEGA-3	OMEGA-6	SODIUM
270	17%	4 g	54 g	4 g	35 mg	5 g	2.6 g	1 g	0.3 g	0.1 g	0.2 g	95 mg

% DAILY VALUE FOR:

VIT A	VIT C	VIT E	VIT B₁	VIT B₂	VIT B₃	VIT B₆	VIT B₁₂	FOLATE	CAL	MAG	POT	SELEN	ZINC
10%	11%	3%	2%	3%	1%	5%	1%	1%	12%	3%	5%	1%	1%

LIGHT ITALIAN WEDDING SOUP

You can make a batch of this soup and freeze the leftovers. Just thaw and enjoy on one of those busy weeknights. The key to great flavor with this soup is using the best chicken broth you can find. As far as the meatballs are concerned, use high-quality ground sirloin that is superlean but fresh, so when you are cooking the meatballs, it will smell like you are grilling a steak. Orzo is a tiny pasta shaped liked rice. If you want to use higher-fiber pasta instead, break some dry whole wheat spaghetti into tiny pieces.

FOOD SYNERGY NOTES | *Dark leafy green vegetables are featured, along with carotene-rich carrots. The dish is topped off with a sprinkle of phytochemicals from the onions.*

Makes 6 servings (12 cups)

¾	pound ground sirloin
¼	cup egg substitute or 1 large egg (omega-3, if available)
¼	cup dry Italian bread crumbs
2	tablespoons grated Parmesan cheese
¼	teaspoon garlic salt
¼	teaspoon ground black pepper
⅛	teaspoon ground oregano or ¼ teaspoon dried leaves, crumbled
1	teaspoon canola or olive oil

8	cups chicken or beef broth
1¼	cups thinly sliced carrots
1¼	cups thinly sliced celery
½	cup thinly sliced green onions
1	teaspoon dried basil, crumbled
½	cup orzo
6	ounces baby spinach or chopped escarole (about 6 cups firmly packed)
	Shredded Parmesan cheese and/or fresh parsley, for garnish (optional)

PER SERVING:

CALORIES	FAT CAL	PROTEIN	CARB	FIBER	CHOLEST	TOTAL FAT	SAT FAT	MONO FAT	POLY FAT	OMEGA-3	OMEGA-6	SODIUM
239	23%	22 g	25 g	4 g	36 mg	6 g	2.7 g	1.5 g	1.1 g	0.3 g	0.7 g	470 mg

In a mixing bowl, place the beef, egg substitute or egg, bread crumbs, cheese, garlic salt, pepper, and oregano and beat on low speed to blend well. Form into about 60 small meatballs about ¾" in diameter.

Heat the oil in a large nonstick skillet over medium-high heat. Add the meatballs and brown them well, turning frequently, for 8 minutes.

In a large saucepan, combine the broth, carrots, celery, onions, and basil and bring to a boil. Reduce the heat to simmer, cover, and cook for 10 minutes, or until the vegetables are almost tender. Add the orzo, spinach or escarole, and meatballs. Cover and simmer for 15 minutes more. Serve each cup of soup with a sprinkling of cheese or parsley, if desired.

% DAILY VALUE FOR:

VIT A	VIT C	VIT E	VIT B₁	VIT B₂	VIT B₃	FOLATE	CAL	MAG	POT	SELEN	ZINC
147%	18%	7%	22%	28%	11%	28%	11%	13%	20%	1%	35%

JESSIE'S WHITE CHILI

I know most of us think a chili powder– and tomato-free chili is an urban legend, but it really does exist. I've made light versions of a couple different white chili recipes, and this one is by far the best. If pepper triggers heartburn in you or anyone who will be eating this, just delete or reduce the lemon pepper. To keep this recipe light, we use skinless chicken breasts and only a couple teaspoons of canola oil, with just a small handful of reduced-fat tortilla chips and a sprinkle of shredded cheese to garnish each bowl.

FOOD SYNERGY NOTES | *This dish has synergy from the onions and garlic, and the smart fat helps the body absorb the phytochemicals from the plant foods in this dish. It contains a high-antioxidant vegetable—corn—and high-protein and high-fiber beans, all topped off by a light serving of low-fat dairy.*

Makes 8 servings

4	cups chicken broth
1	teaspoon lemon pepper
1	teaspoon cumin seed
4	boneless, skinless chicken breast halves
2	teaspoons canola oil or olive oil
2	teaspoons minced garlic
1¼	cups chopped sweet or mild onion
16	ounces frozen white corn, slightly thawed
7	ounces (1 can) diced green chiles, undrained

½	teaspoon ground cumin
3	tablespoons lime juice
2	cans (15 ounces each) cannellini beans (white kidney beans) or any other white beans, drained and rinsed
6	ounces reduced-fat tortilla chips
1¼	cups (6 ounces) reduced-fat shredded Monterey Jack or regular Jack cheese

PER SERVING:

CALORIES	FAT CAL	PROTEIN	CARB	FIBER	CHOLEST	TOTAL FAT	SAT FAT	MONO FAT	POLY FAT	OMEGA-3	OMEGA-6	SODIUM
404	20%	32 g	50 g	8 g	61 mg	9 g	4 g	2 g	2 g	0.3 g	1 g	630 mg

In a large saucepan over medium-high heat, combine the broth, lemon pepper, and cumin seed and bring to a boil. Add the chicken and reduce the heat to low. Cover and simmer for 20 to 30 minutes, or until no longer pink inside and the juices run clear. Remove the chicken, cut into 1" pieces, and add back to the saucepan.

Meanwhile, in a medium nonstick skillet, heat the oil over medium heat. Add the garlic and onion and cook, stirring frequently, for 5 minutes or until tender. Transfer to the saucepan with the chicken and broth.

Stir in the corn, chiles, ground cumin, lime juice, and beans and bring to a boil. Cook at a gentle boil for 3 minutes, or until the beans are hot.

Put a small handful of tortilla chips into each soup bowl and sprinkle a slightly heaping ⅛ cup of the cheese over the chips. Then ladle a serving of chili into each bowl and serve.

% DAILY VALUE FOR:

VIT A	VIT C	VIT E	VIT B$_1$	VIT B$_2$	VIT B$_3$	VIT B$_6$	VIT B$_{12}$	FOLATE	CAL	MAG	POT	SELEN	ZINC
12%	14%	4%	11%	21%	44%	28%	13%	8%	24%	9%	12%	25%	25%

NOT-SO-KILLER CHILI

FOOD SYNERGY NOTES | *This dish boasts synergy from its garlic and onions, as well as a wealth of antioxidant action from the beans, green pepper, jalapeño, and tomato paste.*

Makes 6 servings (12 cups)

4	slices reduced-fat turkey bacon
8	ounces reduced-fat turkey sausage (such as turkey polska kielbasa), casings removed
1	pound extra-lean ground sirloin (around 6 percent fat)
1½	cups chopped onion
1	green bell pepper (stem, seeds, and membranes removed), chopped
1	tablespoon minced garlic
2	jalapeño chile peppers,* seeded and chopped (wear plastic gloves when handling)

1½	tablespoons chili powder
1	teaspoon dried oregano flakes
8	ounces taco sauce
2	cups beer (nonalcoholic or regular) or water
1	can (12 ounces) low-sodium tomato paste
1	can (16 ounces) pinto beans, rinsed and drained

* Chopped jalapeños are available in jars in some supermarkets.

In a large nonstick skillet, cook the bacon until crisp, then crumble into pieces and set aside. Cut the sausage into bite-size pieces and cook in the same skillet until no longer pink. Set aside.

In the same skillet, combine the ground sirloin, onion, bell pepper, and garlic and cook over medium-high heat until the beef is nicely browned. Stir in the reserved sausage, chile peppers, chili powder, and oregano, then stir in the taco sauce, beer or water, and tomato paste. Bring to a boil, cover, and simmer for 1½ hours, stirring occasionally. Stir in the beans, cover, and simmer for 30 minutes more. Serve each cup of chili with a sprinkling of the reserved bacon.

PER SERVING:

CALORIES	FAT CAL	PROTEIN	CARB	FIBER	CHOLEST	TOTAL FAT	SAT FAT	MONO FAT	POLY FAT	OMEGA-3	OMEGA-6	SODIUM
320	25%	27 g	33 g	7.3 g	72 mg	9 g	3 g	3.4 g	2.1 g	0.3 g	1.5 g	980 mg

% DAILY VALUE FOR:

VIT A	VIT C	VIT E	VIT B₁	VIT B₂	VIT B₃	VIT B₆	VIT B₁₂	FOLATE	CAL	VIT D	MAG	POT	SELEN	ZINC
22%	66%	24%	25%	37%	46%	52%	72%	22%	8%	5%	26%	33%	14%	61%

FARMER'S MARKET PASTA SALAD

This recipe is incredibly flexible, so go ahead and add or substitute whatever vegetables you find this weekend at your farmer's market! A colorful mix of red, yellow, and orange bell peppers is especially attractive. To toast pine nuts, just place them in a small nonstick skillet and cook over medium-low heat, stirring often, until lightly browned. This takes only a few minutes.

This salad maximizes the synergy between tomatoes and broccoli and the synergy of adding some good fat along with your vegetables.

FOOD
SYNERGY
NOTES

Makes 6 servings

8	cups cooked whole wheat–blend rotini, drained	1	cup finely diced bell pepper
½	cup prepared pesto	3	cups lightly cooked and cooled broccoli or cauliflower florets
2	large ripe tomatoes, diced	¼	cup toasted pine nuts (optional)

In a large serving bowl, combine the pasta, pesto, tomatoes, bell pepper, and broccoli or cauliflower and toss to blend well. Sprinkle the toasted pine nuts over the top, if desired. If not serving immediately, cover tightly and keep refrigerated until needed.

PER SERVING:

CALORIES	FAT CAL	PROTEIN	CARB	FIBER	CHOLEST	TOTAL FAT	SAT FAT	MONO FAT	POLY FAT	OMEGA-3	OMEGA-6	SODIUM
350	13%	13 g	63 g	9 g	4 mg	5.4 g	2 g	1 g	0.6 g	0.1 g	0.5 g	163 mg

% DAILY VALUE FOR:

VIT A	VIT C	VIT E	VIT B₁	VIT B₂	VIT B₃	VIT B₆	FOLATE	CAL	MAG	POT	SELEN	ZINC
303%	52%	6%	29%	15%	18%	28%	9%	11%	24%	15%	88%	22%

SWEET PEPPER AND BASIL PASTA SALAD

To develop this dish, I first sautéed yellow and orange bell peppers, sweet onion, garlic, and seasonings in a token tablespoon of olive oil, then I mixed it all with noodles, tossed in some fresh basil, drizzled fresh lemon juice over the top, and voilà! That was the ticket! I later brought a huge bowl of this salad to a barbecue and went home with an empty bowl—always a good sign.

FOOD SYNERGY NOTES | *This salad is based on the synergy in whole grains in the pasta, plus smart fats and phytochemicals in olive oil working with the phytochemicals in the bell peppers, basil, and garlic.*

Makes 10 servings

1	box (16 ounces) multigrain pasta
3	tablespoons olive oil
1	yellow bell pepper, seeded and finely chopped
1	orange or red bell pepper, seeded and finely chopped
1	sweet onion, chopped
1	tablespoon minced garlic
1	teaspoon salt
½	teaspoon ground white pepper
1½	tablespoons chopped fresh oregano or 2 teaspoons dried
1	cup loosely packed fresh basil leaves, coarsely chopped
1	small or ½ large lemon, cut into wedges

Boil the pasta for 12 minutes or just until tender, according to the package directions, and drain. Place in a large serving bowl and drizzle 2 tablespoons of oil over the top. Toss to blend well.

PER SERVING:

CALORIES	FAT CAL	PROTEIN	CARB	FIBER	CHOLEST	TOTAL FAT	SAT FAT	MONO FAT	POLY FAT	OMEGA-3	OMEGA-6	SODIUM
206	22%	7 g	37 g	5 g	0 mg	5 g	0.7 g	3.3 g	0.7 g	0.1 g	0.6 g	237 mg

Heat the remaining 1 tablespoon of oil in a large nonstick skillet over medium heat. Add the bell peppers, onion, and garlic and cook, stirring frequently, for 5 minutes, or until the vegetables are just starting to brown. About midway through, sprinkle with salt, white pepper, and oregano and toss to blend. Let cool completely.

Add the pepper-onion mixture to the pasta and toss to blend. Refrigerate until needed. This can be done a day or two before a party or barbecue.

Right before serving, add the basil to the pasta mixture and drizzle with juice squeezed from the lemon wedges. Toss to blend well. Add more salt and white pepper to taste, if desired.

% DAILY VALUE FOR:

VIT A	VIT C	VIT E	VIT B$_1$	VIT B$_2$	VIT B$_3$	VIT B$_6$	FOLATE	CAL	MAG	POT	SELEN	ZINC
22%	65%	5%	22%	7%	18%	15%	9%	3%	22%	5%	1%	15%

ROASTED PEPPER AND MUSHROOM PASTA SALAD

This light dish is beefed up with roasted vegetables, which add color, flavor, and nutrients to the mix. The end result: a hearty, healthy, fiber-packed pasta salad.

FOOD SYNERGY NOTES | *The smart fats in the canola oil and olive oil enhance absorption of the phytochemicals in the bell pepper. The whole wheat pasta counts as a serving of whole grains, which and may help prevent some cancers and help protect against heart disease and stroke.*

Makes 6 servings

4	cups cooked and cooled whole wheat rotelle pasta (about 2 cups dry)
1	tablespoon canola oil
4	cups sliced cremini or portobello mushrooms (cut portobellos into bite-size pieces)
1	large (or 2 small) red, orange, or yellow bell pepper (stem and seeds removed), cut in half widthwise and sliced into ½" strips
1	red onion (ends and outer skin removed), sliced into ¼"-thick half circles
1½	teaspoons fresh rosemary, finely chopped (optional)
1½	tablespoons parsley
1	tablespoon olive oil
2	tablespoons balsamic vinegar
¾	teaspoon garlic salt
¼	teaspoon freshly ground black pepper

Place the pasta in a medium serving bowl.

Heat the canola oil in a large, nonstick skillet over high heat, add the mushrooms, and cook, stirring frequently, until lightly brown. Add to the pasta.

Start heating an indoor contact grill (like a George Foreman) or broiler.

PER SERVING:

CALORIES	FAT CAL	PROTEIN	CARB	FIBER	CHOLEST	TOTAL FAT	SAT FAT	MONO FAT	POLY FAT	OMEGA-3	OMEGA-6	SODIUM
187	24%	7 g	30 g	4 g	0 mg	5 g	0.6 g	3.2 g	1.2 g	0.3 g	0.9 g	234 mg

Coat the bottom grill plate with canola-oil cooking spray and add the bell pepper and onion, then coat the top grill plate with cooking spray. Lower the top onto the vegetables and cook for 8 to 10 minutes. If using the broiler, cook the vegetables for a few minutes or until they start to blacken in spots, then flip them over to broil the other side for a few minutes more. Add the cooked vegetables to the pasta.

In a small bowl, combine the rosemary, parsley, olive oil, vinegar, garlic salt, and black pepper and whisk to blend. Pour over the pasta salad and toss everything together. Refrigerate until ready to serve.

% DAILY VALUE FOR:

VIT A	VIT C	VIT E	VIT B₁	VIT B₂	VIT B₃	VIT B₆	FOLATE	CAL	VIT D	MAG	POT	SELEN	ZINC
2%	28%	7%	19%	15%	21%	15%	8%	2%	9%	18%	7%	4%	13%

SHRIMP AND RED GRAPEFRUIT SALAD

This salad features a unique combination of ingredients, and the grapefruit-ginger vinaigrette ties it all together. To save prep time, look for grapefruit segments in your grocery's produce section.

FOOD SYNERGY NOTES *We've got a whole lot of synergy going on here: a little citrus synergy plus the fat-containing ingredients (avocados and canola oil) that help the body absorb more of the nutrients in the vegetables, plus plant omega-3s working with fish omega-3s—and a sprinkle of nut synergy to top it all off!*

Makes 4 servings

VINAIGRETTE

¼	cup grapefruit juice	1	tablespoon canola oil
2	teaspoons lime juice	1½	tablespoons flaked or shredded packaged coconut
¼	teaspoon finely grated peeled fresh ginger or ⅛ teaspoon ground ginger		

SALAD

6	cups fresh baby spinach, lightly packed	½	pound cooked large shrimp, shelled and deveined
2	cups red grapefruit segments	½	cup diced jicama (optional)
1	firm ripe avocado, quartered and cut lengthwise into ¼"-thick slices		Salt and ground pepper
		¼	cup lightly toasted pecans, walnuts, or hazelnuts

PER SERVING:

CALORIES	FAT CAL	PROTEIN	CARB	FIBER	CHOLEST	TOTAL FAT	SAT FAT	MONO FAT	POLY FAT	OMEGA-3	OMEGA-6	SODIUM
288	53%	16 g	21 g	7 g	110 mg	17 g	2.6 g	9.8 g	3.8 g	0.7 g	3.1 g	174 mg

To make the vinaigrette: In a jar with a tight-fitting lid, combine the grapefruit juice, lime juice, ginger, oil, and coconut and shake well (or whisk everything together in a medium bowl).

To make the salad: Divide the spinach among four salad bowls. Top decoratively with the grapefruit, avocado, shrimp, and jicama (if using) and sprinkle with salt and pepper to taste. Spoon the vinaigrette evenly over the top of each salad and sprinkle with the nuts.

% DAILY VALUE FOR:

VIT A	VIT C	VIT E	VIT B$_1$	VIT B$_2$	VIT B$_3$	VIT B$_6$	VIT B$_{12}$	FOLATE	CAL	MAG	POT	SELEN	ZINC
57%	94%	20%	18%	19%	22%	29%	35%	35%	9%	30%	26%	43%	22%

MEDITERRANEAN CHICKPEA SALAD

This lovely salad also qualifies as a lacto-vegetarian recipe. Whatever dietary pattern you choose to follow, trust me—this one is a keeper.

FOOD SYNERGY NOTES *Legumes have a synergistic combo of protein and fiber, which helps reduce postmeal hunger. This salad also includes the high-antioxidant tomato and the synergy of low-fat dairy.*

Makes 6 servings

1	can (15 ounces) chickpeas, drained and rinsed	2	tablespoons finely chopped fresh basil
1	cucumber, unpeeled and finely chopped	4	ounces fresh mozzarella, finely chopped or cubed
1	cup grape tomatoes, halved	1	tablespoon olive oil
¼	cup finely chopped sweet onion	2	tablespoons balsamic vinegar
2	teaspoons minced garlic	¼	teaspoon salt
1½	tablespoons finely chopped parsley		

In a medium serving bowl, combine the chickpeas, cucumber, tomatoes, onion, garlic, parsley, basil, and mozzarella. Drizzle with oil and vinegar and sprinkle with salt, then toss all the ingredients well to combine. Cover the bowl and refrigerate at least 1 hour to let the flavors blend.

PER SERVING:

CALORIES	FAT CAL	PROTEIN	CARB	FIBER	CHOLEST	TOTAL FAT	SAT FAT	MONO FAT	POLY FAT	OMEGA-3	OMEGA-6	SODIUM
153	38%	9 g	15 g	2.5 g	10 mg	6.5 g	2.5 g	2 g	0.7 g	0.1 g	0.6 g	197 mg

% DAILY VALUE FOR:

VIT A	VIT C	VIT E	VIT B₁	VIT B₂	VIT B₃	VIT B₆	FOLATE	CAL	MAG	POT	SELEN	ZINC
12%	15%	4%	5%	4%	2%	32%	16%	15%	10%	8%	4%	11%

AVOCADO MANGO SALAD

One of my favorite flavor combinations is avocado and mango, so I started this side salad with those two featured foods. If you don't add any salt to taste, each serving contains just 7 milligrams of sodium. The best part is that you also get a healthy dose of fiber (4 grams) and one of the smart fats—monounsaturated (5 grams). If you prefer, chop the avocado and mango into smaller pieces and enjoy as a salsa with chips, nachos, quesadillas, grilled fish, or chicken!

The avocado represents the smart fat that will boost the nutrients absorbed from the fruits and vegetables.

FOOD
SYNERGY
NOTES

Makes 4 servings (½ cup each)

1	avocado, peeled, pitted, and chopped
1	mango, peeled, seeded, and chopped (at least 1 cup)
1	tablespoon lime juice
⅓	cup finely chopped red or sweet onion

½	jalapeño chile pepper, seeded and finely chopped + more to taste, if desired
2	tablespoons chopped fresh cilantro
	Salt and black pepper (optional)

Place the avocado and mango in a small or medium serving bowl. Drizzle with the lime juice and top with the onion, chile pepper, cilantro, and black pepper and salt to taste (if using). Gently toss to blend well. Cover and refrigerate until ready to serve.

To serve, spoon over lettuce leaves.

PER SERVING:

CALORIES	FAT CAL	PROTEIN	CARB	FIBER	CHOLEST	TOTAL FAT	SAT FAT	MONO FAT	POLY FAT	OMEGA-3	OMEGA-6	SODIUM
114	57%	2 g	12 g	4 g	0 mg	7.3 g	1.3 g	5 g	1 g	0.1 g	0.9 g	6 mg

% DAILY VALUE FOR:

VIT A	VIT C	VIT E	VIT B₁	VIT B₂	VIT B₃	VIT B₆	FOLATE	CAL	MAG	POT	SELEN	ZINC
28%	24%	8%	8%	8%	9%	17%	10%	1%	8%	11%	1%	3%

LESS-FUSS PECAN-CRUSTED CHICKEN SALAD

One helping of this salad is definitely a full meal! No need to serve anything else with it.

FOOD SYNERGY NOTES | *A serving of this dish contains the three Bs (folic acid, vitamin B$_6$, and B$_{12}$), which together may reduce the level of an amino acid that, at high levels, may damage artery linings, leading to heart attack and stroke.*

Makes 4 servings

4	boneless, skinless chicken breasts	1	cup unbleached all-purpose flour
½–1	tablespoon canola oil	12	cups fresh chopped romaine lettuce
½	cup finely chopped pecans	1	cup sliced celery
¾	cup cornflake crumbs	½	cup bottled light balsamic vinaigrette
½	teaspoon salt	½	cup dried cranberries
1	cup low-fat milk or fat-free half-and-half	1	cup drained mandarin orange segments (from a can or jar)
1	large egg (omega-3, if available)	6	tablespoons crumbled blue cheese
¼	cup egg substitute		

Preheat the oven to 450°F.

Pound each chicken breast to about ½" thick. (Cover each breast in waxed paper and pound with a mallet.) Line a baking sheet or 13" × 9" baking dish with foil and coat the bottom with the oil. (If you are using larger chicken breasts, you may need to use a jelly-roll pan.)

PER SERVING:

CALORIES	FAT CAL	PROTEIN	CARB	FIBER	CHOLEST	TOTAL FAT	SAT FAT	MONO FAT	POLY FAT	OMEGA-3	OMEGA-6	SODIUM
371	37%	26 g	32 g	5 g	65 mg	15 g	3.3 g	6.2	3.2	0.4 g	2.8 g	623 mg

In a medium bowl, combine the pecans, cornflake crumbs, and salt. In a large measuring cup, combine the milk or half-and-half, egg, and egg substitute and whisk together well. Place the flour in another medium bowl.

Coat each chicken breast with the flour, dip into the egg mixture, then coat well with the pecan mixture. Place each breast on the baking dish and coat the top with canola-oil cooking spray.

Bake the chicken for 20 to 25 minutes, or until a thermometer in the thickest portion registers 160°F and the juices run clear. Let cool while you proceed to the next step, or cover and refrigerate until you are ready to assemble the salad.

In a large bowl, toss the lettuce and celery with the vinaigrette. Divide among four dinner plates, then arrange the cranberries and oranges on top. Sprinkle with the cheese and arrange one sliced chicken breast on top (in a fan shape, if desired).

% DAILY VALUE FOR:

VIT A	VIT C	VIT E	VIT D	VIT B_1	VIT B_2	VIT B_3	VIT B_6	VIT B_{12}	FOLATE	CAL	MAG	POT	SELEN	ZINC
52%	52%	11%	4%	41%	45%	68%	53%	14%	47%	13%	15%	20%	34%	21%

MEDITERRANEAN PITA SANDWICH

To make more than two sandwiches, just multiply the ingredients. This sandwich can be wrapped well and stored in the refrigerator for up to 2 days.

FOOD SYNERGY NOTES | *Each sandwich features the high-viscous-fiber vegetable eggplant, plus smart fats and phytochemicals from olive oil pesto and walnuts. It includes two Synergy Super Foods: tomatoes and spinach.*

Makes 2

1	small to medium eggplant, cut into ⅓"-thick slices
⅓	cup goat cheese
2	tablespoons toasted walnut pieces
	Ground black pepper

2	pitas, each cut in half
4	teaspoons prepared pesto sauce
1	tomato, sliced thin
12	spinach leaves

Preheat an indoor grill, toaster oven, or oven broiler. Spray both sides of the eggplant with canola- or olive-oil cooking spray, and place on a sheet of foil if using a toaster oven or oven broiler.

If using an indoor grill (like the George Foreman), place the eggplant between the two grill plates. Cook 7 to 8 minutes, or until the eggplant is soft on the inside and lightly brown on the outside.

PER SERVING (2 HALVES):

CALORIES	FAT CAL	PROTEIN	CARB	FIBER	CHOLEST	TOTAL FAT	SAT FAT	MONO FAT	POLY FAT	OMEGA-3	OMEGA-6	SODIUM
255	38%	10 g	32 g	8 g	7 mg	11 g	3 g	4 g	4 g	0.4 g	3 g	426 mg

If using a broiler, place the eggplant about 5" from the broiling unit. Watching carefully, flip the slices over when the tops are nicely brown, then broil until the second side is nicely brown, 7 to 8 minutes total.

In a small bowl, mix the goat cheese with the walnuts and black pepper to taste.

To assemble the sandwiches, spread the bottom inside of each pita half with 1 teaspoon of the pesto, then spread a heaping tablespoon of the cheese mixture over that. Fill each half with at least two slices of eggplant and tomato and a few spinach leaves. If you aren't going to eat the sandwiches right away, wrap well with plastic wrap and refrigerate until needed.

% **DAILY VALUE FOR:**

VIT A	VIT B$_1$	VIT B$_2$	VIT B$_3$	VIT B$_6$	VIT C	VIT E	FOLATE	CAL	MAG	POT	SELEN	ZINC
74%	22%	15%	16%	31%	36%	8%	14%	7%	24%	16%	30%	14%

2-MINUTE TOASTED TOMATO AND CHEESE SANDWICH

Calling all garden or vine-ripened tomatoes! This open-faced sandwich makes a great light breakfast or afternoon snack. It could be a lunch or dinner if you add some fruit or veggies to your meal.

FOOD SYNERGY NOTES | *This sandwich has a serving of whole grains and low-fat dairy (two food groups with synergy), plus the phytochemicals in the tomato, with the fat in the cheese increasing their absorption.*

Makes 1

1 slice whole wheat bread

1 slice reduced-fat or regular Cheddar cheese

½ ripe tomato, thinly sliced

Salt and ground pepper

Place the cheese on the bread slice and put on the baking rack in a toaster oven set to slightly dark toast. By the time the toast is done, the cheese will be bubbly. Top with the tomato, sprinkle with salt and pepper to taste, and cut in half on the diagonal.

PER SERVING:

CALORIES	FAT CAL	PROTEIN	CARB	FIBER	CHOLEST	TOTAL FAT	SAT FAT	MONO FAT	POLY FAT	OMEGA-3	OMEGA-6	SODIUM
164	40%	8 g	16 g	3 g	22 mg	7.7 g	4.5 g	2 g	0.3 g	0.1 g	0.2 g	233 mg

% DAILY VALUE FOR:

VIT A	VIT C	VIT E	VIT D	VIT B₁	VIT B₂	VIT B₃	VIT B₆	VIT B₁₂	FOLATE	CAL	MAG	POT	SELEN	ZINC
16%	23%	5%	1%	14%	17%	10%	7%	7%	4%	18%	5%	6%	6%	9%

DELUXE GRILLED CHEESE SANDWICH

One of the most common ways to enjoy cheese is in a grilled sandwich, so here's a deluxe and healthful rendition of an old favorite.

In this sandwich, you get two whole foods with synergy: dairy and whole wheat. You also can count on the synergy in tomatoes, and you get a serving of plant sterol–enriched margarine, too.

FOOD SYNERGY NOTES

Makes 2

4	slices whole wheat bread
2	teaspoons light plant sterol–enriched margarine
3	ounces fresh mozzarella cheese, thinly sliced, or shredded reduced-fat Swiss, Jarlsberg Lite, or part-skim mozzarella

1	medium vine-ripened tomato, thinly sliced
	Freshly ground pepper
	Salt (optional)
½	cup fresh basil leaves

Heat a large nonstick skillet over medium heat. Coat one side of all four slices of bread with the margarine.

Place two slices spread-side down on the griddle. Top with the cheese, then the tomato, pepper, and salt (if desired) to taste, and basil. Top with the remaining two bread slices, spread-side up.

Grill for 2 to 3 minutes, or until the bottom side is nicely golden. Flip the sandwiches over and grill for 2 to 3 minutes more, until golden. Cut each sandwich diagonally and serve.

PER SERVING:

CALORIES	FAT CAL	PROTEIN	CARB	FIBER	CHOLEST	TOTAL FAT	SAT FAT	MONO FAT	POLY FAT	OMEGA-3	OMEGA-6	SODIUM
273	42%	13 g	26 g	4 g	33 mg	12 g	6.3 g	2 g	1.4 g	0.2 g	1 g	256 mg

% DAILY VALUE FOR:

VIT A	VIT C	VIT E	VIT B$_1$	VIT B$_2$	VIT B$_3$	VIT B$_6$	FOLATE	CAL	MAG	POT	SELEN	ZINC
28%	18%	5%	20%	16%	15%	5%	4%	30%	5%	5%	1%	2%

FRENCH-STYLE HAM AND CHEESE SANDWICH

I tasted a savory treat recently that had crème fraîche, bits of ham, Gruyère cheese, and caramelized onions all sitting on top of a buttery French pastry. Needless to say, it was as rich as it was wonderful. It took my stomach a few hours to recover. Days later, that decadent appetizer inspired me to create a sandwich in its likeness, but lighter.

FOOD SYNERGY NOTES | *Each sandwich gets the equivalent of half an onion! Onions are rich in phytochemicals that help reduce LDL oxidation, and in here you get them sautéed in a small dose of monounsaturated fat. If you enjoy this sandwich on whole grain bread, you'll add the synergy from this group as well (and help protect against heart disease, stroke, insulin resistance, and obesity).*

Makes 2

1	teaspoon extra-virgin olive oil
1	sweet onion, thinly sliced
2	teaspoons light pancake syrup (optional)
4	slices whole grain bread
3	ounces thinly sliced extra-lean ham
2	tablespoons whipped light cream cheese
½	cup shredded Gruyère cheese, firmly packed

Heat the oil in a medium nonstick skillet over medium-high heat. Add the onion and cook for 4 minutes, stirring frequently, or until nicely browned and caramelized. Drizzle with the syrup (if desired) and stir. Set aside to cool.

PER SERVING:

CALORIES	FAT CAL	PROTEIN	CARB	FIBER	CHOLEST	TOTAL FAT	SAT FAT	MONO FAT	POLY FAT	OMEGA-3	OMEGA-6	SODIUM
382	35%	23 g	37 g	6 g	53 mg	15 g	6.5 g	5.5 g	1 g	0.2 g	0.8 g	928 mg

Toast the bread, if desired. Top two of the slices with the ham and spread the reserved onions over the ham. Then spread 1 tablespoon of the cream cheese over each of the remaining two slices of bread. Sprinkle the Gruyère evenly over the top of the cream cheese.

Place all four slices under the toaster oven broiler (or regular broiler) and broil for 3 to 4 minutes, watching carefully, until the cheese starts to bubble. Place the slices with the cheese over the slices with the ham and onions. Cut each sandwich on the diagonal.

% DAILY VALUE FOR:

VIT A	VIT C	VIT E	VIT B₁	VIT B₂	VIT B₃	VIT B₆	VIT B₁₂	FOLATE	CAL	MAG	POT	SELEN	ZINC
15%	14%	7%	60%	31%	28%	31%	31%	9%	35%	10%	12%	21%	27%

Appetizers, Snacks, and Sides

SPICY NUT MIX

These nuts are lovely to munch on as a snack or sprinkle onto green salads or meat entrées—and they're a delicious part of the Porfolio plan.

FOOD
SYNERGY
NOTES

Each nut has a slightly different nutrient portfolio (including antioxidant phytochemicals), but in general, nuts contain mostly monounsaturated fat, and most contribute phytosterols (which in sufficient amounts help lower blood cholesterol, enhance the immune system, and decrease the risk of some cancers). Nuts also contribute some vitamins and minerals we need more of, like vitamin E, potassium, and magnesium. Two forms of vitamin E work best together (alpha- and gamma-tocopherol) and you'll find them in almonds, cashews, and walnuts. Walnuts also contribute plant omega-3s and (as do pecans) phenolic acid.

Makes 12 servings

1	egg white
1½	cups whole almonds
1½	cups whole walnuts, pecans, or cashews
2	tablespoons brown sugar, packed

½	teaspoon seasoning salt
½	teaspoon curry powder
½	teaspoon ground cinnamon
¼	teaspoon ground red pepper (double if you really like it hot)

PER SERVING:

CALORIES	FAT CAL	PROTEIN	CARB	FIBER	CHOLEST	TOTAL FAT	SAT FAT	MONO FAT	POLY FAT	OMEGA-3	OMEGA-6	SODIUM
214	75%	6 g	8 g	3.2 g	0 mg	18 g	1.6 g	7 g	9.1 g	1.4 g	7.7 g	44 mg

Preheat the oven to 250°F. Generously coat a nonstick baking sheet with canola-oil cooking spray.

In a mixing bowl, beat the egg white until foamy. Add the almonds and walnuts and toss well to coat.

In a small measuring cup, combine the brown sugar, salt, curry, cinnamon, and pepper and blend well with a fork. Add to the nuts and stir to combine everything well.

Spread the nuts on the baking sheet and bake for 50 minutes, stirring after 30 minutes. Let cool for 15 minutes, then break into smaller pieces. When completely cool, place in an airtight container and store for up to 1 week.

% DAILY VALUE FOR:

VIT E	VIT B₁	VIT B₂	VIT B₃	VIT B₆	FOLATE	CAL	MAG	POT	SELEN	ZINC
28%	8%	18%	6%	8%	6%	2%	8%	2%	2%	6%

FUN FALL SNACK MIX

With pumpkin spice and dried cranberries, this fruit-and-nut mixture brings you the taste of the fall season and fulfills part of the Portfolio prescription.

FOOD SYNERGY NOTES | *This homemade trail mix includes almonds, which have synergy with other nutrients like vitamin E (also in almonds). It's a nice little snack with protein and fiber, which synergistically help decrease after-meal hunger.*

Makes 10 servings (⅓ cup each)

1	cup dried apricots, finely chopped		1	cup unsalted or lightly salted roasted peanuts
½	cup dried cherries or cranberries		¾	teaspoon pumpkin pie spice
1	cup unsalted or lightly salted roasted almonds		⅓	cup white chocolate chips (optional)

In a gallon-size plastic bag, combine the apricots, cherries or cranberries, almonds, peanuts, spice, and chocolate chips (if using) and seal. Toss the bag around to mix all the ingredients well.

NOTE: *Using the white chocolate chips adds 30 calories, 2 grams of fat, and 1 gram saturated fat to each serving.*

PER SERVING (WITHOUT WHITE CHOCOLATE CHIPS):

CALORIES	FAT CAL	PROTEIN	CARB	FIBER	CHOLEST	TOTAL FAT	SAT FAT	MONO FAT	POLY FAT	OMEGA-3	OMEGA-6	SODIUM
234	53%	8 g	21 g	4.2 g	0 mg	14 g	1.5 g	8.2 g	4 g	0 g	4 g	49 mg

% DAILY VALUE FOR:

VIT A	VIT C	VIT E	VIT B₁	VIT B₂	VIT B₃	VIT B₆	FOLATE	CAL	MAG	POT	SELEN	ZINC
2%	3%	32%	7%	12%	18%	4%	6%	6%	20%	12%	3%	12%

AVOCADO-EDAMAME SALSA

Leave out the olives if your guests or family members don't care for them. This salsa is great with reduced-fat tortilla chips and as a garnish for quesadillas or burritos.

This appetizer or condiment features soy, a whole food with synergy, and another way to work in some fruits (avocado) and vegetables, too. The smart monounsaturated fat from the avocado helps the body absorb the nutrients and phytochemicals from the other plant foods in this dish. There is also synergy with the phytochemicals in garlic and onions.

FOOD SYNERGY NOTES

Makes 4 servings

1 cup frozen petite corn kernels, thawed	¼ cup light vinaigrette salad dressing, such as Kraft Light Italian
1 can (2.25 ounces) sliced ripe olives, drained	½ teaspoon ground black pepper (optional)
½ red bell pepper, finely chopped	1 avocado, finely chopped
⅓ cup finely chopped sweet onion	⅔ cup shelled edamame, thawed
2 teaspoons minced garlic	

In a medium bowl, place the corn, olives, bell pepper, onion, and garlic. Add the dressing and toss to blend. Add the black pepper (if desired). Cover and chill in the refrigerator at least 8 hours or overnight.

Right before serving, stir the avocado and edamame into the corn mixture.

PER SERVING:

CALORIES	FAT CAL	PROTEIN	CARB	FIBER	CHOLEST	TOTAL FAT	SAT FAT	MONO FAT	POLY FAT	OMEGA-3	OMEGA-6	SODIUM
230	49%	7 g	22 g	6 g	0 mg	12.5 g	1.7 g	5.3 g	2.1 g	0.2 g	1.9 g	238 mg

% DAILY VALUE FOR:

VIT A	VIT C	VIT E	VIT B₁	VIT B₂	VIT B₃	VIT B₆	FOLATE	CAL	MAG	POT	SELEN	ZINC
23%	71%	6%	18%	14%	16%	27%	22%	7%	16%	19%	3%	9%

STUFFED GRAPE LEAVES

To make these as healthful as possible, the grape leaves are stuffed with seasoned brown rice instead of white rice. These can be a main dish, side dish, or appetizer. Serve with a green salad or your favorite soup.

FOOD SYNERGY NOTES | *Synergy from whole grains fills the grape leaves, which themselves are rich in nutrients and phytochemicals, enhanced by the small amount of smart fat and phytochemicals from olive oil.*

Makes 8 servings (4 leaves each)

1	cup uncooked brown rice
½	cup chopped onion
3	tablespoons chopped fresh dill
3	tablespoons chopped fresh mint
4	cups low-sodium chicken broth
⅓	cup fresh lemon juice
32	grape leaves, drained and rinsed (8-ounce bottle)
3	tablespoons olive oil or flavored olive oil

Heat a large nonstick saucepan coated with cooking spray over medium-high heat. Add the rice, onion, dill, and mint and cook, stirring frequently, for 3 minutes, or until the onion is soft. Pour in 2 cups of the broth, cover the saucepan, reduce the heat to low, and simmer for 45 minutes, or until the rice is almost cooked. Stir in half the lemon juice and remove the saucepan from the heat.

PER SERVING:

CALORIES	FAT CAL	PROTEIN	CARB	FIBER	CHOLEST	TOTAL FAT	SAT FAT	MONO FAT	POLY FAT	OMEGA-3	OMEGA-6	SODIUM
157	37%	4 g	23 g	1.5 g	2 mg	6.5 g	1.3 g	4.3 g	0.9 g	0.2 g	0.7 g	450 mg

Take one leaf, shiny side down, blot dry with paper towel, and place 1 heaping teaspoon of the rice mixture at the bottom (stem) end of the leaf. Fold both sides of the leaf toward the center, roll up from the broad bottom to the top, and place in a 12" skillet. Repeat with all the leaves, leaving no gaps between the leaves in the skillet (to prevent them from opening while cooking). Sprinkle with the oil and remaining lemon juice.

Pour the remaining 2 cups of broth into the skillet to cover the leaves. Cover and simmer for 1 hour (do not boil, because this will make the stuffing burst out of the leaves). Remove from the heat, uncover, and let cool for 30 minutes. Serve chilled if desired.

% DAILY VALUE FOR:

VIT A	VIT C	VIT E	VIT B$_1$	VIT B$_2$	VIT B$_3$	VIT B$_6$	FOLATE	CAL	MAG	POT	SELEN	ZINC
22%	10%	6%	10%	7%	13%	13%	5%	6%	12%	3%	10%	7%

SUMMER SUCCOTASH

This dish tastes like summer. You can use either frozen corn or kernels cut off the cob if in season.

FOOD SYNERGY NOTES *This side dish boasts the antioxidant power of corn (a high-antioxidant veggie), plus some soy protein and soy synergy (from the edamame) and a touch of tomato phytochemicals and plant sterol–enriched margarine.*

Makes 6 servings

2 cups corn, fresh or frozen	Salt and ground pepper
2 cups shelled edamame (green soybeans)	1 teaspoon plant sterol–enriched margarine or whipped butter (optional)
1 large ripe tomato, chopped	

In a microwave-safe dish, combine the corn and edamame and toss to blend. Microwave on high for 3 to 4 minutes or until the vegetables are hot. Stir in the tomato, salt and pepper to taste, and margarine or whipped butter (if desired).

PER SERVING:

CALORIES	FAT CAL	PROTEIN	CARB	FIBER	CHOLEST	TOTAL FAT	SAT FAT	MONO FAT	POLY FAT	OMEGA-3	OMEGA-6	SODIUM
139	28%	9 g	19 g	4 g	0 mg	4.4 g	0.5 g	0.9 g	2.1 g	0.2 g	1.8 g	13 mg

% DAILY VALUE FOR:

VIT A	VIT C	VIT E	VIT B$_1$	VIT B$_2$	VIT B$_3$	VIT B$_6$	FOLATE	CAL	MAG	POT	SELEN	ZINC
5%	26%	1%	20%	13%	13%	12%	23%	9%	15%	14%	2%	10%

COLESLAW WITH SPICY PEANUT DRESSING

The featured ingredient is a cruciferous vegetable—cabbage—that comes with powerful phytochemicals, and the salad dressing and peanut butter add smart fats that help the body absorb the plant phytochemicals. Each serving also includes a sprinkling of almonds, which bring their own phytochemicals and smart fats.

Makes 5 servings

16 ounces (1 bag) slaw (shredded green cabbage with shredded carrots and red cabbage)

¼ cup smooth natural peanut butter

⅔ cup Newman's Own Lighten Up Low Fat Sesame Ginger Salad Dressing or similar dressing

1 teaspoon seeded and finely chopped jalapeño chile peppers (add more or less if desired; wear plastic gloves while handling)

3 scallions (white and green parts), thinly sliced

¼ cup toasted sliced almonds

Place the slaw in a medium serving bowl.

In a small food processor or mixing bowl, place the peanut butter, dressing, and chile peppers and pulse or blend until blended well.

Drizzle the peanut butter mixture and scallions over the slaw in the bowl and toss to mix. Garnish with the almonds.

PER SERVING:

CALORIES	FAT CAL	PROTEIN	CARB	FIBER	CHOLEST	TOTAL FAT	SAT FAT	MONO FAT	POLY FAT	OMEGA-3	OMEGA-6	SODIUM
167	53%	6 g	12 g	7 g	110 mg	11 g	1.4 g	6.1 g	2.4 g	0.3 g	2.1 g	174 mg

% DAILY VALUE FOR:

VIT A	VIT C	VIT E	VIT B$_1$	VIT B$_2$	VIT B$_3$	VIT B$_6$	FOLATE	CAL	MAG	POT	SELEN	ZINC
10%	47%	10%	6%	6%	3%	14%	15%	5%	11%	7%	2%	5%

TAHINI-DRESSED CHILLED NOODLES

This is a different and delicious way to work in some whole wheat noodles.

Whole grains and the synergy they contribute help protect against heart disease, stroke, diabetes, insulin resistance, and obesity. Each serving also offers some soy synergy and antioxidants and phytochemicals from the red bell pepper or tomatoes.

Makes 4 servings

3	tablespoons tahini (sesame seed paste)
2	tablespoons olive oil
3	tablespoons fat-free or light sour cream
2	teaspoons lemon juice
1	teaspoon Mrs. Dash Extra Spicy Seasoning Blend

3	cups al dente cooked (whole wheat–blend) thin spaghetti (6–7 ounces dry), chilled
	Salt (optional)
1	cup finely chopped red bell pepper or chopped ripe tomato
¼	cup soy nuts or 1 tablespoon toasted sesame seeds

In a medium serving bowl, whisk together the tahini, oil, sour cream, lemon juice, and seasoning blend until smooth. Add the noodles and toss to coat well. Add salt to taste, if desired. Cover and chill until ready to serve. Garnish with bell pepper or tomato and soy nuts or sesame seeds.

PER SERVING:

CALORIES	FAT CAL	PROTEIN	CARB	FIBER	CHOLEST	TOTAL FAT	SAT FAT	MONO FAT	POLY FAT	OMEGA-3	OMEGA-6	SODIUM
327	38%	12 g	41 g	8 g	0 mg	14 g	2.2 g	8 g	3.5 g	0.2 g	3.3 g	22 mg

% DAILY VALUE FOR:

VIT A	VIT C	VIT E	VIT B₁	VIT B₂	VIT B₃	VIT B₆	FOLATE	CAL	MAG	POT	SELEN	ZINC
30%	97%	10%	37%	8%	21%	16%	11%	7%	24%	7%	57%	20%

ROASTED ASPARAGUS SPEARS
WITH SLIVERED GARLIC

Double or triple this recipe if you are making this tasty and beautiful side dish for a large group.

Eating a little good fat along with vegetables helps the body absorb their protective phytochemicals (like those in dark green veggies and tomatoes). This recipe pairs nutrient-packed asparagus with olive oil (considered a smart fat due to its high monounsaturated fat content).

FOOD
SYNERGY
NOTES

Makes 4 servings

24	asparagus spears, ends trimmed (about 1 large bunch)	⅛	teaspoon dried basil
½	whole garlic bulb	⅛	teaspoon coarse salt (optional)
2	teaspoons olive oil	¼	teaspoon freshly ground pepper

Preheat the oven to 425°F. Spread the asparagus in a 13" × 9" baking dish. Remove the skin from individual cloves of the garlic bulb and cut each clove lengthwise into slivers (3 or 4 per clove).

Drizzle the oil over the asparagus. Add the garlic slivers, basil, salt (if desired), and pepper, tossing to combine.

Place the dish in the center of the oven and roast the asparagus for 10 to 12 minutes, or until just tender, tossing after 5 minutes to ensure even baking.

PER SERVING:

CALORIES	FAT CAL	PROTEIN	CARB	FIBER	CHOLEST	TOTAL FAT	SAT FAT	MONO FAT	POLY FAT	OMEGA-3	OMEGA-6	SODIUM
64	34%	3 g	8 g	3 g	0 mg	2.4 g	0.3 g	1.8 g	0.2 g	0 g	0.2 g	2 mg

% DAILY VALUE FOR:

VIT A	VIT C	VIT E	VIT B₁	VIT B₂	VIT B₆	CAL	MAG	POT	SELEN	ZINC
9%	18%	2%	2%	1%	8%	4%	1%	9%	2%	1%

BRUSSELS SPROUTS SAUTÉED WITH PECANS AND SHALLOTS

I wish I could take credit for dreaming up this side dish, but I saw something like it in a deli and reproduced a light version at home. It features Brussels sprouts dressed up with sautéed sliced shallots, minced garlic, toasted pecans, and bacon bits.

FOOD SYNERGY NOTES | *This dish packs the synergy of a cruciferous vegetable plus a little smart fat from canola oil and the phytochemicals in onions and nuts.*

Makes 8 servings

8	cups Brussels sprouts, trimmed and halved	¾	cup pecan pieces, lightly toasted in a nonstick skillet
4	slices turkey bacon	2	teaspoons brown sugar
1	tablespoon canola oil		Salt and ground pepper (optional)
1	cup sliced shallots		
1	teaspoon minced garlic		

Steam the Brussels sprouts by microwaving on high in a covered dish with a few tablespoons of water for 6 minutes, or until just barely tender. Drain and set aside.

PER SERVING:

CALORIES	FAT CAL	PROTEIN	CARB	FIBER	CHOLEST	TOTAL FAT	SAT FAT	MONO FAT	POLY FAT	OMEGA-3	OMEGA-6	SODIUM
170	47%	6 g	16 g	4 g	6 mg	9 g	1.3 g	2.5 g	2 g	0.5 g	1 g	117 mg

Meanwhile, in a large nonstick skillet coated with canola-oil cooking spray, cook the bacon over medium-high heat, flipping often, until crisp. Cool on a paper towel, then chop into small pieces. Set aside.

Add the oil to the same pan and heat over medium-high heat. Add the shallots and cook, stirring frequently, for 2 minutes. Add the garlic and cook for 1 to 2 minutes more, or until the shallots are golden. Stir in the Brussels sprouts and cook for 1 to 2 minutes, or until the sprouts begin to brown.

Sprinkle the pecans and sugar over the top and stir to blend. Reduce the heat to medium-low and continue to cook for another minute, stirring occasionally. Add salt and pepper to taste, if desired. Transfer to a serving bowl and sprinkle with the reserved bacon.

% DAILY VALUE FOR:

VIT A	VIT C	VIT E	VIT B$_1$	VIT B$_2$	VIT B$_3$	VIT B$_6$	FOLATE	CAL	MAG	POT	SELEN	ZINC
14%	102%	8%	12%	8%	5%	21%	15%	5%	8%	12%	3%	8%

QUICK SPINACH ITALIANO

You can whip up this side dish in about 5 minutes. It's an easy way to add a serving of vegetables instead of the usual side salad.

FOOD SYNERGY NOTES | *The synergy of dark green leafy vegetables along with a little smart fat (olive oil) is in this dish.*

Makes 4 servings

1½ tablespoons olive oil	Salt (optional)
2 teaspoons bottled minced garlic	Freshly ground black pepper
1 pound frozen chopped spinach, partially thawed	2 tablespoons shredded Parmesan cheese

Heat the oil in a large nonstick skillet over medium heat until hot but not smoking. Add the garlic and cook, stirring frequently, for 30 seconds.

Stir in the spinach and cook, stirring frequently, for a few minutes, or until heated through. Add salt (if desired) and pepper to taste, then sprinkle the cheese over the top.

PER SERVING:

CALORIES	FAT CAL	PROTEIN	CARB	FIBER	CHOLEST	TOTAL FAT	SAT FAT	MONO FAT	POLY FAT	OMEGA-3	OMEGA-6	SODIUM
92	59%	5 g	5 g	4 g	1 mg	6 g	1.5 g	4 g	0.6 g	0.2 g	0.4 g	84 mg

% DAILY VALUE FOR:

VIT A	VIT C	VIT E	VIT B$_1$	VIT B$_2$	VIT B$_3$	VIT B$_6$	FOLATE	CAL	MAG	POT	SELEN	ZINC
126%	37%	12%	9%	16%	4%	14%	34%	16%	21%	32%	3%	6%

STOVETOP SPANAKORIZO (SPINACH AND RICE)

I tweaked this Greek side-dish recipe by using less oil to lower the calories and switching to brown rice to increase the fiber and other nutrients.

Loaded with nutrients from brown rice, onions, spinach, and tomato sauce, the olive oil enhances the availability of many of them.

FOOD SYNERGY NOTES

Makes 6 servings

2	tablespoons extra-virgin olive oil
2	small sweet onions, chopped (about 1½ cups)
20	ounces frozen chopped spinach, slightly thawed
⅓	cup white wine or chicken or vegetable broth
1½	cups tomato sauce or bottled marinara sauce
2	cups water
¾	teaspoon dried dillweed
1	teaspoon chopped parsley
⅔	cup uncooked brown rice
	Salt (optional)
	Ground black pepper
¼	cup crumbled Gorgonzola or feta cheese

Heat the oil in a large nonstick skillet or saucepan over medium-high heat. Add the onions and cook, stirring frequently, for 3 to 4 minutes, or until soft and lightly brown. Add the spinach and wine or broth and cook, stirring frequently, for a few minutes. Stir in the tomato or marinara sauce, water, dillweed, parsley, and rice and bring to a boil.

Reduce the heat to low, cover the pan, and simmer for 45 to 50 minutes, or until the rice is tender. Add salt (if using) and pepper to taste.

Add a sprinkling of cheese over each serving.

PER SERVING:

CALORIES	FAT CAL	PROTEIN	CARB	FIBER	CHOLEST	TOTAL FAT	SAT FAT	MONO FAT	POLY FAT	OMEGA-3	OMEGA-6	SODIUM
215	28%	7 g	32 g	6 g	4 mg	6.7 g	1.8 g	3.8 g	0.8 g	0.2 g	0.6 g	500 mg

% DAILY VALUE FOR:

VIT A	VIT C	VIT E	VIT B₁	VIT B₂	VIT B₃	VIT B₆	FOLATE	CAL	MAG	POT	SELEN	ZINC
115%	46%	17%	21%	19%	16%	31%	33%	15%	32%	19%	12%	14%

SAVORY BARLEY

If you want to use homemade or canned broth, just substitute 3 cups of broth for the water and broth powder called for below. This is a great base recipe to use in any other recipe calling for cooked barley, which adds so much flavor along with all its fiber and nutritional attributes.

FOOD SYNERGY NOTES | *This is a great basic dish to enjoy the food synergy and fiber in barley, and each serving will also include ⅛ cup of chopped onion and all the phytochemicals that come with it.*

Makes 4 servings

1   cup pearl barley

3   cups water

1   tablespoon chicken broth powder

1   teaspoon garlic-and-herb salt-free seasoning blend

½   cup chopped onion

In a medium saucepan, place the barley, water, broth powder, seasoning, and onion and stir to blend. Bring to a boil. Reduce the heat to a simmer, cover with a tight-fitting lid, and cook for 1 hour, or until all the liquid is absorbed.

Serve immediately or let cool, then keep in the refrigerator for use in recipes that call for cooked barley.

PER SERVING:

CALORIES	FAT CAL	PROTEIN	CARB	FIBER	CHOLEST	TOTAL FAT	SAT FAT	MONO FAT	POLY FAT	OMEGA-3	OMEGA-6	SODIUM
195	4%	6 g	43 g	8.5 g	0 mg	0.8 g	0.2 g	0.2 g	0.3 g	0.1 g	0.3 g	580 mg

% DAILY VALUE FOR:

VIT C	VIT E	VIT B₁	VIT B₂	VIT B₃	VIT B₆	FOLATE	CAL	MAG	POT	SELEN	ZINC
3%	1%	11%	7%	18%	14%	5%	3%	14%	6%	36%	14%

BARLEY MUSHROOM BAKE

This is a delicious way to introduce your family to the whole grain barley. It is worth the time it takes to bake this dish. You might want to double the recipe if you have a family of four or more, especially because leftovers taste great the next day, too.

High-viscous-fiber barley is the base of this dish. It includes some plant omega-3s and monounsaturated fat from canola oil and pine nuts, plus phytochemicals from onions and mushrooms.

FOOD SYNERGY NOTES

Makes 4 servings

1½	tablespoons canola oil
1	yellow or white onion, chopped
1	cup pearl barley
¼	cup pine nuts
3	green onions, thinly sliced
1	cup sliced cremini mushrooms
½	cup chopped fresh parsley
¼	teaspoon salt (optional)
⅛	teaspoon ground pepper
2	cans (14 ounces each) vegetable broth

Preheat the oven to 350°F.

Heat the oil in a large ovenproof saucepan over medium-high heat. Stir in the yellow or white onion, barley, and pine nuts. Cook and stir for 3 to 4 minutes, or until the barley is lightly browned. Mix in the green onions, mushrooms, parsley, salt (if desired), pepper, and broth.

Bake uncovered for 1 hour 15 minutes, or until the liquid is absorbed and the barley is tender.

PER SERVING:

CALORIES	FAT CAL	PROTEIN	CARB	FIBER	CHOLEST	TOTAL FAT	SAT FAT	MONO FAT	POLY FAT	OMEGA-3	OMEGA-6	SODIUM
335	27%	10 g	53 g	11 g	0 mg	10 g	1.2 g	4.8 g	3.7 g	0.6 g	3.1 g	390 mg

% DAILY VALUE FOR:

VIT A	VIT C	VIT E	VIT B₁	VIT B₂	VIT B₃	VIT B₆	FOLATE	CAL	MAG	POT	SELEN	ZINC
15%	15%	11%	20%	16%	25%	20%	11%	6%	23%	12%	41%	22%

BARLEY EGGPLANT BAKE

The trick here is cooking the barley ahead of time so that all you have to do is assemble this dish and pop it in the microwave oven.

FOOD SYNERGY NOTES | *This recipe includes whole grain barley, plus the viscous-fiber vegetable eggplant. It also contains some low-fat dairy plus monounsaturated fat and phytochemical-rich onions.*

Makes 3 servings

3	cups cooked pearl barley
¾	cup thinly sliced sweet or yellow onion
1	small eggplant, cut into ¼"-thick slices
3	teaspoons extra-virgin olive oil (flavored works well)

1½	teaspoons garlic-and-herb salt-free seasoning blend
	Ground black pepper
3	ounces reduced-fat Cheddar cheese (¾ cup shredded or 4 thin slices)

Spoon the barley evenly into the bottom of a microwave-safe 9" deep-dish pie plate (or similar casserole dish). Spread half the onion evenly over the barley. Layer the eggplant to cover the barley completely. Drizzle with the oil and sprinkle with the seasoning blend and black pepper. Spread the remaining onion slices over the top of the eggplant. Cover with a microwave-safe cover and cook on high for 12 minutes, or until the eggplant is soft and cooked throughout.

Layer the cheese over the top and cook on high, covered or uncovered, for 1 minute longer, just until the cheese is nicely melted.

PER SERVING:

CALORIES	FAT CAL	PROTEIN	CARB	FIBER	CHOLEST	TOTAL FAT	SAT FAT	MONO FAT	POLY FAT	OMEGA-3	OMEGA-6	SODIUM
350	26%	13 g	56 g	9 g	15 mg	10 g	3.8 g	3.7 g	0.9 g	0.1 g	0.8 g	179 mg

% DAILY VALUE FOR:

VIT A	VIT C	VIT E	VIT B₁	VIT B₂	VIT B₃	VIT B₆	FOLATE	CAL	MAG	POT	SELEN	ZINC
9%	8%	6%	19%	12%	27%	25%	12%	24%	16%	12%	26%	19%

MAPLE ROASTED SQUASH WITH APPLE FILLING

You're getting two whole foods with synergy in this side dish: vegetables and apples with skin. The margarine adds plant sterols, too (part of the Portfolio plan).

Makes 8 servings

4	acorn squash, halved lengthwise and seeded
	Salt and freshly ground black pepper
8	teaspoons plant sterol–enriched margarine or whipped butter
4	tablespoons maple syrup or 8 tablespoons light pancake syrup
3	apples, cored and diced
2	tablespoons finely chopped assorted fresh herbs (thyme, rosemary, parsley) or 2 teaspoons dry herbs

Preheat the oven to 450°F.

Place the squash cut-side up on a baking pan. Season insides with salt and pepper to taste.

Place 1 teaspoon of the margarine or whipped butter and ½ tablespoon of maple syrup (or 1 tablespoon light syrup) into the bowl of each squash half. Add the apples and sprinkle the herbs over the top.

Roast until tender about 1 hour, or until nicely browned, spooning syrup from the squash bowl over the top of the apples about every 20 minutes.

PER SERVING:

CALORIES	FAT CAL	PROTEIN	CARB	FIBER	CHOLEST	TOTAL FAT	SAT FAT	MONO FAT	POLY FAT	OMEGA-3	OMEGA-6	SODIUM
175	12%	2 g	41 g	6 g	0 mg	2.3 g	0.3 g	0.6 g	1.2 g	0.2 g	1 g	7 mg

% DAILY VALUE FOR:

VIT A	VIT C	VIT E	VIT B₁	VIT B₂	VIT B₃	VIT B₆	FOLATE	CAL	MAG	POT	SELEN	ZINC
19%	38%	7%	29%	3%	11%	28%	10%	8%	23%	25%	3%	9%

BARLEY-STUFFED TOMATOES

FOOD SYNERGY NOTES | *This side dish features the high-viscous-fiber whole grain barley; the antioxidant-rich tomato; and a nut rich in phytochemicals and plant omega-3s.*

Makes 9 servings

½	cup pearl barley, uncooked		¼	teaspoon salt (optional)
2¾	cups vegetable broth (use less-sodium broth if desired)*		¼	teaspoon ground pepper + more to taste
9	small red tomatoes, washed and halved vertically		2	green onions (white and green parts), finely chopped
½	cup shredded Romano or Parmesan cheese		¼	cup toasted pine nuts**
1	teaspoon dried oregano		¼	cup shredded Parmesan cheese (optional)

Preheat the oven to 375°F.

In a medium saucepan, combine the barley and broth and bring to a boil over high heat. Reduce the heat and simmer, covered, for 45 minutes, or until the moisture is absorbed and the barley is just tender. Let cool.

Hollow out the tomato halves and chop the insides, then spoon the insides into a small bowl after draining any excess liquid. Set aside the tomato halves.

PER SERVING:

CALORIES	FAT CAL	PROTEIN	CARB	FIBER	CHOLEST	TOTAL FAT	SAT FAT	MONO FAT	POLY FAT	OMEGA-3	OMEGA-6	SODIUM
99	29%	5 g	15 g	3.5 g	3 mg	3.2 g	0.8 g	0.8 g	1.2 g	0.2 g	1 g	182 mg

In a large bowl, mix the reserved barley, the ½ cup Romano or Parmesan, oregano, chopped tomato, salt (if desired), pepper, onions, and pine nuts. Fill each tomato half with a spoonful of the mixture and place in a 13" × 9" baking dish. Sprinkle the ¼ cup Parmesan, if using, evenly over the top of each tomato, if desired. Bake uncovered for 30 minutes, or until the tomatoes are soft but still slightly firm and the cheese is lightly browned on top.

Beef broth can be used in place of vegetable broth. If you use low-sodium broth, it will reduce the sodium per serving significantly.

** *To toast pine nuts, add them to a small non-stick skillet and heat over medium heat, stirring frequently, for 6 to 8 minutes, or until golden brown.*

% DAILY VALUE FOR:

VIT A	VIT C	VIT E	VIT B₁	VIT B₂	VIT B₃	VIT B₆	FOLATE	CAL	MAG	POT	SELEN	ZINC
13%	24%	3%	10%	6%	9%	8%	5%	3%	9%	8	9%	6%

BAKED BUTTERNUT MACARONI

For 8 to 12 servings, just double the ingredients and use a 13" × 9" baking dish.

FOOD SYNERGY NOTES *Two kinds of squash, butternut and acorn, provide an assortment of carotenes and vitamins, many of which offer synergy together. Each serving also contributes some low-fat dairy and about 2 whole grain servings.*

Makes 6 servings

1	medium butternut squash, halved lengthwise and seeded, or 1 pound frozen butternut cubes
1	medium acorn squash (1½ pounds), halved lengthwise and seeded
2	teaspoons olive oil
	Freshly ground black pepper
	Salt (optional)
1	cup fat-free half-and-half or whole milk

	Freshly ground nutmeg
8	cups cooked whole grain–blend macaroni or penne pasta
⅔	cup shredded Parmesan cheese
⅓	cup part-skim ricotta cheese
2	tablespoons whipped butter
¼	cup plain or seasoned dry bread crumbs
¼	cup ground gingersnap cookies

Place the butternut squash halves cut-side down on a microwaveable baking dish or plate and microwave on high power for 8 minutes, or until tender. If using frozen squash, place in a microwaveable dish and microwave for 4 minutes, or until tender. Then place the acorn squash cut-side down on a microwaveable baking dish or plate and microwave for 8 minutes, or until tender.

Preheat the oven broiler. Coat a foil-lined jelly-roll pan and a 9" × 9" baking dish with canola-oil cooking spray.

PER SERVING:

CALORIES	FAT CAL	PROTEIN	CARB	FIBER	CHOLEST	TOTAL FAT	SAT FAT	MONO FAT	POLY FAT	OMEGA-3	OMEGA-6	SODIUM
428	19%	18 g	74 g	8 g	17 mg	9 g	4 g	4 g	1 g	0.2 g	0.8 g	266 mg

Cut the squash flesh into cubes, discarding the skins. Add the cubes to a large bowl and drizzle with the oil. Spread on the prepared jelly-roll pan, season with the pepper and salt (if desired) to taste, and broil for 3 to 4 minutes, or until lightly browned in some areas. Reduce the oven temperature to 350°F.

In a food processor, combine the squash and half-and-half or milk and process until smooth. Add the nutmeg and pulse briefly to blend well. Pour into a large bowl and stir in the pasta and Parmesan. Pour into the prepared baking dish. Dot with the ricotta.

Add the butter to a small nonstick saucepan and cook over medium heat, stirring constantly, until nicely brown (it will smell like caramel). Add the bread crumbs and cookies and stir to combine. Sprinkle evenly over the pasta mixture. Bake for 30 minutes, or until heated through.

% DAILY VALUE FOR:

VIT A	VIT C	VIT E	VIT B$_1$	VIT B$_2$	VIT B$_3$	VIT B$_6$	VIT B$_{12}$	FOLATE	CAL	VIT D	MAG	POT	SELEN	ZINC
63%	17%	6%	38%	20%	20%	28%	7%	12%	24%	3%	31%	15%	101%	28%

Main Dishes

PORTOBELLO TACOS

FOOD SYNERGY NOTES | *This dish has synergy, being a vegetarian option to a high-fat entrée, and each taco has a serving of a low-fat dairy. Plus, the phytochemicals from the mushrooms, olive oil, onion, zucchini, and tomato-based salsa contribute synergy.*

Makes 4 servings

About 4 medium portobello mushrooms, stems removed and cut into ½"-thick pieces	Salt and ground pepper
2 teaspoons dried oregano	8 corn or flour tortillas
1½ tablespoons olive oil	1 cup (4 ounces) shredded reduced-fat Monterey Jack cheese
3 medium zucchini, cut into ½"-thick pieces	½ cup prepared salsa
1 medium red onion, halved and sliced ¼" thick	

Preheat the oven to 425°F. Line a jelly-roll pan with nonstick foil.

In a large bowl, combine the mushrooms, oregano, oil, zucchini, and onion. Season to taste with salt and pepper and toss to blend well.

Spoon the mixture evenly onto the jelly-roll pan. Roast the vegetables for 30 minutes, tossing occasionally.

Soften the tortillas by wrapping them in a damp cloth or paper towel and heating them in the microwave oven for 1 minute or warming them in a non-stick skillet (use a little canola-oil cooking spray, if you like).

Divide the mushroom mixture, cheese, and salsa among the tortillas and roll up.

PER SERVING:

CALORIES	FAT CAL	PROTEIN	CARB	FIBER	CHOLEST	TOTAL FAT	SAT FAT	MONO FAT	POLY FAT	OMEGA-3	OMEGA-6	SODIUM
299	39%	14 g	37 g	6.2 g	20 mg	13 g	5 g	4.4 g	1.3 g	0.1 g	1.2 g	333 mg

% DAILY VALUE FOR:

VIT A	VIT C	VIT E	VIT B₁	VIT B₂	VIT B₃	VIT B₆	VIT B₁₂	FOLATE	CAL	MAG	POT	SELEN	ZINC
19%	25%	8%	21%	48%	30%	28%	11%	26%	32%	24%	24%	17%	36%

PORTOBELLO MUSHROOM BURGER
WITH GARLIC MAYONNAISE

I'm a portobello mushroom lover, and I've grilled or broiled my fair share of them over the years. To make garlic mayonnaise, combine 1 tablespoon of light mayonnaise with ½ teaspoon of minced garlic, plus a splash of lemon juice and Worcestershire, if you like.

Another vegetarian alternative to a meat-laden meal, this sandwich boasts whole grain synergy from the bun.

FOOD
SYNERGY
NOTES

Makes 2

2	portobello mushrooms (about 3½" wide), cleaned and stems removed
1	tablespoon low-fat bottled marinade
2	large, thin slices reduced-fat Jack cheese (about 2 ounces)

2	leaves fresh romaine lettuce
2	multigrain or whole wheat hamburger buns
4	tomato slices
1	tablespoon garlic mayonnaise

Preheat the toaster oven to 400°F or heat the grill. Place the mushrooms on a sheet of foil, round-side down, and drizzle the marinade evenly over the top. Bake for 10 to 12 minutes a side or cook directly on a hot grill for 8 to 10 minutes a side, or until tender. Place the cheese on top and continue to bake or grill briefly to melt the cheese.

Assemble your sandwich by placing the lettuce leaf and tomato on the bottom half of each bun. Top with the cheese-topped mushroom and spread the top bun lightly with half of the garlic mayonnaise, then place on top of the mushroom (the lettuce keeps the bottom bun from getting soggy).

PER BURGER:

CALORIES	FAT CAL	PROTEIN	CARB	FIBER	CHOLEST	TOTAL FAT	SAT FAT	MONO FAT	POLY FAT	OMEGA-3	OMEGA-6	SODIUM
246	31%	14 g	31 g	5.5 g	22 mg	8.5 g	4 g	2 g	2 g	0.2 g	1.1 g	810 mg

% DAILY VALUE FOR:

VIT A	VIT C	VIT E	VIT B₁	VIT B₂	VIT B₃	VIT B₆	VIT B₁₂	FOLATE	CAL	MAG	POT	SELEN	ZINC
21%	22%	6%	20%	49%	35%	17%	11%	11%	26%	18%	17%	50%	37%

BAKED BEEF MEATBALLS (WITH SPINACH) AND TOMATO SAUCE

Because these meatballs are lean, they can be dressed up with a light crumb coating. I pair these meatballs with a homemade tomato sauce, but you can serve them with a sauce of your choosing.

FOOD SYNERGY NOTES | *This savory dish features two Synergy Super Foods—spinach and tomatoes. Serve it over a whole grain pasta, and you'll have three stars on your plate.*

Makes 30 meatballs (5 main-dish servings) and 4 cups sauce

SAUCE

4	teaspoons extra-virgin olive oil
1	can (28 ounces) whole peeled or diced tomatoes in juice
1	can (6 ounces) low-sodium tomato paste + 3–6 ounces more if necessary to thicken
½	cup light or nonalcoholic beer or wine or broth

1½	teaspoons Italian seasoning
1	teaspoon garlic powder
1½	teaspoons chopped parsley
¾	teaspoon salt (optional)
⅛	teaspoon freshly ground black pepper or white pepper

MEATBALLS

1½	pounds super-lean ground beef (around 6% fat)
1½	cups (10-ounce box) frozen spinach, thawed and drained
½	cup grated or shredded Parmesan cheese
1	large beaten egg (omega-3, if available) or ¼ cup egg substitute

1½	teaspoons Italian seasoning
1½	teaspoons parsley
1	teaspoon garlic powder
½	teaspoon salt
¾	cup seasoned or plain dry bread crumbs

PER SERVING:

CALORIES	FAT CAL	PROTEIN	CARB	FIBER	CHOLEST	TOTAL FAT	SAT FAT	MONO FAT	POLY FAT	OMEGA-3	OMEGA-6	SODIUM
337	32%	26 g	31 g	5.3 g	33 mg	12 g	3.7 g	5.8 g	1 g	0.3 g	0.4 g	990 mg

Preheat the oven to 400°F.

To make the sauce: Add the oil to a large nonstick saucepan or skillet over medium heat. Add the tomatoes; tomato paste; beer, wine, or broth; Italian seasoning; garlic powder; parsley; salt, if desired; and pepper. Use a potato masher to crush the tomatoes while the mixture heats up. When the mixture comes to a gentle boil, reduce the heat to low and continue to simmer, covered, for about 30 minutes.

To make the meatballs: In a large mixing bowl, combine the beef, spinach, Parmesan cheese, egg, Italian seasoning, parsley, garlic powder, salt, and ¼ cup of the bread crumbs. Using your hands or a standing mixer, mix all ingredients together until nicely blended.

Place the remaining ½ cup bread crumbs in a small bowl. Shape meatballs using a cookie scoop to measure exactly ⅛ cup. Roll each in the bread crumbs and lightly coat with canola-oil cooking spray. Place each in a mini muffin cup (or on a nonstick jelly-roll pan). Bake for 20 minutes, or until the meatballs are cooked throughout and nicely brown on the outside. Serve with the pizza sauce as either an appetizer or entrée.

% DAILY VALUE FOR:

VIT A	VIT C	VIT E	VIT B$_1$	VIT B$_2$	VIT B$_3$	VIT B$_6$	VIT B$_{12}$	FOLATE	CAL	VIT D	MAG	POT	SELEN	ZINC
89%	62%	22%	21%	58%	51%	40%	91%	25%	18%	8%	28%	34%	5%	63%

SAUSAGE AND SAFFRON RICE

If fresh chile peppers aren't available, substitute ½ teaspoon crushed red pepper.

FOOD SYNERGY NOTES | *This dish starts with the whole grain synergy of brown rice and ends with the synergy in soy protein (from the vegetarian sausage); the phytochemicals and smart fat in olive oil; and the phytochemicals in the chile peppers, garlic and onions, and tomato.*

Makes 4 servings

1	tablespoon olive oil	5–6	ounces vegetarian sausage, cut into ½" slices
1	small red chile pepper, stemmed, seeded, and finely minced (optional) (wear plastic gloves when handling)	1	cup diced vine-ripened tomato
		2	bay leaves
2	teaspoons minced garlic	¼	cup chopped green onions
1	cup long-grain brown rice		Salt and freshly ground black pepper
1¾	cups vegetable broth		
	Pinch of saffron threads		

Heat the oil in a medium nonstick saucepan over medium-high heat. Add the chile pepper (if desired) and garlic and cook, stirring frequently, for 1 minute. Stir in the rice and let it brown in the oil for 1 minute. Stir in the broth, saffron, sausage, tomato, and bay leaves. Bring to a boil.

Reduce the heat to simmer, cover, and cook for 35 to 40 minutes, or until the rice is tender. Let the mixture sit in the covered saucepan for 10 minutes. Stir in the onions and season to taste with salt and pepper.

PER SERVING:

CALORIES	FAT CAL	PROTEIN	CARB	FIBER	CHOLEST	TOTAL FAT	SAT FAT	MONO FAT	POLY FAT	OMEGA-3	OMEGA-6	SODIUM
291	23%	14 g	43 g	5 g	0 mg	7.6 g	0.5 g	3 g	4.1 g	0.4 g	3.7 g	620 mg

% DAILY VALUE FOR:

VIT A	VIT C	VIT E	VIT B$_1$	VIT B$_2$	VIT B$_3$	VIT B$_6$	FOLATE	CAL	MAG	POT	SELEN	ZINC
60%	46%	11%	95%	19%	47%	46%	6%	5%	27%	9%	25%	19%

PORTFOLIO PESTO

Pesto purists might prefer to blend the pesto and then stir in the edamame, but I like blending them together for a thicker pesto, then using it as a spread for bread and sandwiches.

I call this Portfolio Pesto because it incorporates almonds and soy (two of the Portfolio plan prescription foods). It also includes the phytochemicals and monounsaturated fat from olive oil.

FOOD
SYNERGY
NOTES

Makes 7 servings (1¾ cups)

3	cups lightly packed fresh basil leaves	½	cup shredded Parmesan cheese
4	tablespoons extra-virgin olive oil	1	teaspoon minced garlic
⅓	cup double-strength chicken or vegetable broth		Dash of salt (optional)
			Dash of ground pepper
½	cup roasted almonds	1	cup shelled edamame (cooked green soybeans)

In a food processor, combine the basil, oil, broth, almonds, cheese, garlic, salt (if desired), and pepper and pulse, scraping the sides of the bowl after 5 seconds, until well blended, about 10 seconds. Stir in the edamame.

Cover and store in the refrigerator until needed. The top of the pesto will turn light brown due to being exposed to oxygen. If you want to avoid this, you can squeeze some lemon juice over the top before covering and storing.

When you're ready to use the pesto in a hot pasta dish, warm it up in a small nonstick saucepan or skillet, adding more broth as needed for your desired consistency. Toss with about 3 cups of cooked noodles. If using for a cold dish, just spoon or spread as needed.

PER ¼ CUP (PREPARED WITHOUT SALT):

CALORIES	FAT CAL	PROTEIN	CARB	FIBER	CHOLEST	TOTAL FAT	SAT FAT	MONO SAT	POLY FAT	OMEGA-3	OMEGA-6	SODIUM
196	70%	9 g	7 g	3.5 g	3 mg	14.5 g	2.4 g	9 g	3 g	0.3 g	2.6 g	123 mg

% DAILY VALUE FOR:

VIT A	VIT C	VIT E	VIT B$_1$	VIT B$_2$	VIT B$_3$	VIT B$_6$	VIT B$_{12}$	FOLATE	CAL	MAG	POT	SELEN	ZINC
11%	19%	26%	15%	21%	9%	4%	1%	19%	16%	13%	12%	2%	7%

HOMEMADE PIZZA SAUCE

I love this stuff! It's a thick, full-flavored sauce that works great on pizza, but it also works well anywhere you would put a marinara sauce.

FOOD SYNERGY NOTES | *The added olive oil contributes the "good" fat that helps your body absorb the protective phytochemicals, like the lycopene in tomatoes.*

Makes 10 servings (5 cups)

4	teaspoons olive oil
28	ounces whole peeled tomatoes (canned in tomato juice)
1	can (12 ounces) tomato paste
1	teaspoon garlic powder

½	tablespoon parsley flakes
½	tablespoon Italian seasoning
¾	teaspoon salt
⅛	teaspoon white pepper

In a large nonstick saucepan, combine the oil, tomatoes, tomato paste, garlic powder, parsley, seasoning, salt, and pepper. Use a potato masher to break the tomatoes into smaller pieces. Cover and cook over medium-low heat for 40 to 50 minutes, or until the sauce is thick.

PER ¼ CUP (PREPARED WITHOUT SALT):

CALORIES	FAT CAL	PROTEIN	CARB	FIBER	CHOLEST	TOTAL FAT	SAT FAT	MONO SAT	POLY FAT	OMEGA-3	OMEGA-6	SODIUM
196	70%	9 g	7 g	3.5 g	3 mg	14.5 g	2.4 g	9 g	3 g	0.3 g	2.6 g	123 mg

% DAILY VALUE FOR:

VIT A	VIT C	VIT E	VIT B₁	VIT B₂	VIT B₃	VIT B₆	VIT B₁₂	FOLATE	CAL	MAG	POT	SELEN	ZINC
11%	19%	26%	15%	21%	9%	4%	1%	19%	16%	13%	12%	2%	7%

BUTTERNUT SQUASH RAVIOLI
WITH LEMON CREAM SAUCE

This dish is fabulous with a side of broccoli or asparagus spears. I had a pasta dish similar to this at a fabulous Italian restaurant and immediately went home and tried to reproduce it—this comes close!

Butternut squash is a phytochemical-rich veggie bursting with carotenes and vitamin C. We've added some plant sterol–enriched margarine and other synergy-rich vegetables like broccoli.

FOOD
SYNERGY
NOTES

Makes 4 servings

8	ounces fresh or frozen butternut squash ravioli
3	tablespoons plant sterol–enriched margarine
4	tablespoons lemon curd
2	teaspoons Wondra quick-mixing flour

⅔	cup fat-free half-and-half
	Ground white pepper
4	cups steamed asparagus or broccoli spears, cooked until just tender

In a large pot of salted boiling water, cook the ravioli according to package instructions for 10 minutes, or until tender but still firm to the bite. Drain well and transfer to a serving bowl.

Melt the margarine in a small nonstick saucepan over medium heat. Reduce the heat to low and whisk in the lemon curd. When smooth, whisk in the flour, then the half-and-half. Continue to cook over low heat, whisking frequently, for 2 minutes, or until it starts to boil. Pour over the reserved ravioli and toss gently to coat well. Season with pepper to taste. Serve with the asparagus or broccoli.

PER SERVING:

CALORIES	FAT CAL	PROTEIN	CARB	FIBER	CHOLEST	TOTAL FAT	SAT FAT	MONO FAT	POLY FAT	OMEGA-3	OMEGA-6	SODIUM
423	20%	16 g	73 g	11 g	5 mg	9.2 g	2 g	3.6 g	3.1 g	0.6 g	2 g	189 mg

% DAILY VALUE FOR:

VIT A	VIT C	VIT E	VIT B₁	VIT B₂	VIT B₃	VIT B₆	VIT B₁₂	FOLATE	CAL	MAG	POT	SELEN	ZINC
214%	196%	16%	40%	42%	31%	37%	7%	50%	33%	37%	32%	48%	24%

LIGHT SPINACH AND ARTICHOKE HEART ALFREDO

One of the most popular appetizers at the Cheesecake Factory is the Hot Spinach and Cheese Dip. The savory combination of white sauce, cheeses, artichoke hearts, spinach, garlic, and other seasonings really hits the spot. Turns out this dip makes a mighty wonderful pasta sauce, too. You can make a batch and keep the sauce in the refrigerator. Just heat some up and stir in some pasta—easy and delicious.

FOOD SYNERGY NOTES | *This entrée includes the synergy of whole grains, garlic and onions, carotene-rich spinach, lower-fat dairy products, and plant sterol–enriched margarine.*

Makes 6 servings

8	cups low-sodium chicken broth or water
4	cups dried multigrain pasta
1	tablespoon plant sterol–enriched margarine
2	cups whole milk
4	tablespoons Wondra quick-mixing flour
⅛	teaspoon ground nutmeg
½	cup shredded Parmesan cheese
	Salt and ground white pepper (optional)

1	tablespoon minced or chopped garlic
¼	cup chopped green onions
1	package (10 ounces) frozen chopped spinach, thawed and gently squeezed of excess water
1	can (14 ounces) artichoke hearts (water packed), drained and chopped
1	cup shredded part-skim mozzarella cheese

Bring the broth or water to a boil in a large saucepan. Add the pasta and bring to a rapid boil. Cook uncovered, stirring frequently, for 13 to 15 minutes, or until cooked to desired doneness. Drain.

PER SERVING:

CALORIES	FAT CAL	PROTEIN	CARB	FIBER	CHOLEST	TOTAL FAT	SAT FAT	MONO FAT	POLY FAT	OMEGA-3	OMEGA-6	SODIUM
472	23%	28 g	69 g	9 g	31 mg	12 g	6.3 g	2.8 g	1.2 g	0.3 g	0.8 g	464 mg

Meanwhile, make the sauce. Melt the margarine in a medium nonstick saucepan. Stir in ⅓ cup of the milk, the flour, and the nutmeg. Slowly stir in the remaining milk. Bring to a gentle boil over medium-high heat. Reduce the heat to medium-low and continue to gently boil, stirring constantly until the sauce thickens (about 4 minutes). Stir in the Parmesan and season to taste with salt and pepper, if desired.

In a large nonstick saucepan, combine the garlic, green onions, spinach, artichokes, hot Alfredo sauce, and mozzarella and stir with a spoon to blend. Bring to a gentle boil over medium heat. Reduce the heat to low, cover, and continue to cook for a couple minutes to blend the flavors. Stir in the cooked pasta and serve hot.

NOTE: *Another way to cook this dish is to pour the hot Alfredo sauce into a large mixing bowl and stir in the garlic, green onions, spinach, artichoke hearts, mozzarella, and pasta. Spoon into a 13" × 9" baking pan coated with canola-oil cooking spray. Bake in a 375°F oven for 30 minutes or until bubbling.*

% DAILY VALUE FOR:

VIT A	VIT C	VIT E	VIT B$_1$	VIT B$_2$	VIT B$_3$	VIT B$_6$	VIT B$_{12}$	FOLATE	CAL	MAG	POT	SELEN	ZINC
68%	22%	7%	43%	40%	32%	27%	23%	31%	44%	52%	17%	11%	40%

PENNE WITH CREAMY TOMATO VODKA SAUCE

Barilla makes a wonderful multigrain pasta. Loaded with a wealth of nutritional benefits, its taste and texture are remarkably similar to regular pasta.

Makes 6 servings

1	package (16 ounces) multigrain penne pasta	1	teaspoon crushed red pepper (optional)
2	tablespoons extra-virgin olive oil	¾	cup chopped fresh basil
¾	cup chopped sweet onion		Salt and pepper
1	tablespoon minced or chopped garlic	¼	cup vodka
1	can (28 ounces) Italian-style diced tomatoes	1	cup fat-free half-and-half
		1	cup low-fat or whole milk
		½	cup grated Parmesan cheese

In a large pot, bring lightly salted water to a boil. Add the pasta and cook for 8 to 10 minutes, or until al dente. Drain the pasta in a colander.

Meanwhile, heat the oil in a large nonstick skillet over medium heat. Add the onion and garlic and cook, stirring frequently, for 2 to 3 minutes, or until tender. Stir in the tomatoes, red pepper (if desired), basil, and salt and pepper to taste. Bring to a gentle boil, then reduce the heat to a simmer and cook for 10 minutes more.

Stir in the vodka and simmer for 10 minutes more. Stir in the half-and-half and milk and simmer another 10 minutes. Toss the sauce with the hot pasta and sprinkle with the cheese.

PER SERVING:

CALORIES	FAT CAL	PROTEIN	CARB	FIBER	CHOLEST	TOTAL FAT	SAT FAT	MONO FAT	POLY FAT	OMEGA-3	OMEGA-6	SODIUM
478	16%	20 g	79 g	8.1 g	10 mg	8.5 g	2.5 g	4.6 g	1 g	0.1 g	0.8 g	708 mg

% DAILY VALUE FOR:

VIT A	VIT C	VIT E	VIT B₁	VIT B₂	VIT B₃	VIT B₆	VIT B₁₂	FOLATE	CAL	MAG	POT	SELEN	ZINC
15%	28%	5%	42%	28%	27%	27%	10%	15%	37%	44%	14%	8%	28%

MARGI'S TORTELLINI AND SHRIMP SAUTÉ

When shopping for frozen tortellini, choose brands with around 5 grams of fat or less per 1⅓-cup serving.

The fish omega-3s may have synergy with the plant omega-3s from the canola oil, and the tomatoes have synergy with the fatty acids from both the shrimp and canola oil.

FOOD SYNERGY NOTES

Makes 4 servings

9½ ounces (half of a 19-ounce bag) frozen or fresh cheese tortellini	2 cups halved cherry tomatoes
2 tablespoons canola oil	1 cup coarsely chopped fresh basil, loosely packed
1½ cups coarsely chopped sweet onion	Salt and ground pepper (optional)
1 tablespoon minced garlic	
3 cups (15 ounces) cooked large shrimp	

Fill a large saucepan with water 4" deep and bring to a boil. Add the tortellini and cook according to package directions until just tender. Drain in a colander.

Meanwhile, heat the oil in a large nonstick skillet over medium-high heat. Add the onion and cook, stirring frequently, for 4 minutes. Stir in the garlic and continue cooking, stirring frequently, for 2 minutes more. Stir in the shrimp and tomatoes and cook for 2 minutes more, stirring often. Add the basil and tortellini and cook, stirring, for 1 minute more to allow the flavors to combine. Season to taste with salt and pepper, if desired.

PER SERVING:

CALORIES	FAT CAL	PROTEIN	CARB	FIBER	CHOLEST	TOTAL FAT	SAT FAT	OMEGA-3	OMEGA-6	SODIUM
360	27%	31.5 g	34.5 g	3.5 g	230 mg	10.5 g	2.3 g	1.1g	1.7 g	434 mg

% DAILY VALUE FOR:

VIT A	VIT C	VIT E	VIT D	VIT B₁	VIT B₂	VIT B₃	VIT B₆	VIT B₁₂	FOLATE	CAL	MAG	POT	SELEN	ZINC
25%	44%	16%	76%	11%	9%	25%	24%	66%	9%	16%	19%	16%	78%	25%

EASY MU SHU SHRIMP

This dish literally comes together in 10 minutes! With stir-fry becoming an increasingly popular dish, I've found prechopped bags of Asian veggies widely available in both the fresh and frozen sections of many grocery stores. If Napa cabbage isn't available, regular cabbage works well, too.

FOOD SYNERGY NOTES | *This dish has the synergy of plant omega-3s with fish omega-3s, vegetables with some smart fat (canola oil), and cruciferous vegetables. If you use whole wheat tortillas, you also have the synergy of whole grains.*

Makes 6 servings

1	tablespoon canola oil
1	bag (16 ounces) chopped Asian vegetables
2	teaspoons bottled minced garlic
2	cups frozen cooked shrimp, tail off; thawed, shredded roasted chicken or pork; or diced tofu
3	cups shredded Chinese or Napa cabbage, packed

2	large eggs (omega-3, if available), beaten with 2 teaspoons water
	Freshly ground black pepper
3	tablespoons bottled hoisin sauce
6	whole wheat flour tortillas

Heat the oil in the middle of a nonstick wok or large nonstick skillet over medium-high heat. Add the vegetables and garlic and cook, stirring frequently, for 2 minutes.

PER SERVING (WITH SHRIMP):

CALORIES	FAT CAL	PROTEIN	CARB	FIBER	CHOLEST	TOTAL FAT	SAT FAT	MONO FAT	POLY FAT	OMEGA-3	OMEGA-6	SODIUM
215	23%	18 g	29 g	6 g	163 mg	5.5 g	1 g	2.3 g	1.6 g	0.5 g	1.1 g	460 mg

Add the meat and cabbage and cook, stirring frequently, for 2 minutes more. Push the mixture around the sides of the wok or skillet to make a 4"-wide opening in the center.

Pour in the eggs and cook for 1 minute. Meanwhile, grind some black pepper lightly over the top. Toss the mixture together to finish cooking the eggs, about 1 minute more. Drizzle with the hoisin and toss to blend well.

Soften the tortillas by heating briefly in the microwave oven. Place some of the vegetable mixture in the center of each tortilla and roll up like a burrito.

% DAILY VALUE FOR:

VIT A	VIT C	VIT E	VIT D	VIT B$_1$	VIT B$_2$	VIT B$_3$	VIT B$_6$	VIT B$_{12}$	FOLATE	CAL	MAG	POT	SELEN	ZINC
33%	48%	13%	38%	16%	21%	19%	25%	36%	16%	11%	21%	21%	46%	23%

COCONUT FRIED RICE

To add another flavor boost to this dish, cook the rice in low-sodium chicken broth instead of water (unless you want to keep this a lacto-ovo-vegetarian dish). Feel free to add a tablespoon (or more to taste) of chopped red chile peppers along with the tomato for some heat.

FOOD SYNERGY NOTES *This dish starts with the food synergy in brown rice (a whole grain) and adds in the synergy of tomato phytochemicals in the presence of some smart fat— omega-3s in eggs and canola oil, plus the fish omega-3s in shrimp—and the combination of garlic and onions.*

Makes 4 servings

2	large eggs (omega-3, if available)
¼	cup egg substitute
1	tablespoon canola oil
1	onion, finely chopped
2–3	teaspoons minced garlic
½	teaspoon salt (optional)
½	teaspoon ground black pepper
2	tablespoons ketchup
1	cup finely diced tomato
¼	cup low-fat milk
	Pinch of saffron

	Pinch of curry powder
¼	teaspoon coconut extract
4	cups cooked brown rice
8	ounces or more frozen, cooked, shelled, and deveined shrimp, thawed (or diced tofu; or cooked shredded or diced chicken, beef, or pork if desired), optional
½	cup chopped green onions
¼	cup chopped fresh cilantro leaves

In a medium bowl, place the eggs and egg substitute and beat with a fork until well blended. Coat a large nonstick wok or skillet with cooking spray and place over medium-high heat. Pour in the egg mixture and either scramble or cook like an omelet. Set aside. If you made an omelet, cut it into shreds.

PER SERVING (WITHOUT SHRIMP):

CALORIES	FAT CAL	PROTEIN	CARB	FIBER	CHOLEST	TOTAL FAT	SAT FAT	MONO FAT	POLY FAT	OMEGA-3	OMEGA-6	SODIUM
350	21%	12 g	59 g	6 g	107 mg	8 g	1.5 g	3.9 g	2.2 g	0.4 g	1.8 g	181 mg

Add the oil to the wok or skillet and heat over medium-high heat. Add the onion and garlic and cook, stirring constantly, for 2 to 3 minutes, or until golden. Add the salt (if desired), pepper, ketchup, and tomato and continue to cook for 1 to 2 minutes. Meanwhile, in a 1-quart measuring cup, add the milk, saffron, curry, and coconut extract and stir to blend.

Add the rice, shrimp (if desired), and coconut-milk mixture to the wok with the onion mixture and continue to cook, stirring constantly, for 2 minutes, or until heated through. Stir in the reserved eggs. Divide among 4 bowls and garnish with the green onions and cilantro.

% DAILY VALUE FOR:

VIT A	VIT C	VIT E	VIT D	VIT B$_1$	VIT B$_2$	VIT B$_3$	VIT B$_6$	VIT B$_{12}$	FOLATE	CAL	MAG	POT	SELEN	ZINC
16%	29%	14%	12%	26%	41%	26%	41%	18%	15%	9%	33%	14%	51%	24%

FAST ITALIAN-STYLE FISH
WITH EVEN FASTER LEMON SAUCE

This recipe uses thin fish fillets (like orange roughy or sole), but you can use thicker types (like bass or halibut) if you cut them in half lengthwise. The lemon sauce is pretty powerful, so a light drizzle will do. And if you like, you can always just serve the fish with a sliced lemon.

FOOD SYNERGY NOTES | *This super-easy recipe features fish, a Synergy Super Food that experts recommend we eat at least twice a week.*

Makes 4 servings

FISH

1¼ pounds thin fish fillets (sole, orange roughy, sea bass, or halibut)

1½ cups dry Italian-style bread crumbs

1½ teaspoons ground sage

2 teaspoons Old Bay Seasoning

2 large eggs (omega-3, if available)

2 teaspoons water

4 teaspoons extra-virgin olive oil or canola oil

SAUCE (OPTIONAL)

2 tablespoons lemon curd

2 tablespoons fat-free half-and-half or low-fat milk thickened with ¾ teaspoon cornstarch

1 tablespoon finely chopped Italian or regular parsley (optional)

PER SERVING (WITH LEMON SAUCE):

CALORIES	FAT CAL	PROTEIN	CARB	FIBER	CHOLEST	TOTAL FAT	SAT FAT	MONO FAT	POLY FAT	OMEGA-3	OMEGA-6	SODIUM
232	27%	29 g	10	6 g	126	7	1.6	4.1	1	0.3 g	1 g	485
(269)	(30%)		(17) g		(138) mg	(9) g	(1.8) g	(4.5) g	(2) g			(501) mg

To make the fish: Pat the fish dry with paper towels and set aside on a piece of waxed paper.

In a medium bowl, whisk together the bread crumbs, sage, and seasoning.

In another medium bowl, whisk together the eggs, water, and oil.

Coat a large nonstick skillet with olive-oil spray and place over medium-high heat. Quickly dip each fillet in the egg wash and then the crumb mixture, making sure plenty of crumbs stick. Place the coated fish in the skillet and repeat with the remaining fillets. When all are in the pan, coat the tops with the cooking spray.

Cook for 4 minutes, or until the bottoms are nice and brown, then flip the fish over and cook for 3 minutes more to brown the other side, or until the fish flakes easily. Remove to a serving dish and cover with a sheet of foil to keep warm.

To make the sauce: In a small nonstick saucepan, combine the lemon curd and half-and-half or thickened milk and bring to a gentle boil over medium heat, stirring frequently, for 1 minute, or until smooth and slightly thickened. Remove from the heat.

Drizzle 1 tablespoon of the lemon sauce over each serving of fish. Sprinkle with a pinch or two of parsley, if you wish.

% DAILY VALUE FOR:

VIT A	VIT C	VIT E	VIT B₁	VIT B₂	VIT B₆	VIT B₁₂	FOLATE	CAL	VIT D	POT	SELEN	ZINC
3%	0%	5%	1%	6%	1%	5%	1%	6%	3%	10%	7%	2%
(6%)	(1%)	(5%)	(2%)	(10%)	(2%)	(7%)	(2%)	(9%)	(6%)	(11%)	(7%)	(3%)

SALMON PECAN PATTIES

To add an interesting flavor, try using your favorite crackers in this recipe, such as whole wheat or even rosemary garlic crackers. Just pulse in a small food processor until fine crumbs form. To toast the pecans, place in a nonstick skillet over medium heat for 2 minutes, until lightly browned and fragrant.

FOOD SYNERGY NOTES | *The fish omega-3s have synergy with the plant omega-3s from the egg and canola oil. Each serving has some synergy from onion phytochemicals and nuts.*

Makes 3 servings (2 large patties each)

1	can (14.75 ounces) salmon	3	tablespoons chopped parsley
1	medium onion, chopped	1	teaspoon ground mustard
1	large egg (omega-3, if available), beaten	⅔	cup cracker crumbs
2	tablespoons egg substitute	¼	cup toasted pecan pieces
		2	teaspoons canola or olive oil

Drain the salmon, picking out any pieces of bones or skin, and flake what is left. Place the salmon flakes in a large mixing bowl.

Coat a small nonstick skillet with canola-oil cooking spray and heat over medium-high heat. Add the onion and cook, stirring frequently, until golden and tender.

PER SERVING:

CALORIES	FAT CAL	PROTEIN	CARB	FIBER	CHOLEST	TOTAL FAT	SAT FAT	MONO FAT	POLY FAT	OMEGA-3	OMEGA-6	SODIUM
376	48%	26 g	22 g	5 g	124 mg	20 g	3.1 g	10 g	6.3 g	2 g	4 g	192 mg

Add the onions to the salmon in the mixing bowl, along with the egg, egg substitute, parsley, mustard, and ⅓ cup of the crackers and beat on low speed to blend. Add the pecans and briefly beat on low speed until mixed. Shape into 6 patties about ½" thick. Press both sides of each patty into the remaining ⅓ cup of cracker crumbs to lightly coat.

Heat the oil in a large nonstick skillet over medium heat and spread evenly in the pan. Cook the patties for 10 minutes, or until nicely browned on both sides.

% DAILY VALUE FOR:

VIT A	VIT C	VIT E	VIT B$_1$	VIT B$_2$	VIT B$_3$	VIT B$_6$	VIT B$_{12}$	FOLATE	CAL	MAG	POT	SELEN	ZINC
10%	16%	16%	33%	59%	62%	71%	108%	17%	6%	22%	22%	80%	24%

SEASONED SALMON WITH LEMON-CAPER SAUCE

When I want to fix salmon fast, this is one of the recipes I grab. It takes 5 minutes to put together and 10 minutes to broil the salmon! And it tastes terrific—can't ask for much more than that.

Makes 4 servings

SALMON

1	pound salmon fillet	1/8–1/4	teaspoon freshly ground pepper
2	teaspoons canola oil	1/4–1/2	teaspoon garlic powder
1/8	teaspoon salt	1/2	teaspoon dried dillweed

SAUCE

1/2	cup fat-free or light sour cream	1/2	teaspoon finely chopped lemon peel (optional)
1	tablespoon drained capers		
2	teaspoons lemon juice		

Preheat the broiler. Line a 9" round baking pan or baking dish with foil. Coat the foil with canola-oil cooking spray.

To make the salmon: Rinse and dry the salmon well. Place skin-side down on the prepared pan. Brush the top (flesh side) with the oil. Sprinkle the salt and pepper evenly over the salmon, then sprinkle the garlic powder and dillweed evenly over the top.

PER SERVING:

CALORIES	FAT CAL	PROTEIN	CARB	FIBER	CHOLEST	TOTAL FAT	SAT FAT	OMEGA-3	OMEGA-6	SODIUM
191	36%	24 g	5 g	0.1 g	65 mg	7.5 g	1.4 g	2.1 g	1 g	206 mg

Place under the broiler (about 6" from the heat) for 5 minutes. Flip the salmon over (skin-side up now) and broil for 5 minutes longer, or until the fish is opaque.

Peel off the skin (it comes off easily) and discard. Serve the salmon with seasoned-side up (spoon any juices and seasoning in the bottom of the pan over the top of the salmon).

To make the sauce: While the salmon is broiling, in a small food processor, combine the sour cream, capers, lemon juice, and lemon peel (if desired), and pulse for 5 seconds to blend well. Alternatively, finely chop the capers and, in a small serving bowl, blend with the sour cream, lemon juice, and lemon peel (if desired).

% DAILY VALUE FOR:

VIT A	VIT C	VIT E	VIT D	VIT B$_1$	VIT B$_2$	VIT B$_3$	VIT B$_6$	VIT B$_{12}$	FOLATE	CAL	MAG	POT	SELEN	ZINC
2%	2%	11%	119%	21%	38%	47%	62%	108%	6%	7%	10%	18%	72%	9%

ORANGE-MANGO CHICKEN

The almonds in this recipe provide a great hit of crunchy flavor. If you prefer flavored almonds, go for it! They'll work just as well in this dish. If you don't have Chinese rice wine on hand, a splash of vodka makes a handy substitution.

FOOD SYNERGY NOTES | *This Asian-style entrée features two foods that are rich in one of the carotenes that have synergy—orange juice has lutein, and mango has beta-carotene. The little bit of canola oil contributes plant omega-3s and monounsaturated fat. If served over brown rice, you will add a high-synergy whole grain into the mix as well.*

Makes 3 servings

2	teaspoons low-sodium soy sauce
1	teaspoon cornstarch
1	pound boneless, skinless chicken breast, cut into 1" cubes
⅓	cup fresh orange juice
2	tablespoons Chinese rice wine
1	tablespoon bottled hoisin sauce
2	teaspoons sugar
2	teaspoons bottled tomato-based chili sauce
¾	teaspoon minced garlic

2	teaspoons canola oil
2	teaspoons cornstarch dissolved in 1 tablespoon water
3	green onions, thinly sliced on a diagonal
1	mango, cut into bite-size pieces (about 1 cup)
3	tablespoons chopped toasted almonds
	Cooked brown rice (optional)

PER SERVING:

CALORIES	FAT CAL	PROTEIN	CARB	FIBER	CHOLEST	TOTAL FAT	SAT FAT	MONO FAT	POLY FAT	OMEGA-3	OMEGA-6	SODIUM
284	17%	36 g	21.5 g	2 g	88 mg	5.5 g	0.8 g	2.3 g	2.4 g	0.4 g	2 g	347 mg

In a medium bowl, combine the soy sauce and cornstarch. Add the chicken and stir to coat. Set aside for 10 minutes.

Meanwhile, in a 2-cup measuring cup, place the orange juice, wine, hoisin sauce, sugar, chili sauce, and garlic and stir to blend and dissolve the sugar.

Heat a large nonstick skillet or wok over high heat. Once it is hot (a few minutes, depending on your stove and pan), add the oil and swirl the pan to coat the bottom well. Add the reserved chicken and cook, stirring constantly, for 4 minutes, or until no longer pink and the juices run clear. Add the orange juice sauce and bring to a gentle boil. Stir in the cornstarch, onions, and mango and cook, stirring constantly, until the sauce thickens (about 20 seconds).

Sprinkle with the almonds and serve over cooked brown rice (if desired).

% DAILY VALUE FOR:

VIT A	VIT C	VIT E	VIT B₁	VIT B₂	VIT B₃	VIT B₆	VIT B₁₂	FOLATE	CAL	MAG	POT	SELEN	ZINC
35%	44%	21%	16%	22%	126%	71%	24%	7%	5%	24%	18%	50%	19%

STUFFED CHICKEN BREAST

Sprinkled inside and over the top of the stuffed chicken is a bright-green mixture of chopped parsley, spinach, and garlic, plus a wee bit of olive oil. The chicken is baked in individual foil pouches and briefly broiled to add color.

FOOD SYNERGY NOTES | *This elegant entrée features one of the leaner protein sources (skinless chicken breast) and fills it with a powerful antioxidant mixture.*

Makes 4 small or 2 large servings

2	boneless, skinless whole chicken breasts or 4 chicken breast halves	2	teaspoons minced garlic
⅓	cup goat cheese	2	teaspoons lemon-flavored olive oil or extra-virgin olive oil
½	cup drained roasted red bell pepper strips (from a jar)		Salt and ground pepper (optional)
½	cup chopped fresh parsley		
½	cup chopped fresh or frozen spinach		

Preheat the oven to 400°F.

Wash and dry the chicken well. Lay each whole or half breast on its own large sheet of foil coated with canola-oil cooking spray. Spread the cheese over the chicken, dividing it evenly among the pieces. Top with the pepper strips.

PER SMALL SERVING:

CALORIES	FAT CAL	PROTEIN	CARB	FIBER	CHOLEST	TOTAL FAT	SAT FAT	MONO FAT	POLY FAT	OMEGA-3	OMEGA-6	SODIUM
200	32%	30 g	4 g	1.2 g	88 mg	7.2 g	3.2 g	3 g	1 g	0.1 g	0.9 g	218 mg

In a small food processor, combine the parsley, spinach, garlic, and oil and pulse to blend (or use an electric mixer). Add salt and pepper to taste, if desired. Spread half the mixture over the pepper strips, then fold the chicken over to create a stuffed breast. Top each with the remaining parsley mixture. Completely wrap with the foil. Place in a 9" × 9" baking dish.

Bake for 45 minutes. Open the pouches to uncover the chicken and broil, if desired, for a minute or two to lightly brown the top.

% DAILY VALUE FOR:

VIT A	VIT C	VIT E	VIT B$_1$	VIT B$_2$	VIT B$_3$	VIT B$_6$	VIT B$_{12}$	FOLATE	CAL	VIT D	MAG	POT	SELEN	ZINC
29%	32%	5%	9%	18%	93%	50%	19%	6%	6%	7%	13%	11%	38%	14%

KALE QUICHE

Kale is a super nutrient-packed leafy green veggie that most of us don't know what to do with. So I tried using it in a crustless quiche, and it worked out very nicely. When preparing kale, make sure to discard the tough stems before cooking.

FOOD SYNERGY NOTES | *Working in any of the dark-green leafy veggies or cruciferous vegetables is always a good thing—and kale is a member of both distinguished groups and rich in the antioxidant vitamin C and carotene phytochemicals as well. Omega-3 eggs will increase the smart fats and omega-3s, and there is even some low-fat dairy in each serving.*

Makes 4 servings

6	cups shredded kale leaves		½	teaspoon garlic powder
2	tablespoons shredded Parmesan cheese		½	teaspoon onion powder or ¼ cup finely chopped onion
2	tablespoons dry bread crumbs, seasoned or unseasoned		¼	teaspoon hot-pepper sauce
2	large eggs (omega-3, if available)		⅔	cup shredded reduced-fat sharp Cheddar cheese
½	cup egg substitute		⅓	cup shredded Gruyère or Jarlsberg Lite cheese
1½	cups fat-free half-and-half			
¼	teaspoon salt (optional)			

PER SERVING:

CALORIES	FAT CAL	PROTEIN	CARB	FIBER	CHOLEST	TOTAL FAT	SAT FAT	MONO FAT	POLY FAT	OMEGA-3	OMEGA-6	SODIUM
296	32%	25 g	25 g	3 g	134 mg	10.5 g	5.6 g	2.3 g	1.2 g	0.3 g	0.7 g	570 mg

Preheat the oven to 350°F. Coat the inside of a 9"-deep pie plate with canola-oil cooking spray.

Heat a large nonstick skillet over medium-high heat. Rinse the kale and place the leaves directly into the hot pan (with plenty of water still on the leaves). Cook, stirring frequently, for 3 minutes, or until the leaves start to soften. Turn off the heat and set the kale aside to cool.

In a small bowl, combine the Parmesan and bread crumbs, then pour into the prepared pie plate and tilt to coat the inside of the plate with the mixture.

In a mixing bowl, beat the eggs, egg substitute, half-and-half, salt (if desired), garlic powder, onion powder or onion, and hot-pepper sauce on medium speed until smooth.

Sprinkle the cheeses and reserved kale evenly into the bottom of the pie plate. Pour in the egg mixture and stir lightly with a fork to mix the ingredients together.

Bake for 40 to 45 minutes, until the edges are browned and puffy and the center is set.

% DAILY VALUE FOR:

VIT A	VIT C	VIT E	VIT B$_1$	VIT B$_2$	VIT B$_3$	VIT B$_6$	VIT B$_{12}$	FOLATE	CAL	MAG	POT	SELEN	ZINC
164%	162%	10%	17%	99%	9%	32%	41%	17%	69%	21%	25%	26%	39%

GARDEN SUN-DRIED TOMATO LASAGNA

I call this garden lasagna because I think it will work well with whatever you have in your garden or crisper. Consider it a "designer" recipe. The key to more healthful lasagna is switching to low-fat dairy ingredients and incorporating as many high-nutrient veggies as possible. If you can find part whole wheat lasagna pasta, go for it. Otherwise, just use the semolina flour lasagna noodles and take comfort in knowing you are still getting 5 grams of fiber per serving due to all the vegetables and tomatoes! I love to use fresh pasta sheets available in places like Whole Foods supermarkets; if you prefer, use Barilla Oven Ready Lasagne (use 3½ sheets per layer and 11 sheets per recipe).

FOOD SYNERGY NOTES | *This lasagna pairs the tomato with olive oil and broccoli for a couple different types of synergy.*

Makes 12 servings

1	container (15 ounces) part-skim ricotta cheese
¼	cup egg substitute or 1 large egg (omega-3 egg, if available), lightly beaten
¼	cup low-fat milk
4	green onions, white and part of green, chopped
1½	teaspoons garlic powder
1½	teaspoon Italian seasoning
9	long sheets fresh pasta (about 9 ounces)
5	cups raw broccoli florets, cut into bite-size pieces, slightly cooked in microwave
½	cup shredded Parmesan cheese
1	cup pizza or marinara sauce
½	cup red or white wine or water
1	cup fresh basil leaves, washed and drained
1½	cups shredded part-skim mozzarella
½	cup shredded reduced-fat sharp Cheddar cheese
⅓	cup well-drained julienned sun-dried tomatoes
3	vine-ripened tomatoes, cut into ⅓" slices
1	teaspoon chicken broth powder blended with ⅓ cup hot water

PER SERVING:

CALORIES	FAT CAL	PROTEIN	CARB	FIBER	CHOLEST	TOTAL FAT	SAT FAT	MONO FAT	POLY FAT	OMEGA-3	OMEGA-6	SODIUM
215	35%	15 g	21 g	3 g	39 mg	7.7 g	4.5 g	2 g	0.6 g	0.2 g	0.4 g	384 mg

Preheat the oven to 400°F. Coat a 13" × 9" baking dish with canola- or olive-oil cooking spray.

In a 4- to 8-cup measure, combine the ricotta cheese, egg substitute or egg, milk, onions, and ¾ teaspoon each of the garlic powder and Italian seasoning and stir until blended.

Line the baking dish with three of the sheets of the pasta. Spread with half of the ricotta mixture and top with the broccoli. Sprinkle with ¼ cup of the Parmesan.

Top with three more pasta sheets. Blend 1 cup of the pizza sauce with the wine or water and pour over the pasta. Lay basil evenly over the top, then sprinkle 1 cup of the mozzarella and ¼ cup of the Cheddar over the top.

Top with the remaining three pasta sheets. Spread with the remaining ricotta mixture and top evenly with the sun-dried tomatoes. Lay the fresh tomato slices over this, and sprinkle with the remaining ¼ cup Parmesan, ½ cup mozzarella, and ¼ cup Cheddar. Sprinkle the remaining ¾ teaspoon each of garlic powder and Italian seasoning over the top. Pour the chicken broth mixture evenly over the top. Cover with foil and bake for 1 hour.

% DAILY VALUE FOR:

VIT A	VIT C	VIT E	VIT B₁	VIT B₂	VIT B₃	VIT B₆	VIT B₁₂	FOLATE	CAL	MAG	POT	SELEN	ZINC
33%	50%	4%	19%	32%	9%	10%	17%	19%	32%	11%	10%	19%	19%

EGGPLANT NAPOLEON

FOOD SYNERGY NOTES | *You get the synergy between calcium and vitamin D with each serving (28 percent Daily Value for vitamin D, 52 percent for calcium), which also includes synergy from the phytochemicals in the onion and a serving of low-fat dairy.*

Makes 2 main-dish or 4 side-dish servings

1	eggplant
1½	tablespoons melted plant sterol–enriched margarine
1½	teaspoons garlic-and-herb salt-free seasoning blend
¾	block light firm tofu, sliced ¼" thick
½	red onion, thinly sliced (keep slices intact, if possible)

3	ounces fresh or low-moisture, part-skim mozzarella, sliced, or ¾ cup shredded
4	tablespoons shredded Parmesan cheese
1	teaspoon red pepper flakes (optional)
4	strips roasted red bell pepper
	Salt (optional)

Trim the top and bottom off the eggplant, then cut into ⅓"-thick slices. Coat both sides generously with the margarine and place on foil. Broil in a toaster oven or oven about 5" from the heat for 4 to 5 minutes, watching carefully to avoid burning. Flip the slices over and sprinkle with the seasoning blend. Broil for 3 to 4 minutes more or until lightly brown.

PER MAIN-DISH SERVING:

CALORIES	FAT CAL	PROTEIN	CARB	FIBER	CHOLEST	TOTAL FAT	SAT FAT	MONO FAT	POLY FAT	OMEGA-3	OMEGA-6	SODIUM
350	38%	30 g	24 g	8 g	30 mg	15 g	7 g	4.5 g	3.5 g	0.4 g	3 g	649 mg

Assemble the napoleons in a 9" × 9" microwave-safe baking dish by laying 4 eggplant slices in the dish. Top each slice with a slice of tofu, then a slice of onion, a slice of mozzarella (or 3 tablespoons shredded mozzarella), 1 tablespoon of Parmesan, a light sprinkle of crushed red pepper (if desired), 1 strip of the roasted red pepper, another tofu slice, and finally another eggplant slice. Seasson to taste with salt if desired.

Microwave on high, uncovered, for 6 minutes, or until heated throughout and the cheese melts.

% DAILY VALUE FOR:

VIT A	VIT C	VIT E	VIT B₁	VIT B₂	VIT B₃	VIT B₆	VIT B₁₂	FOLATE	CAL	MAG	POT	SELEN	ZINC
53%	30%	11%	21%	29%	14%	24%	22%	16%	52%	23%	23%	6%	33%

SAVORY SUMMER TART

FOOD SYNERGY NOTES | *Each serving has synergy from phytochemicals in onions and garlic plus a little omega-3 from the eggs, low-fat dairy, and smart fat, along with the phytochemicals in tomatoes.*

Makes 6 servings

CRUST

½ cup ground wheat crackers (about eight 2½"-square crackers)

1 teaspoon garlic-and-herb salt-free seasoning blend

2 tablespoons shredded Parmesan cheese

1½ teaspoons olive oil

FILLING

1 tablespoon olive oil

1¼ cups chopped red bell pepper

1 cup chopped red onion

2 teaspoons minced garlic

¼ cup chopped fresh basil

2 large eggs (omega-3, if available)

½ cup egg substitute

1 cup fat-free half-and-half

½ teaspoon salt

½ teaspoon ground white pepper

2 cups reduced-fat shredded Monterey Jack cheese

¼ cup shredded Parmesan cheese

3 Roma or plum tomatoes, sliced ¼" thick

PER SERVING:

CALORIES	FAT CAL	PROTEIN	CARB	FIBER	CHOLEST	TOTAL FAT	SAT FAT	MONO FAT	POLY FAT	OMEGA-3	OMEGA-6	SODIUM
304	39%	22 g	23 g	4 g	102 mg	13 g	7.9 g	3.5 g	1.5 g	0.2 g	1.2 g	686 mg

Preheat the oven to 425°F.

To make the crust: In a small food processor or a mixer, place the crackers, seasoning blend, and cheese and pulse to combine. Coat a 9" deep-dish pie plate generously with the olive oil. Add the crumb mixture and tilt to distribute evenly over the bottom and partway up the sides. Bake for 8 to 10 minutes. Remove from the oven and set aside.

To make the filling: Heat the oil in a large nonstick skillet over medium-high heat. Add the bell pepper, onion, and garlic and cook, stirring frequently, for 5 minutes, or until lightly browned. Stir in the basil.

In a large mixing bowl, combine the eggs, egg substitute, half-and-half, salt, and white pepper. Beat on medium-low speed to combine.

Stir in the vegetable mixture and the Jack and Parmesan cheeses. Pour into the reserved crust. Place the tomatoes on top in a circular pattern. Bake for 40 to 45 minutes, or until brown on top and nicely set in the middle. Let stand 5 minutes before serving.

% DAILY VALUE FOR:

VIT A	VIT C	VIT E	VIT B$_1$	VIT B$_2$	VIT B$_3$	VIT B$_6$	VIT B$_{12}$	FOLATE	CAL	MAG	POT	SELEN	ZINC
40%	91%	16%	13%	29%	7%	14%	31%	20%	56%	13%	25%	21%	16%

TUNA GRUYÈRE TART

FOOD SYNERGY NOTES | *When you enjoy this diner tart, you'll also benefit from 4 Synergy Super Foods (fish, whole grains, olive oil, and tomatoes). The onion and cheese add even more synergy to the mix.*

Makes 8 servings

CRUST

¾ cup whole wheat pastry flour or regular whole wheat flour

¾ cup unbleached all-purpose flour

¾ teaspoon salt

1 tablespoon light pancake syrup

5 tablespoons canola oil

3 tablespoons low-fat buttermilk

FILLING

3 tablespoons Dijon mustard

1 sweet onion, thinly sliced

1 can (12 ounces) chunk light tuna in water, drained well

1 cup shredded Gruyère cheese

3 tomatoes, sliced into ½" circles

1 cup fat-free half-and-half or whole milk

1 large egg (omega-3, if available)

½ teaspoon salt (optional)

½ teaspoon ground pepper + more if desired

Preheat the oven to 400°F.

To make the crust: In a medium bowl, combine the flours and salt and blend well with an electric mixer on low speed.

PER SERVING:

CALORIES	FAT CAL	PROTEIN	CARB	FIBER	CHOLEST	TOTAL FAT	SAT FAT	MONO FAT	POLY FAT	OMEGA-3	OMEGA-6	SODIUM
310	39%	19 g	28 g	3 g	51 mg	14 g	3.5 g	7 g	3.5 g	1.2 g	2.3 g	573 mg

Add the syrup and oil and beat on low speed until the mixture looks blended and crumbly. Pour in the buttermilk and mix for 15 seconds, or just until the dough is moist and holds together well. Stir in another teaspoon or two of buttermilk if the dough seems too dry.

Using your hands, press the dough evenly into a 10" deep-dish pie plate. If the dough is a little thicker around the rim, pinch it into scallops or make the rim double thickness and press around it with a fork.

To make the filling: Spread the mustard over the bottom of the crust. Place the onion over the mustard. Sprinkle with half the tuna. Spread ½ cup of the cheese on top of this layer, then sprinkle the remaining tuna on top. Sprinkle the remaining ½ cup of cheese over the tuna, then cover with a layer of tomatoes placed as closely together as possible.

In a separate bowl, lightly beat together the half-and-half or milk, egg, salt (if using), and pepper until blended. Pour into the pie crust. Bake for 45 to 50 minutes, or until the filling looks firm and the crust is lightly browned. Cool for 15 minutes before serving.

% DAILY VALUE FOR:

VIT A	VIT C	VIT E	VIT B$_1$	VIT B$_2$	VIT B$_3$	VIT B$_6$	VIT B$_{12}$	FOLATE	CAL	VIT D	MAG	POT	SELEN	ZINC
16%	12%	15%	19%	26%	13%	12%	15%	11%	26%	15%	13%	10%	31%	19%

Drinks

LEMON-GINGER ICED GREEN TEA

FOOD SYNERGY NOTES | *First you get the phytochemicals from green tea, and then you get a little burst of citrus synergy from the lemon peel and juice.*

Makes 5 or more servings (1⅓ cups)

2	cups water		1½	teaspoons grated lemon peel
1	cup Splenda		6	green tea bags
1	teaspoon ground ginger		4	teaspoons fresh lemon juice

In a medium saucepan, place the water, Splenda, ginger, and lemon peel and bring to a boil over medium heat. Reduce the heat so it sustains a gentle boil and cook for 7 to 8 minutes. Remove from the heat and add the tea bags. Steep for 10 minutes, stirring or dunking the bags often.

Remove the tea bags and stir the lemon juice into the tea syrup. Cover and refrigerate for up to 2 weeks.

To make a cup of iced tea, pour ¼ cup of the syrup into a tall glass and stir in ¾ cup of sparkling or seltzer water or club soda. Add ice cubes and enjoy!

NUTRITIONAL ANALYSIS: THIS IS A 0-CALORIE BEVERAGE.

PEACH PLEASURE ICED TEA

You can make a pitcher or make this yummy tea glass by glass. You can use your favorite black tea; I suggest Paradise brand Tropical Tea, available (in decaf, too) at Trader Joe's and other fine stores.

You get the phytochemicals in black tea and some nutrients from the peach nectar.

Makes 4 servings

4	cups brewed and chilled black tea, regular or decaf
2	cups peach nectar

4   cups ice cubes

Pour 1 cup of the tea into a glass. Stir in ½ cup of peach nectar and add 1 cup of ice cubes. Repeat with the remaining ingredients to make three more servings.

PER SERVING:

CALORIES	TOTAL FAT	PROTEIN	CARB	FIBER	CHOLEST	OMEGA-3s	OMEGA-6s	SODIUM
67	0%	0.3 g	17 g	0.8 g	0 mg	0 g	0 g	9 mg

% DAILY VALUE FOR:

VIT A	VIT C	VIT B$_2$	VIT B$_3$	VIT B$_6$	CAL	MAG	POT	ZINC
5%	9%	2%	3%	1%	1%	2%	1%	1%

STRAWBERRY LIGHT LEMONADE

You can adjust the Splenda and sugar, adding more or less depending on your taste preference. If you have superfine sugar, use it; it will dissolve in the water faster.

FOOD SYNERGY NOTES | *This beverage packs 2 grams of fiber in a glass along with the synergy from berries and a daily supply of vitamin C.*

Makes 4 servings

2	cups sliced or halved strawberries	12	tablespoons freshly squeezed lemon juice
5	tablespoons superfine or granulated sugar	2⅔	cups club soda, mineral water, or seltzer per glass
8	tablespoons Splenda		

In a blender or small food processor, combine the strawberries and 1 tablespoon of the sugar and puree.

Spoon 3 tablespoons of the puree into each of the 4 glasses, then add 2 tablespoons of the Splenda and 1 tablespoon of the remaining sugar into each glass. Add 3 tablespoons of the lemon juice to each glass, then stir to blend well. Stir in about ⅔ cup of the club soda, mineral water, or seltzer into each glass, add some ice, and serve.

PER SERVING:

CALORIES	FAT CAL	PROTEIN	CARB	FIBER	CHOLEST	TOTAL FAT	SAT FAT	MONO FAT	POLY FAT	OMEGA-3	OMEGA-6	SODIUM
84	3%	1 g	22 g	2 g	0 mg	0.3 g	0 g	0 g	0.2 g	0.1 g	0.1 g	1 mg

% DAILY VALUE FOR:

VIT C	VIT E	VIT B₁	VIT B₂	VIT B₃	VIT B₆	FOLATE	CAL	MAG	POT	SELEN	ZINC
91%	1%	3%	6%	2%	6%	5%	1%	3%	6%	1%	2%

APPENDIX A

NUTRITIONAL PROFILE OF RECIPES

	CALORIES/SERVING				
	<150	**151–300**	**301–450**	**<500 MG SODIUM/ SERVING**	**>4 G FIBER/ SERVING**
Breakfast, Baked Goods, and Sweet Treats					
Edamame-Spinach Scramble			X	X	X
Breakfast Panini with Roasted Red Pepper Spread			X		X
Breakfast Sausage Casserole			X	X	X
Vegetarian Sausage-and-Sage Gravy	X			X	
Easy Sweet Potato Harvest Rolls	X			X	
Lemon-Rosemary Rolls		X		X	
Apple Oat Muffins	X			X	
Strawberry-Orange Spread	X			X	
Vanilla-Cherry-Almond Granola		X		X	X
Orange-Cranberry Oatmeal		X		X	X
Blueberry-Vanilla-Walnut Almost-Instant Oatmeal		X		X	X
Lemon-Blueberry Buttermilk Pancakes		X			X
Best Swedish Pancakes		X		X	
Hot Apple-Blueberry Cobbler with Walnut-Butter Streusel		X		X	
Light and Luscious Berry Grunt		X		X	X
Berry Easy Topping	X			X	
Three-Grain Buttermilk Waffles		X		X	X
Fruit and Cream Crisp		X		X	X
10-Minute Spiced Apple Wedges with Caramel Sauce		X		X	

	CALORIES/SERVING				
	<150	151–300	301–450	<500 MG SODIUM/ SERVING	>4 G FIBER/ SERVING
Soups, Salads, and Sandwiches					
Light Italian Wedding Soup		X		X	
Jessie's White Chili			X		X
Not-So-Killer Chili			X		X
Farmer's Market Pasta Salad			X	X	X
Sweet Pepper and Basil Pasta Salad		X		X	X
Roasted Pepper and Mushroom Pasta Salad		X		X	
Shrimp and Red Grapefruit Salad		X		X	X
Mediterranean Chickpea Salad		X		X	
Avocado Mango Salad	X			X	
Less-Fuss Pecan-Crusted Chicken Salad			X		X
Mediterranean Pita Sandwich		X		X	X
2-Minute Toasted Tomato and Cheese Sandwich		X		X	
Deluxe Grilled Cheese Sandwich		X		X	
French-Style Ham and Cheese Sandwich			X		X
Appetizers, Snacks, and Sides					
Spicy Nut Mix		X		X	X
Fun Fall Snack Mix		X		X	X
Avocado-Edamame Salsa		X		X	X
Stuffed Grape Leaves		X		X	
Summer Succotash	X			X	

	CALORIES/SERVING				
	<150	151–300	301–450	<500 MG SODIUM/ SERVING	>4 G FIBER/ SERVING
Appetizers, Snacks, and Sides (cont.)					
Coleslaw with Spicy Peanut Dressing		X		X	X
Tahini-Dressed Chilled Noodles			X	X	X
Roasted Asparagus Spears with Slivered Garlic	X			X	
Brussels Sprouts Sautéed with Pecans and Shallots		X		X	
Quick Spinach Italiano	X			X	
Stovetop Spanakorizo		X			X
Savory Barley		X			X
Barley Mushroom Bake			X	X	X
Barley Eggplant Bake			X	X	X
Barley-Stuffed Tomatoes	X			X	
Maple Roasted Squash with Apple Filling		X		X	X
Baked Butternut Macaroni			X	X	X
Main Dishes					
Portobello Tacos		X		X	X
Portobello Mushroom Burger with Garlic Mayonnaise		X			X
Baked Beef Meatballs (with Spinach) and Homemade Pizza Sauce			X		X
Sausage and Saffron Rice		X			X
Portfolio Pesto		X		X	
Homemade Pizza Sauce		X		X	

	CALORIES/SERVING				
	<150	151–300	301–450	<500 MG SODIUM/ SERVING	>4 G FIBER/ SERVING
Main Dishes *(cont.)*					
Butternut Squash Ravioli with Lemon Cream Sauce			X	X	X
Light Spinach and Artichoke Heart Alfredo				X	X
Penne with Creamy Tomato Vodka Sauce					X
Margi's Tortellini and Shrimp Sauté			X	X	
Easy Mu Shu Shrimp		X		X	X
Coconut Fried Rice			X	X	X
Fast Italian-Style Fish with Even Faster Lemon Sauce		X		X	X
Salmon Pecan Patties			X	X	X
Seasoned Salmon with Lemon-Caper Sauce		X		X	
Orange-Mango Chicken		X		X	
Stuffed Chicken Breast		X		X	
Kale Quiche		X			
Garden Sun-Dried Tomato Lasagna		X		X	
Eggplant Napoleon			X		X
Savory Summer Tart			X		
Tuna Gruyère Tart			X		
Drinks					
Lemon-Ginger Iced Green Tea	X			X	
Peach Pleasure Iced Tea	X			X	
Strawberry Light Lemonade	X			X	

APPENDIX B

NUTRIENT DENSITY OF COMMON FOODS

TOP 10 FOLIC ACID–RICH FOODS (NOT INCLUDING ORGAN MEATS OR VEAL)

RANK	FOOD	FOLATE (MCG)
#1	Brewer's yeast, 1 Tbsp	313
#2	Lentils, ½ c, cooked	179
#3	Romaine lettuce, 2 c	152
#4	Okra, ½ c, cooked	134
#5	Black beans, ½ c, cooked	128
#6	Black-eyed peas, ½ c, cooked	120
#7	Spinach, 2 c, fresh	218
#8	Kidney beans, ½ c, cooked	115
#9	Broccoli, chopped, 1 c, cooked	104
#10	Spinach, ½ c, cooked	103

TOP 10 B_6-RICH FOODS (NOT INCLUDING ORGAN MEATS OR VEAL)

RANK	FOOD	VITAMAIN B_6 (MG)
#1	Banana, 1	0.7
#2	Salmon, 3.5 oz, cooked	0.65
#3	Light-meat chicken, 3.5 oz, cooked	0.63
#4	Herring, 3.5 oz, cooked	0.52
#5	Light-meat turkey, 3.5 oz, cooked	0.5
#6	Pork (lean), 3.5 oz, cooked	0.47
#7	Baked potato with skin, 1	0.42
#8	Prune juice, ¾ c	0.42
#9	Halibut, 3.5 oz, cooked	0.4
#10	Shrimp, 3.5 oz cooked	0.4

TOP 10 B$_{12}$-RICH FOODS (NOT INCLUDING ORGAN MEATS OR VEAL)

RANK	FOOD (3.5 OZ COOKED)	VITAMIN B$_{12}$ (MCG)
#1	Clams (steamed)	99
#2	Oysters	27
#3	Herring	10
#4	Crab	9
#5	Trout	5
#6	Pollock	3.7
#7	Catfish	2.8
#8	Salmon	2.8
#9	Beef	2.5
#10	Lamb	2.4

TOP VITAMIN E FOODS

FOOD	VITAMIN E (IU)
Sunflower seeds, ¼ c	27
Almonds, ¼ c	12
Hazelnuts/filberts, ¼ c	10
Peanut butter, 2 Tbsp	5
Swiss chard, 1 c, cooked	4.9
Canola oil, 1 Tbsp	4.4
Mustard greens, 1 c, cooked	4.2
Peanuts, ¼ c	4.2
Brazil nuts, ¼ c	4
Broccoli, 1 c, cooked	3.9
Wheat germ, toasted, 2 Tbsp	3.8
Mango slices, 1 c	2.8
Spinach, cooked, 1c	2.7
Tomato sauce, ½ c	2.6
Papaya cubes, 1 c	2.3
Blueberries, frozen, 1 c	2.3
Pistachios, ¼ c	2

THE EASY-TO-FIND VITAMIN: C (TOP 40 FOODS)

FOOD	VITAMIN C (MG)
Orange juice, fresh, 1 c	124
Broccoli, 1c, cooked from fresh	124
Brussels sprouts, 1 c, cooked	96
Grapefruit juice, fresh, 1 c	94
Papaya cubes, 1 c	86
Strawberry halves, 1 c	86
Kiwifruit, 1 whole	74
Red bell pepper, chopped, ¼ c raw	71
Cantaloupe cubes, 1 c	68
Tomato-vegetable juice, 1 c	67
Mango, 1 whole	57
Cauliflower, 1 c, cooked	54
Kale, 1 c cooked	54
Orange, small, 1 whole	51
Collard greens, cooked from frozen	44
Tomato juice, 1 c	44
Grapefruit half (pink/red)	41
Butternut squash, 1 c, cooked	36
Beet greens, 1 c, cooked	36
Mustard greens, 1 c, cooked	34
Green bell pepper, chopped, ¼ c	33
Raspberries, fresh, 1 c	30
Blackberries, fresh, 1 c	30
Pineapple juice, 1 c	30
Watermelon cubes, 2 c	28
Romaine lettuce, 2 c	26
Red cabbage, ½ c, cooked	26
Pineapple cubes, fresh, 1 c	24
Spinach, 1 c, cooked from frozen	24
Collard greens, 1 c, cooked from fresh	24
Clams, 3.5 oz, steamed	22

(continued)

THE EASY-TO-FIND VITAMIN: C (TOP 40 FOODS) *(cont.)*

FOOD	VITAMIN C (MG)
Okra, 1 c, cooked	22
Loose-leaf lettuce, 2 c	20
Grapes, 1 c	17
Tomatoes, chopped, ½ c	17
Baked potato with skin, 1 (122 g)	16
Tomato sauce, ½ c	16
Soybeans, green, ½ c, cooked	15
Sweet potato, 1 small baked	15
Oysters, Pacific, 3.5 oz, cooked	13

TOP CALCIUM-RICH FOODS

The suggested daily calcium intake is very doable with foods, as long as you like and tolerate dairy. Here are some of the top calcium-rich foods I found.

FOOD	CALCIUM (MG)
Low-fat yogurt, 1 c	448
Sardines with bones, 3.5 oz	380
Fat-free milk, 1 c	300
Cheese, 1 oz	200–270
Blackstrap molasses, 1 Tbsp	175
Cottage cheese, ½ c	153
Spinach, ½ c, cooked	140
Tofu, ½ c	138
Green soybeans, ½ c, cooked	130
Soy nuts, ½ c	119
Butternut squash, 1 c, cooked	100
Collard greens, ½ c, cooked	100

SO MANY MAGNESIUM-RICH FOODS . . . SO LITTLE TIME

The Daily Reference Intakes (DRIs) for magnesium are:

   420 mg/day for men ages 31+; 400 for men ages 19–30

   320 mg/day for women ages 31+; 310 for women ages 19–30

FOOD	MAGNESIUM (MG)
Pumpkin seeds, ¼ c, roasted	303
Swiss chard, 1 c, cooked	150
Spinach, 1 c, cooked	132
Tofu, ½ c	128
Almonds, ¼ c	119
Soynuts, ¼ c, roasted	98
Hazelnuts, ¼ c	96
Okra, 1 c, cooked	92
Chocolate, unsweetened, 1 oz	88
Brazil nuts, ¼ c	83
Soybeans, green, ½ c, cooked	83
Sunflower seeds, ¼ c, shelled	82 (average; range is 42–118 mg)
Cashews, ¼ c	79
Artichoke, 1, cooked	72
Peanuts, ¼ c	63
Black beans, ½ c, cooked	60
Oatmeal, 1 c, cooked	56
Cocoa powder, 2 Tbsp	54
Navy beans, ½ c, cooked	52
Artichoke hearts, ½ c, cooked	50
Lima beans, baby, ½ c, cooked	50
Whole wheat bread, 2 slices	48
Spinach, raw leaves, 2 c	48
Wheat germ, 2 Tbsp	45
Low-fat yogurt, 1 c	43
Crab, 3.5 oz, cooked	43

(continued)

SO MANY MAGNESIUM-RICH FOODS . . . SO LITTLE TIME *(cont.)*

FOOD	MAGNESIUM (MG)
Whole wheat pasta, 1 c, cooked	42
Brown rice, ½ c, cooked	42
Kidney beans, ½ c, cooked	40
Oysters, 3.5 oz, cooked	39
Shrimp, 3.5 oz, cooked	34
Baked potato with skin, 1	33
Light-meat chicken, 3.5 oz, cooked	29
Fat-free milk, 1 c	28
Grapefruit juice, 1 c	27
Orange juice, 1 c	27
Tomato juice or tomato-vegetable juice, 1 c	27
Light-meat turkey, 3.5 oz, cooked	26
Dark-meat chicken/turkey, 3.5 oz, roasted	24

TOP ZINC-RICH FOODS

FOOD	ZINC (MG)
Oysters, 3.5 oz, cooked	39
Beef pot roast, 3.5 oz, cooked	8.5
Crab (Alaskan King), 3.5 oz, cooked	7.6
Sirloin steak, 3.5 oz, broiled	6.5
Ground beef, 3.5 oz, cooked	5.5
Dark-meat turkey, 3.5 oz, cooked	4.5
Crab (blue), 3.5 oz, cooked	4.2
Pumpkin seeds, ¼ c, roasted	4.2
Lamb, 3.5 oz, cooked	4
Dark-meat chicken, 3.5 oz, cooked	2.9
Clams, 3.5 oz, steamed	2.7
Light-meat turkey, 3.5 oz, cooked	2.1
Soynuts, ¼ c	2.1
Almonds, ¼ c	2
Pecans/peanuts, ¼ c	1.8
Sunflower seeds, ¼ c	1.7
Brazil nuts/cashews, ¼ c	1.6
Light-meat chicken, 3.5 oz, cooked	1.3
Lentils, ½ c, cooked	1.3
Black-eyed peas, ½ c, cooked	1.2
Split peas, ½ c, cooked	1.2
Oatmeal, ½ c, cooked	1.2
Whole wheat pasta, 1 c, cooked	1.1
Whole wheat bread, 2 slices	1.1
Tofu, ½ c	1
Fat-free milk, 1 c	1

TOP POTASSIUM-RICH FOODS

FOOD	POTASSIUM (MG)
Beet greens, 1 c, cooked	1,308
Swiss chard, 1 c, cooked	960
Clams, 3.5 oz, cooked	628
Soy nuts (roasted soybeans), ¼ c	588
Low-fat yogurt, 1 c	573
Tomato juice, 1 c	534
Prune juice, ¾ c	530
Okra, 1 c, cooked	514
Blackstrap molasses, 1 Tbsp	511
Baked potato with skin, 1	510
Kiwifruit, 2 whole	504
Brussels sprouts, 1 c, cooked	498
Cantaloupe cubes, 1 c	494
Orange juice, 1 c	484
Lima beans, ½ c, baked	477
Banana, 1	467
Pumpkin seeds, ¼ c, roasted	457
Tomato sauce, canned, ½ c	454
Fish, 3.5 oz, cooked	380–450 (range)
Collard greens, 1 c, cooked	426
Artichoke, 1, cooked	425
Fat-free milk, 1 c	407
Sardines, 3.5 oz	397
Grapefruit juice, 1 c	388
Navy beans, ½ c, cooked	384
Lentils, ½ c, cooked	365
Papaya cubes, 1 c	360
Kidney beans, ½ c, cooked	357
Watermelon cubes, 2 c	352
Pistachios, ¼ c	350
Grape juice, 1 c	334
Cherries, 1 c	324

FOOD	POTASSIUM (MG)
Beef, 3.5 oz, cooked	323
Black-eyed peas, ½ c, cooked	319
Prunes, 5	317
Black beans, ½ c, cooked	305
Avocado, ¼	301
Peanuts, ¼ c	276
Almonds, ¼ c	268

APPENDIX C

PHYTOCHEMICALS, FOOD SOURCES, AND POTENTIAL HEALTH BENEFITS

CATEGORY/ GROUP	SPECIFIC PHYTOCHEMICALS	FOOD SOURCES	POTENTIAL HEALTH BENEFITS AND ACTIONS
Polyphenols			
BIOFLAVONOIDS/FLAVONOIDS			
	Anthocyanins, proanthocyanidins	Blueberries and other berries like blackberries, cranberries, elderberries, and raspberries. Also found in grapes, grape seed, eggplant, red cabbage, black and green teas, wine	Enhances collagen integrity and structure; strengthens blood vessel walls by reducing activity of compounds (metalloproteinases) that break down collagen and elastin.[1] Anti-inflammatory action through antioxidant effects.[1] Antioxidant: possibly the most potent antioxidants yet discovered. Cancer protection: In lab studies, anthocyanins inhibit growth of lung, colon, and leukemia cancer cells; thought to have a general effect on cancer protection via reducing oxidative stress.
	Catechins/ tannins	Apple juice; grapes; cocoa; lentils; black-eyed peas; black, green, and white teas	Antioxidant. Reduces heart disease risk.[2] Protects against cancer development: Catechins/ tannins are thought to have a general effect on cancer protection via reducing oxidative stress but not specific anticancer activity.[3]

CATEGORY/ GROUP	SPECIFIC PHYTOCHEMICALS	FOOD SOURCES	POTENTIAL HEALTH BENEFITS AND ACTIONS
BIOFLAVONOIDS/FLAVONOIDS (CONTINUED)			
	Ellagic acid	Berries, particularly raspberries and strawberries; apples; cranberries; grapes; walnuts	Antioxidant. Protects against cancer-causing agents in diet and environment:[1, 4] According to the American Institute for Cancer Research, ellagic acid helps the body deactivate specific carcinogens and slows cancer-cell reproduction. In animals, it inhibited development of colon, esophageal, liver, lung, and skin cancers stemming from a variety of carcinogens. Emerging evidence suggests it has the ability to improve patient response to chemotherapy.[3]
	Hesperitin, hesperidin	Pulps and rinds of citrus fruits	Antiviral effects.[1, 4] Antihistamine properties. Strengthens blood vessel walls (by reducing activity of compounds—metalloproteinases—that break down collagen and elastin). Reduces edema (hesperidin in combination with the flavonoid diosmin[3])
	Kaempferol	Strawberries, broccoli, endive, kale, leeks, radishes, red cabbage	Anticancer effects.[1] May help dilate blood vessels.[1]
	Naringin	Citrus fruits (grapefruit)	Antioxidant. Lowers serum cholesterol and triglycerides.[3]

CATEGORY/ GROUP	SPECIFIC PHYTOCHEMICALS	FOOD SOURCES	POTENTIAL HEALTH BENEFITS AND ACTIONS
BIOFLAVONOIDS/FLAVONOIDS (CONTINUED)			
	Rutin (breakdown product of quercetin; see below)	Apricots, citrus fruits, rhubarb, parsley, tomatoes, buckwheat, tea	Antioxidant.[1] Promotes healthy circulation. Forms of rutin used to treat blood vessel diseases including varicose veins, hemmorhoids, and certain eye diseases.[3] Protects against cell damage and arterial plaque formation caused by LDL cholesterol.[1]
	Quercetin	Apples, pears, tea, cherries, grapes, strawberries, kale, lettuce, tomatoes, potatoes, onions (also scallions, leeks, and chives), fresh oregano, red cabbage	Strong antioxidant.[1, 4] May have antiviral and anti-inflammatory action, according to the AICR. Possible antihistamine action: Quercetin-containing foods have been associated with lower risk of airway diseases.[1, 4] May help reduce asthma risk.[2] Helps protect blood vessels from damage caused by diabetes.[4] Inhibits growth of bacteria known to cause gastritis and peptic ulcer disease.[1] Possible anticancer activity: may be especially protective against breast, ovarian, and endometrial cancers, according to AICR. In lab studies, it has been shown to inhibit tumor angiogenesis (creation of new blood vessels associated with the tumor).

CATEGORY/ GROUP	SPECIFIC PHYTOCHEMICALS	FOOD SOURCES	POTENTIAL HEALTH BENEFITS AND ACTIONS
PHENOLIC ACIDS			
	Hydroxycinnamic acids: caffeic acid, chlorogenic acid, ellagic acid	Blueberries, kiwifruit, plums, cherries, blackberries, cranberries, cranberry juice, soy, strawberries, grapes, guava, walnuts, mango, rhubarb, tea	Antioxidant. Antiviral effect.[1] Cancer protection: inhibits formation of carcinogens. Ellagic acid has been shown to increase production of two detoxification proteins that help destroy carcinogens.
	Ferulic acid	Whole grains and cereals, oats, soybeans, peanuts, tomatoes, beer, raspberries	Antioxidant: inhibits inflammation and cancer growth.[1,4]
	Hydroxybenzoic acids: protocatechuic acid, gallic acid	Black currant, nuts, tea, red wine	Antioxidant: prevents activation of potential carcinogens and helps rid the body of others.[1]
	Capsaicin	Chile peppers (the hotter the pepper the more the capsaicin)	Ingredient in topical ointments for pain relief of minor aches, sprains, and arthritis.[3] Possible anticancer effect: may contribute to death of cancer cells while inflicting no harm to surrounding healthy cells. This is still preliminary and in the lab stage.[1,4]
	P-coumaric	Coffee, blueberries, carrots, tomatoes, green peppers, strawberries, pineapple, garlic, basil, turmeric	Antioxidant. Prevents cell damage by carcinogens. May reduce colon cancer risk.
	Resveratrol	Grape skins and seeds, red wine, and dealcoholized red wine; found in lesser amounts in blueberries, nuts, and peanuts	Antioxidant: may reduce cardiovascular disease risk. Protection from heart disease. Numerous potent anticancer effects.[1,4]

CATEGORY/ GROUP	SPECIFIC PHYTOCHEMICALS	FOOD SOURCES	POTENTIAL HEALTH BENEFITS AND ACTIONS
PHYTOSTEROLS			
	Plant sterol/stanol esters	Brussels sprouts, legumes, rye bread, whole wheat (bran, germ), seeds (sunflower, sesame), nuts (almonds, cashews, macadamia, peanuts), oils (canola, corn, olive), Benecol and Take Control spreads	Decreases total and LDL cholesterol levels.[3] Reduces risk for certain cancers,[1, 2, 4] including breast and prostate. Effectively treats benign prostatic hyperplasia.[3]
	Beta-sitosterol	Buckwheat, rice bran, wheat germ, soybeans, peanuts, corn oils	
	Campesterol, stigmasterol	Buckwheat	
PHYTOESTROGENS ISOFLAVONES			
	Genistein, daidzein, glycitein	Alfalfa sprouts, red clover, chickpeas, peanuts, various legumes, soybeans, fermented soy foods (miso, tofu, tempeh)	Antioxidant. Inhibits atherosclerosis development.[1–4] Prevents arterial plaque formation.[4] Promotes healthy bones; may protect against osteoporosis.[2, 3] *May decrease certain menopausal symptoms[2, 3] (inconclusive evidence).
LIGNANS			
	Lariciresinol, matairesinol, pinoresinol, secoisolarici-resinol, to name a few (others can also be metabolized to the mammalian lignans)	Ground flaxseed, sesame seeds and paste, nuts (almonds, pistachios, sunflower seeds), soybeans, garlic, winter squash, dried fruits (apricots, prunes, dates), peaches, oranges, red wine, green tea, mung beans and mung bean sprouts, broccoli, cabbage, collards, green beans, sweet potatoes, raspberries and strawberries, rye bread	Promotes favorable estrogen metabolism. May help lower risk of hormone-dependent cancers (breast, endometrial, ovarian, prostate).[3, 4] May promote healthy bones and protect against osteoporosis (not all data agree). May protect against heart disease.[4]

CATEGORY/ GROUP	SPECIFIC PHYTOCHEMICALS	FOOD SOURCES	POTENTIAL HEALTH BENEFITS AND ACTIONS
Terpenes			
CAROTENOIDS			
	Alpha-carotene, beta-carotene, gamma-carotene	Orange and yellow produce such as carrots and cantaloupe; dark green vegetables like broccoli and red peppers; umbelliferous vegetables (parsley, carrots, celery, parsnip, fennel, chervil, dill, coriander)	Antioxidant effects (against limited number of oxygen radicals). May help reduce risk for many types of cancer.[1, 2, 4]
	Lutein	Dark green leafy veggies such as broccoli, mustard and collard greens, kale, romaine lettuce, and spinach. Green peppers, corn, avocados, oranges, tomatoes, and parsley	Antioxidant. Increases macular pigment density, which may lower the risk for macular degeneration. Possible cancer protection.[2]
	Lycopene	Tomatoes and tomato products, red peppers, watermelon, guava, red and pink grapefruit	Antioxidant: may reduce cataract risk and possibly heart disease. Cancer protection, especially breast, prostate, colon, stomach, and lung cancers and possibly skin cancer, according to epidemiological studies.
LIMONOIDS			
	D-limonene, pinene	Parsley, citrus peel	Cancer protection: decreases activity of enzymes involved in cancer cell formation. Stimulates enzymes that detoxify carcinogens.[1, 2]
Organosulfur			
GLUCOSINOLATES DITHIOLTHIONE			
	Sulforaphane	Cruciferous vegetables, especially broccoli	Antioxidant; can help reduce cancer risk.[1, 2, 4] Stimulates enzymes that detoxify carcinogens. Anti-inflammatory actions. Antithrombosis (antiplatelet) effects.[1-4]

CATEGORY/ GROUP	SPECIFIC PHYTOCHEMICALS	FOOD SOURCES	POTENTIAL HEALTH BENEFITS AND ACTIONS
INDOLES			
	Indole-3-carbinol (I3C)	Cruciferous vegetables (cabbage, cauliflower, Brussels sprouts), rutabaga, mustard greens	Stimulates enzymes that detoxify carcinogens.
ALLIUM			
	Allicin, allyl sulfide	Onions, leeks, garlic, chives, shallots	Anti-inflammatory actions. Components in allium vegetables have slowed the development of cancer in several stages and at various sites (animal studies).

Antinutrients

CATEGORY/ GROUP	SPECIFIC PHYTOCHEMICALS	FOOD SOURCES	POTENTIAL HEALTH BENEFITS AND ACTIONS
SAPONINS			
		Alpha sprouts, legumes, spinach, tomatoes, spinach, oats, potatoes, whole grains	Fights fungal and viral infections.[1, 4] Helps prevent cancer development.[1, 4] Binds with bile and decreases cholesterol levels.[4]
PROTEASE INHIBITORS			
	Trypsin inhibitors	Broccoli, cucumbers, radishes, spinach, legumes, soybeans	Evidence of anticancer effects found in humans.[1, 3, 4]
PHYTIC ACIDS			
	Inositol hexaphosphate (IP6)	Whole grains and cereals, nuts, soybeans, legumes	Binds with metals. Cancer protection.[1, 2, 4]

After most of the potential health benefits/actions, you will see a number. This number denotes whether the evidence tends to be based on:

[1] Experimental conditions performed in a laboratory

[2] Epidemiological studies in human populations

[3] Studies in humans

[4] Studies in animals

INDEX

Apples *(cont.)*
    10-Minute Spiced Apple Wedges with
        Caramel Sauce, 261
Arterial plaque
    from LDL cholesterol, 5–6, 51
    reducing, with
        B vitamins, 48
        food synergy, 210
        HDL cholesterol, 11
        omega-3s, 143
        soy, <u>107</u>
        statins, <u>14</u>
        vegetables, 120–21
Artichoke hearts
    Light Spinach and Artichoke Heart Alfredo,
        314–15
Asian cuisine, 183–87
Asparagus
    Roasted Asparagus Spears with Slivered
        Garlic, 293
Atherosclerosis
    HDL cholesterol preventing, <u>11</u>
    from homocysteine, 9
Avocados
    Avocado-Edamame Salsa, 287
    Avocado Mango Salad, 275

B

Baked goods
    Apple Oat Muffins, 244–45
    Easy Sweet Potato Harvest Rolls, 241
    Lemon-Rosemary Rolls, 242–43
    reducing saturated fat from, <u>152</u>
Baking fish, <u>203</u>
Barley
    Barley Eggplant Bake, 300
    Barley Mushroom Bake, 299
    Barley-Stuffed Tomatoes, 302–3
    for blood pressure reduction, 102
    Savory Barley, 298
Basil
    Portfolio Pesto, 311
    Sweet Pepper and Basil Pasta Salad, 268–69

Beans
    as add-in ingredient, 103, 105, 108
    for cancer prevention, <u>31</u>, <u>180</u>
    for diabetes control, 108, <u>180</u>, <u>181</u>
    gas from, <u>181</u>
    for heart protection, <u>180–81</u>
    Jessie's White Chili, 264–65
    Mediterranean Chickpea Salad, 274
    in Mediterranean diet, 158, <u>159</u>
    Not-So-Killer Chili, 266
    nutrients in, 105, <u>180</u>
    preparing, <u>181</u>
Beef
    Baked Beef Meatballs (with Spinach) and
        Tomato Sauce, 308–9
    reducing saturated fat from, <u>152</u>
Beer, homocysteine unaffected by, 10
Benecol, for cholesterol reduction, 5, 111, 166
Berries
    Berry Easy Topping, 258
    buying and storing, <u>75</u>
    health benefits from, <u>74</u>
    Light and Luscious Berry Grunt, 256–57
    nutrients in, <u>74–75</u>
Beta-carotene
    causing lung cancer in smokers, 44–45
    for colon cancer prevention, 84
    sources of, 24, <u>52</u>, <u>53</u>, <u>84–85</u>
    vitamins C and E with, for LDL cholesterol
        reduction, 52
Beverages. *See* Drinks
Blackberries
    Light and Luscious Berry Grunt, 256–57
Bladder cancer, <u>22</u>, <u>74</u>, <u>80</u>
Blood clots
    omega-3s preventing, 55, 143
    strokes and, 15
Blood lipids. *See also* Cholesterol; Triglycerides
    review of, <u>167</u>
Blood pressure. *See also* High blood pressure
    diet affecting, 19–20, 55, <u>106</u>
    readings
        schedule for, 18–19
        understanding, 15, 18

Buckwheat, in diabetes diet, 41

Burgers

Portobello Mushroom Burger with Garlic
Mayonnaise, 307

soy and veggie, 178

Butter, reducing saturated fat from, 153

Buttermilk

Lemon-Blueberry Buttermilk Pancakes,
250–51

Three-Grain Buttermilk Waffles, 259

Butternut squash

Baked Butternut Macaroni, 304–5

Butternut Squash Ravioli with Lemon
Cream Sauce, 313

B vitamins. *See also* Folic acid; Vitamin B$_6$ and
B$_{12}$

deficiency of, 96

for homocysteine reduction, 9, 10

in meal combinations, 50–51

recommended intake of, 47

sources of, 48, 113, 203

for stroke prevention, 18

C

Cabbage

Coleslaw with Spicy Peanut Dressing, 291

Calcium

for blood pressure reduction, 19, 20

for bone health, 64, 122, 123, 127

for cancer prevention, 60, 206

in DASH diet, 175

food sources of, 352

cereal products, 64

dairy products, 122, 123, 123, 130, 131, 206

vs. supplements, 127

for PMS, 61

vitamin D and

for bone mass, 58–60

for PMS, ix, x, 206

for weight control, 128

Calorie control

for reducing diabetes risk, 39

whole foods for, 95

Cancer

bladder, 22, 74, 80

breast (*see* Breast cancer)

cervical, 80

colon (*see* Colon cancer)

colorectal (*see* Colorectal cancer)

contributors to, 22–23, 22, 24, 82

diet and nutrition, 23, 24–25, 28

obesity, 28–30, 28

saturated fat, 33, 40, 151, 154

trans fats, 147

endometrial, 33, 80

esophageal, 74, 89, 90, 103

fast facts about, 22

laryngeal, 89, 103

liver, 80–81

lung (*see* Lung cancer)

non-Hodgkin's lymphoma, 82–83

oral, 103

ovarian, 31, 72, 89, 134–35

pancreatic, 119, 180

pharyngeal, 103

preventing, with

alcohol avoidance, 31

beans, 31, 180

berries, 74

broccoli, 80–81

calcium and vitamin D, 60

catechins, 72

conjugated linoleic acid, 33

exercise, 30

fish, 31

flavonoids, 76

flaxseed, 30, 32–33, 114, 114, 115

folic acid, 34

food synergy, 69, 211–13

fruits and vegetables, 22, 31, 118–20, 155,
211, 212

isoflavones, 76

low-fat diet, 31

olive oil, 161

omega-3s, 31, 55, 114, 115, 143–44

organosulfurs, 85, 89–90

quercetin, 87

soy, 106
tea, 134–35, 185, 199, 200
tofu and tea, 140
tomatoes, 77, 78
vitamin D, 34–35
weight loss, 31
whole grains, 31, 103
prostate (*see* Prostate cancer)
rectal, 33, 184
skin, 22, 74, 78–79, 90
stomach, 89, 90, 103
vitamin E and, 45
Candida vaginitis, yogurt for, 125
Canola oil, 145, 203
Capers
Seasoned Salmon with Lemon-Caper Sauce,
326–27
Caramel
10-Minute Spiced Apple Wedges with
Caramel Sauce, 261
Carbohydrates
in diabetes diet, 37
limiting
for improving HDL cholesterol, 13
for triglycerides reduction, 8
Cardiovascular disease. *See also* Heart disease
vitamin E and, 45
Carotenoids
in DASH diet, 175
in diabetes diet, 41
family of, 77, 82–85
sources of, 24, 84–85, 204, 362
Catechins, 72, 73, 119, 133, 199
Cereals
calcium in, 64
vitamin D–fortified, 62
Cervical cancer, 80
Cheese
Deluxe Grilled Cheese Sandwich, 281
French-Style Ham and Cheese Sandwich,
282–83
healthy cooking with, 130–31
nutrients in, 129–31, 132
reducing saturated fat from, 152

Tuna Gruyère Tart, 340–41
2-Minute Toasted Tomato and Cheese
Sandwich, 280
varieties of, 129, 130–31, 132
Cherries
alfalfa sprouts and, for cholesterol reduction,
139
Vanilla-Cherry-Almond Granola, 247
Chicken
Jessie's White Chili, 264–65
Less-Fuss Pecan-Crusted Chicken Salad,
276–77
Orange-Mango Chicken, 328–29
Stuffed Chicken Breast, 330–31
Chickpeas
Mediterranean Chickpea Salad, 274
Chili
Jessie's White Chili, 264–65
Not-So-Killer Chili, 266
Chocolate, for heart health, 69–70
Cholesterol, blood. *See also* HDL cholesterol;
LDL cholesterol
high, health risks from, 3, 5, 16
lowering, with
alfalfa sprouts and cherries, 139
barley, 2, 102
beans, 180
fish and olive oil, 149
food synergy, 210
garlic, 86
garlic and fish oil, 150
good fats, 5, 109
grapefruit, 73, 76
green tea, 134
low-saturated-fat diet, 5, 154
Mediterranean diet, 162–63
nuts, 3, 109, 110, 112, 113, 166, 167, 169,
172, 174, 197, 198
oats, 2, 99, 102
omega-3, vitamin E, and niacin,
55–56
omega-6s, 145
plant sterol–enriched margarine, 3, 5, 166,
167, 169, 173

food combinations for, 137–41, 147–50

good fats and, 147–50

health benefits from, x, xii, 1

how to use, xii–xiv

importance of, x–xi

in Mediterranean diet, 160, 162

research on, xi, 43–44, 190

summary of

    for cancer protection, 211–13

    for diabetes prevention, 213–14

    for heart disease prevention, 207, 210

    for stroke prevention, 211

    for weight loss, 214–17

Fractures, preventing, 58, 59, 60

Free radicals

    apples fighting, 118–19

    cancer development and, 23–24, 71

    cell damage from, 71

    food synergy and, 213

Fruits. *See also specific fruits*

    in Asian cuisine, 186

    with beta-carotene and vitamins E and C, 52

    for cancer prevention, 22, 26, 31, 118–20, 212

    with carotenoids, 84

    in DASH diet, 175, 176, 176, 177

    dried

        energy density of, 121, 122

        Fun Fall Snack Mix, 286

    Fruit and Cream Crisp, 260

    general health benefits from, 117, 118

    for heart disease prevention, 3, 120, 207

    with high ORAC values, 117

    improving longevity, 154

    in Mediterranean diet, 158, 159, 160

    nutrients in, 117–18, 117

    recommended servings of, 117

    for stroke prevention, 17

    for weight loss, 119, 121–22, 216

G

Gamma-tocopherol, 45, 46, 49

Garlic

    components of, 86

    fish oil and, for cholesterol reduction, 150

health benefits from, 86–87, 89–90

onions and, for heart disease prevention,
    140–41

Portobello Mushroom Burger with Garlic
    Mayonnaise, 307

preparing, 88

recommended intake of, 87

Roasted Asparagus Spears with Slivered
    Garlic, 293

Garlic supplements, 86

Gas, from beans, 181

Gastrointestinal health

    onions for, 87

    yogurt for, 124–25

Genetics, cancer and, 22

Gestational diabetes, 37

Ginger

    Lemon-Ginger Iced Green Tea, 342

Gluten, in whole grains, 104–5

Glycemic index

    in diabetes diet, 37–38

    triglyceride reduction and, 8

Glycemic load

    affecting HDL cholesterol, 13

    in diabetes diet, 38

Granola

    Vanilla-Cherry-Almond Granola, 247

Grapefruit

    drug interactions and, 76

    health benefits from, 73, 76

    nutrients in, 204–5

    Shrimp and Red Grapefruit Salad, 272–73

Grape leaves

    Stuffed Grape Leaves, 288–89

Gravy

    Vegetarian Sausage-and-Sage Gravy, 240

Grilling fish, 202–3

Grunt

    Light and Luscious Berry Grunt, 256–57

H

Ham

    French-Style Ham and Cheese Sandwich,
    282–83

HDL cholesterol
   fast facts about, 11
   for heart disease prevention, 10–11
   improving, with
      diet and lifestyle, 12–13
      garlic, 86–87
      green tea, 134
      monounsaturated fats, 55, 142, 198
      omega-3s, 143
   ranges of, 167
   trans fats decreasing, 147
Heart attacks
   LDL cholesterol and, 6, 51
   Mediterranean diet reducing, 102
   risk factors for, 3–4, 5, 6
   six steps to, 4
Heart disease
   in China, 184
   CRP levels and, 14
   death rate from, 2
   diabetes and, 35, 213
   nuts reducing death from, 110
   preventing, with
      beans, 180–81
      broccoli, 81
      B vitamins, 47–48
      catechins, 72
      cholesterol reduction, 5–7
      fiber, 2
      fish and olive oil, 149
      food synergy guidelines, 207, 210
      fruits and vegetables, 120
      garlic, 87
      garlic and onions, 140–41
      homocysteine reduction, 9–10
      increased HDL cholesterol, 10–13
      isoflavones, 76–77
      lifestyle changes, 4
      low-saturated-fat diet plus fruits and
         vegetables, 154
      nuts, 3, 113, 172, 174
      omega-3s, 56, 114, 143, 144
      omega-6s, 146
      onions, 87

organosulfurs, 85
      plant sterol–enriched margarine, 3
      smart fats, 55
      soy, 2, 106–7
      tea, 134
      tomatoes, 78
      triglycerides reduction, 7–9
      vitamin E and lycopene, 50, 51
      whole grains, 98–99, 102
   risk factors for, 2, 5, 6, 8, 24, 40, 147, 173
Heart failure, vitamin E and, 45
Heart health, flavonoids for, 69–70
Hemorrhagic stroke, 15
High blood pressure. *See also* Blood pressure
   controlling or lowering, with
      barley, 102
      calcium, 19, 20
      dairy products, 127, 206
      DASH diet, 173–77, 206
      fish and olive oil, 149
      food synergy guidelines, 211
      magnesium, 19, 20
      Mediterranean diet, 163
      monounsaturated fats, 142
      oats, 100
      omega-3s, 143
      potassium, 19–20, 66
      vegetable protein, 20
      weight loss, 40
   health risks from, 3, 15, 16, 173–74
   measurements indicating, 15, 18–19
   salt sensitivity and, 19, 20–21, 175, 176
High-fat diets
   cancer risk from, 24–25, 26, 33
   diabetes risk from, 39
   increasing PMS symptoms, 61
Homocysteine
   high
      causes of, 10
      health risks from, 9
   lowering, with
      B vitamins, 10, 47–48
      folic acid, 9, 18
      garlic, 87

Hot flashes, soy and, 106
Hunger
    inability to recognize, 216
    leptin and, 215
    yogurt reducing, 126
Hyperglycemia, 108
Hyperinsulinemia, 108
Hypertension. *See* High blood pressure

I

Ice cream, reducing saturated fat from, 153
Immune function
    nuts for, 197
    sesame seeds and vitamin E for, 54
    yogurt for, 124
    zinc for, 66
Inflammation
    CRP test measuring, 14
    reducing, with
        broccoli, 81
        food synergy guidelines, 210
        Mediterranean diet, 162
        olive oil, 161
        omega-3s and -6s, 149
Insulin
    foods steadying, 94, 98, 113, 214
    role of, 36
Insulin resistance, 39, 40, 108
Insulin sensitivity
    dietary fat affecting, 39, 142
    fiber improving, 38
Iron absorption, Vitamin C and, x
Ischemic stroke, 15, 17
Isoflavones
    health benefits from, 76–77, 185
    in soy, 26, 76, 77, 106, 185

J

Joint pain, broccoli reducing, 81
Juice, citrus
    for improving HDL cholesterol, 12
    nutrients in, 204–5

K

Kale
    Kale Quiche, 332–33
Kidney disease, from diabetes, 108, 173, 214

L

Laryngeal cancer, 89, 103
Lasagna
    Garden Sun-Dried Tomato Lasagna, 334–35
LDL cholesterol
    CRP levels and, 14
    diabetes and, 37
    heart disease risk from, 5–6, 51
    lowering, with
        alfalfa sprouts and cherries, 139
        citrus and soy, 205
        dietary changes, 6–7
        fiber, 102, 170
        fish and olive oil, 149
        food synergy, 51, 52, 54, 207
        garlic, 86
        garlic and fish oil, 150
        green tea, 134
        Mediterranean diet, 162–63
        monounsaturated fats, 37, 55, 142
        nuts, 113, 172, 198
        oats, 100, 102
        omega-3s, 143
        omega-6s, 145
        plant sterols, 168, 201
        PortfolioEatingPlan, 166, 169, 170
        soy protein, 107, 172
        vitamin E and lycopene, 51
    ranges of, 167
    saturated fats increasing, 5, 39–40, 39, 147,
        151
    trans fats increasing, 147
Lemonade
    Strawberry Light Lemonade, 344
Lemon curd
    Butternut Squash Ravioli with Lemon
        Cream Sauce, 313

Smart fats (*cont.*)
    in recipes, 141–42
    vitamins and, 54–58
    in whole foods, 93
Smoking
    beta-carotene and, 44–45
    homocysteine levels and, 10
Smoking cessation, for improving HDL
    cholesterol, <u>13</u>
Smoothies, 32, <u>63</u>, 205, 206
Snacks
    Fun Fall Snack Mix, 286
    high-synergy, 218, 231–32
    Spicy Nut Mix, 284–85
Sodium. *See also* Salt
    blood pressure and, <u>16</u>, 19
    overconsumption of, 95
    restricted, in DASH diet, 175, 176
Soups
    Jessie's White Chili, 264–65
    Light Italian Wedding Soup, 262–63
    miso, 185
    Not-So-Killer Chili, 266
Soy
    in Asian cuisine, 184–85, 187
    breast cancer and, 26–27, 184
    calcium and, for bone mass, 64
    calcium-fortified, 64–65, <u>65</u>
    for cholesterol reduction, 2
    citrus and, for cholesterol improvement,
      205
    components of, <u>106</u>
    in diabetes diet, 41
    flaxseed and, for breast cancer, 139–40
    for improving HDL cholesterol, <u>13</u>
    isoflavones in, 26, 76–77, <u>77</u>, <u>106</u>, 185
    for stroke prevention, 211
Soybeans. *See* Edamame
Soy burgers, <u>178</u>
Soy protein, in PortfolioEatingPlan, 166, 167,
    171–72, <u>172</u>, 173
Spinach
    Baked Beef Meatballs (with Spinach) and
      Tomato Sauce, 308–9

Breakfast Panini with Roasted Red Pepper
    Spread, 236–37
Edamame-Spinach Scramble, 234–35
Light Italian Wedding Soup, 262–63
Light Spinach and Artichoke Heart Alfredo,
    314–15
Quick Spinach Italiano, 296
raw, 193
Stovetop Spanakorizo (Spinach and Rice),
    297
Spreads
    Portfolio Pesto, 311
    Strawberry-Orange Spread, 246
Squash
    Baked Butternut Macaroni, 304–5
    Butternut Squash Ravioli with Lemon
      Cream Sauce, 313
    Maple Roasted Squash with Apple Filling,
      301
Statins, 2, <u>14</u>, <u>168</u>
Stomach cancer, 89, 90, 103
Stomach ulcers, broccoli preventing, <u>81</u>
Strawberries
    Strawberry Light Lemonade, 344
    Strawberry-Orange Spread, 246
Stroke
    blood clots and, 15
    cause of, 14–15
    preventing, with
      carotenoids, 83
      folic acid, <u>18</u>
      food synergy, 211
      Mediterranean diet, 102
      onions, <u>87</u>
      soy, 211
      whole grains, 102–3, 211
    risk factors for
      free radical damage, 24
      high blood pressure, 15, <u>16</u>, 18–21, 173
      high cholesterol, 6, 40, 147
      high homocysteine, 9
      high triglycerides, 8
      reducing, <u>16–17</u>
    types of, 15

Succotash
Summer Succotash, 290
Sugar, in diabetes diet, 40
Sun exposure, vitamin D from, 35, _59_, 123, 127
Supplements, vs. foods, 46, 91
Sweet potatoes
Easy Sweet Potato Harvest Rolls, 241
Synergy Super Foods, 189–90, _208–9_, 217, 218.
See also Menus, sample

T

Tacos
Portobello Tacos, 306
Tahini
Tahini-Dressed Chilled Noodles, 292
Take Control, for cholesterol reduction, 3, 5, 111, 166, 173, 201
Tarts
Savory Summer Tart, 338–39
Tuna Gruyère Tart, 340–41
Tea
in Asian cuisine, 185–86, 187
for cancer prevention, 72, 134–35, 185, 199
components of, _73_, 132–33, 134, 199
for heart disease prevention, 134
iced, _133_
Lemon-Ginger Iced Green Tea, 342
Peach Pleasure Iced Tea, 343
tips for drinking, 200
tofu and, for cancer prevention, 140
types of, 186, 199–200
for weight loss, 135, 199, 217
TIA (transient ischemic attack), 15
Tofu
tea and, for cancer prevention, 140
uses for, 187
Tomatoes
Baked Beef Meatballs (with Spinach) and Tomato Sauce, 308–9
broccoli and, for prostate cancer, ix, 138–39, 211
Farmer's Market Pasta Salad, 267

Garden Sun-Dried Tomato Lasagna, 334–35
health benefits from, _78–79_
Homemade Pizza Sauce, 312
lycopene in, 28, 77, _78_, 82, _83_, 139
Mediterranean Chickpea Salad, 274
Penne with Creamy Tomato Vodka Sauce, 316
preparing, _79_
Savory Summer Tart, 338–39
2-Minute Toasted Tomato and Cheese Sandwich, 280
Topping
Berry Easy Topping, 258
Tortellini
Margi's Tortellini and Shrimp Sauté, 317
Trail mix, 199
Trans fats
characteristics of, 147
harmful effects of, 147, 151
limiting
with diabetes, 39
for LDL cholesterol reduction, 6
omega-6s replacing, 146
whole foods eliminating, 93
Transient ischemic attack (TIA), 15
Triglycerides
high
with diabetes, 37
from excess calories, 7–8
health risks from, 8
from obesity, _13_
leptin and, _215_
lowering, 8–9, 37, 55, 76, 143, 150, 210
ranges of, 8, _167_
Tuna
Tuna Gruyère Tart, 340–41
Type 1 diabetes, 36
Type 2 diabetes. *See* Diabetes

U

Ulcers, stomach, broccoli preventing, _81_

V

Hot Apple-Blueberry Cobbler with Walnut-
    Butter Streusel, 254–55
Weight control
    dairy products for, 128
    whole grains for, 98
Weight gain, breast cancer and, 26
Weight loss
    calorie control for, 39
    for cancer prevention, 31
    for diabetes prevention, 38, 40
    energy density of foods and, 121–22
    fat restriction for, 39
    foods for
        beans, 109
        dairy products, 128, 217
        fruits and vegetables, 119, 121–22, 216
        green tea, 135, 199, 217
        whole grains, 216
    for improving HDL cholesterol, 13
    for LDL cholesterol reduction, 6
    for stroke prevention, 16
    vegetarian diet for, 179, 217
Whole foods
    beans, 103, 105, 108–9
    benefits of eating, 92–96, 191
    dairy products, 122–32
    definition of, 91
    flaxseed, 103, 114–16
    fruits and vegetables, 116–22
    nuts, 103, 109–13
    tea, 132–35
    tips for eating, 192
    vs. unhealthful foods, 92
    whole grains, 96–103
Whole Foods Market, 94
Whole grains. See also specific whole grains
    characteristics of, 104–5
    daily servings of, 194–95

in DASH diet, 175, 176
health benefits from, 31, 94–95, 97, 98–99,
    102–3, 211
in Mediterranean diet, 158, 159
nutrients in, 97, 191
refining of, 96
sources of, 96–97
switching to, 191, 193
for weight loss, 216
Wine
    in Mediterranean diet, 158, 159
    red, vitamin E and, 53–54

Y

Yeast infections, yogurt for, 125
Yogurt
    for diarrhea, 125
    flavoring, 126
    frozen, reducing saturated fat from, 153
    for gastrointestinal health, 124–25
    for immune system, 124
    as probiotic, 124
    for reducing hunger, 126
    in smoothies and drinks, 63
    as substitute ingredient, 126
    for vaginal yeast infections, 125
    vitamin D–fortified, 62, 63, 127

Z

Zeaxanthin
    in oranges, 204
    for preventing non-Hodgkin's lymphoma,
        82–83
Zinc
    for immune function, 66
    sources of, 66, 355

Conversion Chart

These equivalents have been slightly rounded to make measuring easier.

VOLUME MEASUREMENTS

U.S.	Imperial	Metric
¼ tsp	–	1 ml
½ tsp	–	2 ml
1 tsp	–	5 ml
1 Tbsp	–	15 ml
2 Tbsp (1 oz)	1 fl oz	30 ml
¼ cup (2 oz)	2 fl oz	60 ml
⅓ cup (3 oz)	3 fl oz	80 ml
½ cup (4 oz)	4 fl oz	120 ml
⅔ cup (5 oz)	5 fl oz	160 ml
¾ cup (6 oz)	6 fl oz	180 ml
1 cup (8 oz)	8 fl oz	240 ml

WEIGHT MEASUREMENTS

U.S.	Metric
1 oz	30 g
2 oz	60 g
4 oz (¼ lb)	115 g
5 oz (⅓ lb)	145 g
6 oz	170 g
7 oz	200 g
8 oz (½ lb)	230 g
10 oz	285 g
12 oz (¾ lb)	340 g
14 oz	400 g
16 oz (1 lb)	455 g
2.2 lb	1 kg

LENGTH MEASUREMENTS

U.S.	Metric
¼"	0.6 cm
½"	1.25 cm
1"	2.5 cm
2"	5 cm
4"	11 cm
6"	15 cm
8"	20 cm
10"	25 cm
12" (1')	30 cm

PAN SIZES

U.S.	Metric
8" cake pan	20 × 4 cm sandwich or cake tin
9" cake pan	23 × 3.5 cm sandwich or cake tin
11" × 7" baking pan	28 × 18 cm baking tin
13" × 9" baking pan	32.5 × 23 cm baking tin
15" × 10" baking pan	38 × 25.5 cm baking tin (Swiss roll tin)
1½ qt baking dish	1.5 liter baking dish
2 qt baking dish	2 liter baking dish
2 qt rectangular baking dish	30 × 19 cm baking dish
9" pie plate	22 × 4 or 23 × 4 cm pie plate
7" or 8" springform pan	18 or 20 cm springform or loose-bottom cake tin
9" × 5" loaf pan	23 × 13 cm or 2 lb narrow loaf tin or pâté tin

TEMPERATURES

Fahrenheit	Centigrade	Gas
140°	60°	–
160°	70°	–
180°	80°	–
225°	105°	¼
250°	120°	½
275°	135°	1
300°	150°	2
325°	160°	3
350°	180°	4
375°	190°	5
400°	200°	6
425°	220°	7
450°	230°	8
475°	245°	9
500°	260°	–